RADIOTHERAPY

Edited by **Cem Onal**

Radiotherapy
http://dx.doi.org/10.5772/63695
Edited by Cem Onal

Contributors

Robert Michael Hermann, Mirko Nitsche, Frank Bruns, Wenyong Tan, Xianming Li, Yong Dai, Joseph John Bevelacqua, Viktoras Rudzianskas, Rita Kupcinskaite-Noreikiene, Ahmad Esmaili, Seyed Amirreza Dastyar, Despina Katsochi, Papa Dasari, Suk Lee, Kwang Hyeon Kim, Chul Yong Kim, Choi Suk Woo, Jang Bo Shim, Yuan Jie Cao, Kyung Hwan Chang, Ryohei Sasaki, Yasuo Ejima, Takeaki Ishihara, Daisuke Miyawaki, Kenichiro Kakutani, Kotaro Nishida, Junichiro Inoue, Yoshitada Sakai, Tianyuan Wang, Mei Ying Lim, Yuanshui Zheng, Hiroaki Akasaka, Yasuyuki Shimizu, Ryuichi Yada, Saki Osuga, Yuki Wakahara, Masao Nakayama, Naritoshi Mukumoto, Momčilo M. Pejović, Milić M. Pejovic, Kenji Yoshida

Published by InTech

Janeza Trdine 9, 51000 Rijeka, Croatia

Publishing Process Manager Andrea Koric
Technical Editor SPi Global
Cover InTech Design team

First published May, 2017
Printed in Croatia
Legal deposit, Croatia: National and University Library in Zagreb

Additional hard copies can be obtained from orders@intechopen.com

Radiotherapy, Edited by Cem Onal
p. cm.
Print ISBN 978-953-51-3149-6
Online ISBN 978-953-51-3150-2

For EU product safety concerns:
IN TECH d.o.o., Prolaz Marije Krucifikse Kozulić 3, 51000 Rijeka, Croatia,
info@intechopen.com or visit our website at intechopen.com.

Meet the editor

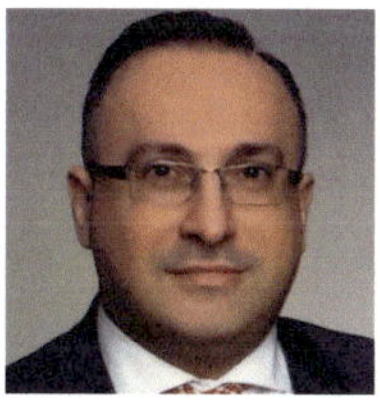

Dr. Cem Onal is the founder physician of Baskent University Adana Dr. Turgut Noyan Research and Treatment Center, Department of Radiation Oncology, and he is still serving as a professor at the same institute. His main areas of interest are prostate cancer, breast cancer, and gynecological malignancies. He has great experience in prostate cancer treatments especially IMRT and IGRT, gynecological tumor brachytherapy, stereotactic radiotherapy, and radiosurgery. He has approximately 100 international and national papers published in different journals. Also, he has approximately 200 international and national abstracts presented at different scientific meetings. He is peer-reviewing in 40 journals. He is giving lectures about new radiotherapy facilities in different course programs conducted by the Turkish Society for Radiation Oncology.

Contents

Preface

It is my pleasure to present the book entitled *Radiotherapy*. This book meets the experience of several researchers who dedicate many hours a day to not only treat patients but also assess the physical aspects of newer radiotherapy facilities.

This book comprises both clinical and physical aspects of radiotherapy modalities. Radiotherapy plays a key role in the treatment of many cancer types. Almost two-thirds of all cancer patients receive some form of radiation therapy during the course of treatment, predominantly with external beam photon therapy. There are three major aspects of radiotherapy delivery strategies: definitive radiotherapy, adjuvant radiotherapy (either with or without concurrent chemotherapy), and neoadjuvant radiotherapy (either with or without concurrent chemotherapy). Highly conformal techniques such as intensity-modulated radiotherapy with image guidance allow precise delivery of higher doses of radiation within the target volume. With increasing technical advances, higher doses per fraction are used for both first-line treatment and re-irradiation for many tumor types, which have a potential to increase local control and survival in most cases. Advances in radiation therapy have contributed to improvements in long-term outcomes for cancer patients. For example, a 5-year survival of cancer has increased to approximately 68% in adults and 83% in children.

The book is divided into three sections with 14 chapters. The first section encompasses new treatment strategies for bone metastasis, lung cancer, and gynecological tumors. Two hot topics, re-irradiation in head and neck cancer and clinical outcomes of simultaneous integrated boost technique, which changes the current practice, are depicted with clinical studies. Treatment outcomes of a rare entity—heel spur irradiation—are also discussed in detail. Long-term survivors are at increased risk to develop treatment-induced side effects, such as radiogenic second cancer, complications of the cardiovascular and central nervous systems, fertility problems, and other toxicities. In other sections, the late effects of radiotherapy are discussed. In the last section, physical parameters of new radiotherapy techniques are discussed in detail.

This book is intended to bring forward the many advancements in the field of radiation oncology. There are many valuable contributions from radiation oncology physicians and medical physicists who are experts in their fields. I would like to thank all contributors for their kind efforts in preparation of this book.

Cem Onal MD
Professor
Baskent University Faculty of Medicine
Dr. Turgut Noyan Research and Treatment Center
Adana, Turkey

Section 1

Clinical Aspects

Chapter 1

New Paradigms of Radiotherapy for Bone Metastasis

Yasuo Ejima, Takeaki Ishihara, Daisuke Miyawaki,
Kenichiro Kakutani, Kotaro Nishida, Junichiro Inoue,
Yoshitada Sakai, Tianyuan Wang and Ryohei Sasaki

Additional information is available at the end of the chapter

http://dx.doi.org/10.5772/66939

Abstract

Proper care of patients with bone metastasis requires interdisciplinary treatments. Radiotherapy (RT) plays a central role in the management of painful bone metastasis. External beam RT can provide rapid successful palliation of painful bone metastasis in 50–80% of patients, is associated with very few adverse effects and leads to complete pain relief at the treated site in up to one-third of patients. Intensity-modulated RT (IMRT) or stereotactic body RT (SBRT) enables the delivery of higher doses to the target tumor while minimizing the dose to adjacent organs. Reirradiation using IMRT or SBRT is a valuable option for the management of bone metastases. A multidisciplinary team, especially one consisting of a spinal surgeon and rehabilitation physician, is particularly useful for treating patients with spinal bone metastases characterized by spinal instability. Rehabilitation intervention which increases the physical activity level and prevents deconditioning is important. Future developments in surgical procedures and RT will likely improve the management protocols for bone metastases and technology to reduce metal artifacts in radiation planning might improve the efficacy and safety of combination therapy.

Keywords: spinal metastases, intensity-modulated radiotherapy, rehabilitation, multidisciplinary team, stereotactic body radiotherapy

1. Introduction

Bone metastases are a common manifestation of malignancies that can cause severe and debilitating effects, including pain, spinal cord compression, hypercalcemia and pathologic fractures. Proper care of patients with bone metastasis requires interdisciplinary treatments delivered by orthopedic surgeons, radiation oncologists, rehabilitation specialists, medical oncologists, pain medicine specialists, radiologists and palliative care professionals. Radiotherapy (RT) has played a central role for palliation of painful bone metastasis, leading to complete pain relief at the treated site in up to one-third of patients [1]. The role of RT and radiotherapeutic techniques using a multidisciplinary approach for the treatment of bone metastases have been discussed recently.

2. Indications and optimal doses for bone metastases RT

External beam RT (EBRT) continues to be the mainstay treatment for painful, uncomplicated, bone metastases. EBRT can provide rapid successful palliation of painful bone metastasis in 50–80% of patients, is associated with very few adverse effects and leads to complete pain relief at the treated site in up to one-third of patients. Although various fractionation schemes can provide good palliation rates, numerous prospective randomized trials have shown that 30 Gy in 10 fractions, 24 Gy in 6 fractions, 20 Gy in 5 fractions, or 8 Gy in a single fraction provide excellent pain control with minimal side effects (**Table 1**) [2–7]. Longer fractionated courses have the advantage of a lower incidence of repeat irradiation to the same site, whereas single fractions have proved more convenient for patients and caregivers. In addition, repeat irradiation with EBRT might be safe, effective and less commonly necessary in patients with a short life expectancy.

Author	Patients (n)	Dose and fractions	Overall pain relief (%)	Complete response (%)	Acute toxicity (%)	Late toxicity (%)	Repeat treatment rate (%)
BPTWP [2]	775	8 Gy in 1 Fx	78	57	30	2	23
		20 Gy in 5 Fx/30 Gy in 10 Fx	78	58	32	1	10
Foro [3]	160	8 Gy in 1 Fx	75	15	13	NA	28
		30 Gy in 10 Fx	86	13	18	NA	2
Hartsell [4]	898	8 Gy in 1 Fx/30 Gy in 10 Fx	66	15	10	4	18
Nielsen [5]	241	8 Gy in 1 Fx	62	15	35	5	21
		20 Gy in 4 Fx	71	15	35	5	12
Roos [6]	272	8 Gy in 1 Fx	53	26	5	5	29
		20 Gy in 5 Fx	61	27	11	4	24
Steenland [7]	1171	8 Gy in 1 Fx	72	37	Equivalent	4	25
		24 Gy in 6 Fx	69	33	Equivalent	2	7

BPTWP, Bone Pain Trial Working Party; NA, not assessed; Fx, fraction(s).

Table 1. Outcomes of single fraction or multifraction external beam radiotherapy for painful bone metastases.

For metastatic spinal cord compression (MSCC), EBRT is the standard of care. Although a total of 30 Gy in 10 fractions is the most frequently employed fractionation schedule, multiple fractionation schemes have been reported, which undoubtedly reflect the heterogeneity in patient populations and tumor histologies (**Table 2**) [8–11]. In a retrospective study, Rades et al. [11] suggested that dose escalation beyond 30 Gy in 10 fractions did not improve motor function and local control in patients with MSCC who had radioresistant tumors such as renal cell carcinomas, colorectal cancers and malignant melanomas. However, in patients with breast cancer, prostate cancer, myeloma or lymphoma and others who had a favorable prognosis, dose escalation beyond 30 Gy provided better local control and extended overall survival [10]. Therefore, the use of 30 Gy in 10 fractions could be regarded as the standard therapeutic dose for MSCC, although the available evidence is limited. In patients with a favorable survival prognosis, dose escalation beyond 30 Gy might improve local control and overall survival, but it might not improve functional outcome and dose escalation to 40 Gy in 20 fractions might be insufficient against radioresistant tumors.

Author	Study design	State of disease	Dose	Ambulatory rate before treatment (%)	Motor function improvement (%)	Local control	Overall survival
Maranzano [8]	RCT	Unfavorable prognosis	8 Gy in 1 Fx	64	12	NA	4 months (median)
			16 Gy in 2 Fx	67	21	NA	4 months (median)
Rades [9]	Prospective non-RCT	Various tumors	8 Gy in 1 Fx/20 Gy in 4 Fx	61	37	61% at 1 year	23% at 1 year
			30–40 Gy in 10–20 Fx	62	39	81% at 1 year	30% at 1 year
Rades [10]	Matched cohort	Favorable prognosis tumors	30 Gy in 10 Fx	85	40	71% at 2 years	53% at 2 years
			37.5 Gy in 15 Fx/40 Gy in 20 Fx	85	41	92% at 2 years	68% at 2 years
Rades [11]	Retrospective	Radioresistant tumors	30 Gy in 10 Fx	62	18	76% at 1 year	NA
			37.5 Gy in 15 Fx40 Gy in 20 Fx	63	22	80 % at 1 year	NA

RCT, randomized controlled trial; Fx, fraction(s); NA, not assessed.

Table 2. External beam radiotherapy outcomes for metastatic spinal cord compression.

3. Intensity-modulated RT or stereotactic body RT for bone metastases

Recently, intensity-modulated RT (IMRT) or stereotactic body RT (SBRT) has been applied for spinal bone metastases and the development of systemic treatments has improved survival in patients with bone metastasis. However, in such cases, the standard regimens for bone metastases including 30 Gy in 10 fractions, 20 Gy in 5 fractions, or 8 Gy in a single fraction were insufficient for long-term pain management. Therefore, to increase the duration of pain control, it might be necessary to consider more intense RT or treatment regimens.

IMRT delivers high doses to tumor targets while decreasing the dose to organs-at-risk and, therefore, presents a major dosimetric advantage over three-dimensional conformal RT. IMRT took radiation treatment planning and delivery to a higher level by combining technologies. It utilizes movement of the multileaf collimator (MLC) during the actual beam-on time to modulate, or alter, the radiation beam as it leaves the radiation treatment unit. Such beam modulation allows the application of concave dose distributions. The computer system calculates an IMRT plan incorporating several beams, or, alternatively, a moving arc arrangement with the movement of the MLC to create a plan that achieves the radiation-dosing goals (**Figure 1**). On the other hand, SBRT is emerging as an alternative RT technique to deliver dose-escalated radiation to tumor targets. Due to the application of several nonisocentric beams, SBRT delivers highly conformal large radiation dose fractions to target volumes with precision (<1 mm) and steep dose gradients. This allows for planning target volume reductions, thereby minimizing exposure to critical adjacent organs, which produces a toxicity profile comparable with that of conventionally fractionated RT, despite the use of higher doses per fraction (**Figure 2**).

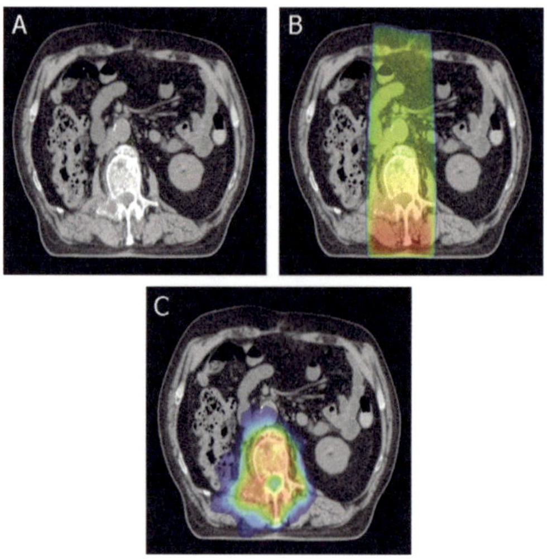

Figure 1. Comparison of radiation dose distributions between conventional radiotherapy and intensity-modulated radiotherapy (IMRT). (A) The osteolytic change in the lumbar vertebral body and infiltration into the spinal canal. (B) The dose distribution of conventional radiotherapy (two-directional anteroposterior-posteroanterior opposed irradiation at 30 Gy in 10 fractions). (C) The distribution of IMRT using volumetric modulated arc therapy (50 Gy in 10 fractions).

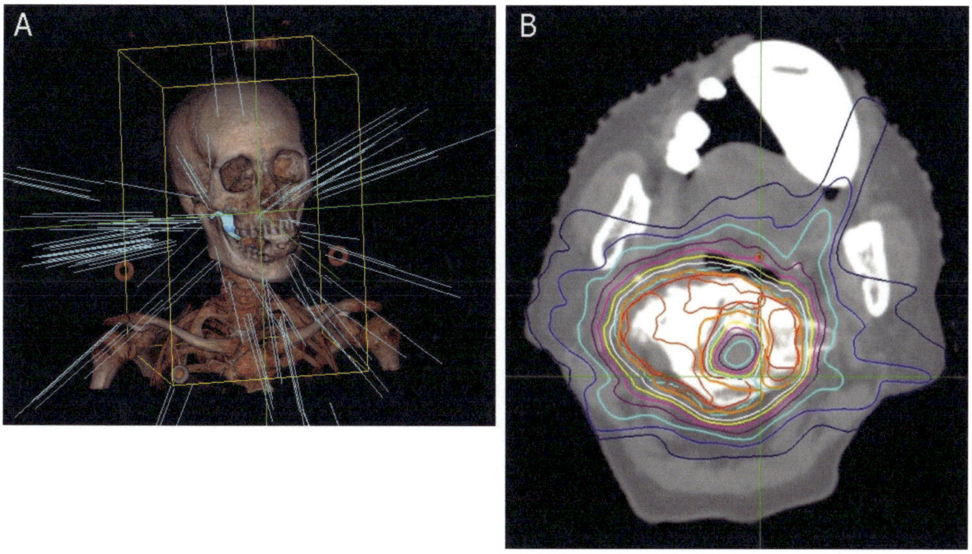

Figure 2. A 70-year-old male patient suffering from lung cancer with cervical vertebral bone metastasis. The schema and dose distribution of SBRT for bone metastasis using CyberKnife treatment system. (A) The blue line indicates the beam directions. (B) Representative dose distribution.

Three important factors should be considered for the decision to utilize IMRT or SBRT. First, IMRT or SBRT must be adapted for the treatment of oligometastasis in the bone. Long-term survival has been noted in patients diagnosed with isolated bone metastasis [12–15]. Therefore, successful control of oligometastasis of the bone due to the delivery of higher doses might contribute to improved treatment outcomes and quality of life (QOL). Second, IMRT or SBRT can be performed for reirradiation of the same site. It is technically difficult to reirradiate the same site using conventional RT. However, with IMRT or SBRT the dose to the spinal cord or adjacent organs can be reduced to within the tolerable range, facilitating reirradiation. Third, IMRT or SBRT can be applied for radioresistant bone metastases. Therefore, when indicating IMRT or SBRT for metastatic bone tumors, oncologists should consider the disease behavior and estimated life expectancy of the patient.

The treatment outcomes of previous studies that utilized IMRT or SBRT for bone metastases [16–19] are compared in **Table 3**. Each study performed IMRT or SBRT using various dose or fractionation protocols because standard regimens have not yet been proposed. The majority of studies demonstrated excellent local control without serious harmful phenomenon such as myelopathy. However, because most previous studies were retrospective and sufficient evidence has not yet been accumulated, any adaptation of IMRT or SBRT to deliver higher doses must be carefully discussed for individual patients. A multidisciplinary team comprising radiation oncologists, orthopedists, medical oncologists, radiologists, rehabilitation physicians and palliative care medicine doctors would be ideal for discussing and deciding treatment options including the application of higher dose RT.

Authors	Machine/type	Dose	LCR	Adverse events
Murai [16]	Tomotherapy/IMRT	40 Gy in 8 fx/48 Gy in 16 fx	84% (1-year)	No radiation-induced myelopathy
Yamada [17]	Linear accelerator/IMRT	18–24 Gy in 1 fx	90%	No radiation-induced myelopathy
Guckenberger [18]	Linear accelerator/SBRT	Median24 Gy in 3 fx	84% (2-year)	No radiation-induced myelopathy
Degen [19]	CyberKnife/SBRT	24 Gy in 1 fx	90%	No radiation-induced myelopathy

IMRT, intensity modulated radiotherapy; SBRT, stereotactic body radiotherapy; LCR, local control rate.

Table 3. Outcomes of IMRT or SBRT in bone metastasis.

4. Assessment of instability due to spinal metastasis: surgery, RT and the combination of both treatments

Oncologic care is improving and the survival rates of patients with various malignancies are increasing. Since the advent of recent technologic advancements in the detection methods used to locate new lesions and metastasis, orthopedic surgeons have been confronted with an increasing number of patients with spinal metastasis. Such patients can develop sudden paraplegia due to pathological fracture or tumor invasion into the spinal canal. Patients with symptomatic spinal metastasis present with severe pain and poor QOL [20].

If a multidisciplinary conference between radiation oncologist, spinal surgeons, physiotherapists and medical oncologists was developed, appropriate treatment strategies could be discussed and implemented. For example, a patient who develops sudden paraplegia sometimes needs urgent treatment including surgical decompression. Therefore, a simple classification method with easily assigned radiographic and patients factors could be helpful to facilitate communication and appropriate referral among the multidisciplinary oncology team, ensuring prompt and optimal treatment decisions.

Most cases of spinal metastasis occur in the vertebral body, intervertebral disc and anterior and/or posterior longitudinal ligament, whereas the involvement of anatomical structures related to spinal motion is rare. Batson's venous plexus and the avalvular vein of the vertebral venous system play an important mechanistic role in the pathology of spinal metastasis. Namely, all cancers with a preference toward bone metastasis, such as bronchial, breast and prostate cancers are disseminated to the spine via these vessels. Consequently, the anterior spinal column is the most frequent site of spinal metastases, with ~80% of lesions appearing in the vertebral body [21].

Instability has been classified as segmental instability, which is mostly the result of trauma or degenerative changes, or component instability, which is caused by tumor invasion in the vertebral body. The type of instability present should be determined when considering the therapeutic management of spinal metastases. Therefore, specific criteria for stability assessments are required. In 2010, Fisher et al. [22] reported a novel classification system for spinal instability in neoplastic disease, which was established using the best evidence provided by systematic reviews and expert opinions. The spine instability neoplastic score (SINS) is a comprehensive classification system based on patient symptoms and radiographic criteria without consideration of neurologic status, histology, or general physical condition. The SINS considers spinal metastasis location, type, pain and lesion quality, spinal alignment, the extent of vertebral body collapse and posterolateral spinal element involvement. Furthermore, the predictive value of the SINS was validated by the analysis of the clinical and radiographic data of 30 patients. The SINS score is categorized into a three-tier system with 0–6 being stable, 7–12 being potentially unstable and 13–18 being unstable [23]. A surgical consultation is recommended for patients with a SINS score greater than 7.

Surgical treatment decisions are broadly based on spinal stability and patient-specific factors including patient health, prognosis and tumor histology [24]. The surgical approach is indicated for pathological fractures and sudden onset of neurological symptoms. The current indications for spinal surgery are radioresistant tumors, progressive neurologic deficits lasting no longer than 24 hours, bone fragments in the spinal canal and spinal instability due to pathologic fracture. In addition, life expectancy should be at least 3 months. Survival duration in patients with bone metastases is largely dependent upon controllability of the primary tumor. Several prognostic scoring systems have been reported in an attempt to indicate the appropriate surgical strategy [24–26]. Tokuhashi et al. [24] and Tomita et al. [25] recommended that patients expected to have a good prognosis should undergo wide excision including total en bloc spondylectomy, those expected to have an intermediate prognosis should undergo marginal or intralesional excision and spinal stabilization (**Figure 3**) and those expected to have a poor prognosis should be managed conservatively. However, it should be emphasized that local spinal pathology, rather than tumor histology, determines the degree of pain or severity of neurologic deficits. The ultimate surgical goals are to obtain good QOL and activity of daily living (ADL) scores by relieving pain and improving neurologic status (**Tables 4** and **5**).

Recently, a prospective analysis of the surgical outcome in 70 patients with symptomatic spinal metastasis was conducted [27]. Laminectomy and posterior stabilization following RT significantly improved the performance status and ADL in >95% of patients, with sustained improvement for at least 6 months in >80%. In a randomized, multicenter, nonblinded trial in 101 patients, Patchell et al. [28] revealed a major breakthrough for surgical treatment followed by RT. They compared the efficacy of surgery followed by RT with that of RT alone. Fifty patients were assigned to surgery followed by RT and 51 to RT alone. Significantly more patients were able to walk after surgery followed by RT (84%) compared with after RT alone (57%). Moreover, the duration of walking ability maintenance was significantly longer in the surgery followed by RT Arm (median, 122 days) compared with the RT alone Arm (median, 13 days).

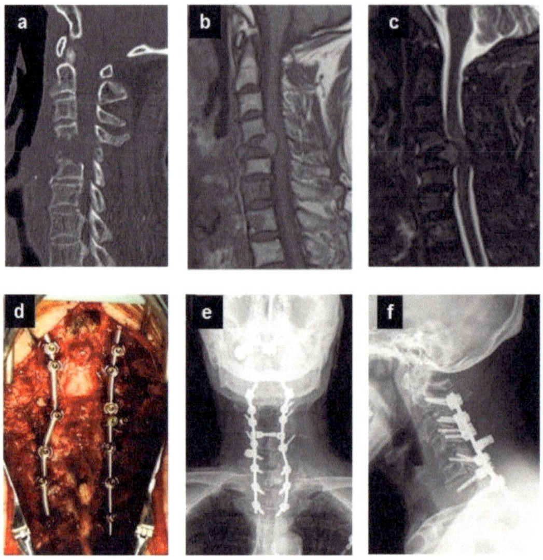

Figure 3. Laminectomy and posterior stabilization in a 76-year-old male with C5 metastasis of thyroid cancer. A patient presented with right deltoid muscle weakness and intractable pain in the right shoulder. The Tomita and Tokuhashi scores were 7 and 9 points, respectively. He underwent combination spinal surgery with a C5 laminectomy and C2 to T2 posterior stabilization, and postoperative conventional radiation therapy (30 Gy in 10 fractions). (a) Preoperative computed tomography. (b) and (c): Preoperative magnetic resonance imaging with T1-weighted and T2-weighted images, respectively. (d): Intraoperative image. (e) and (f): Postoperative radiographs.

	Treatment	Baseline	1 month	3 months	6 months
Median PS	Surgery	4	2	1	1
	Nonsurgery	3	4	4	4
Mean BI	Surgery	43.8 ± 28.0	74.2 ± 26.7	74.9 ± 31.8	82.5 ± 28.1
	Nonsurgery	48.5 ± 31.9	37.9 ± 34.1	35.5 ± 31.0	31.7 ± 10.4

Surgery patients (n = 46), nonsurgery patients (n = 24). PS, Eastern Cooperative Oncology Group Performance Status; BI, Barthel Index.

Table 4. Surgical outcome of performance score and activities of daily life in patients with spinal metastases.

The complication rate after surgery can be as high as 20–30% and this must be weighed against the intended benefits. Postsurgical complication and mortality rates were evaluated in 26,233 patients included in the National Inpatient Sample of United States [29]. The in-hospital mortality rate was 5.6% and the complication rate was 21.9%. Pulmonary (6.7%) and postoperative (5.9%) hemorrhage or hematoma were the most commonly reported complications. Complication rates were higher in older patients and those with comorbidities including hypertension, chronic lung disease and diabetes mellitus; having a single comorbidity increased the risk of in-hospital death by ~4 fold. In a retrospective series of 123 patients treated for spinal metastases, the rate of major wound complications (dehiscence or wound infection) was 32% in the group that underwent RT before surgery, whereas it was 12% in the group of patients first treated using surgery. Therefore, in patients with symptomatic MSCC, postoperative RT appeared to be more beneficial than preoperative RT [30].

	Total	Surgery	Nonsurgery
	No. (%) (n = 70)	No. (%) (n = 46)	No. (%) (n = 24)
PS			
Improved	49 (70.0)	45 (97.8)	4 (16.7)
Unchanged	13 (18.6)	1 (2.2)	12 (50.0)
Deteriorated	8 (11.4)	0 (0.0)	8 (33.3)
Redeteriorated	9 (12.9)	9 (20.0)	0 (0.0)
ADL			
Improved	45 (64.3)	44 (95.7)	1 (4.2)
Unchanged	14 (20.0)	2 (4.3)	12 (50.0)
Deteriorated	11 (15.7)	0 (0.0)	11 (45.8)
Redeteriorated	9 (12.9)	9 (20.5)	0 (0.0)

PS, Eastern Cooperative Oncology Group Performance Status; ADL, activities of daily living.

Table 5. Outcomes of endpoints in patients undergoing surgical treatment and nonsurgical treatment.

In patients with spinal bone metastasis, the goals of spinal surgery are to restore spinal stabilization, preserve neurologic function and provide pain relief. For appropriately indicated patients, spinal surgery can provide significant improvements in both QOL and ADL, possibly leading to the administration of adjuvant systemic therapies.

5. Rehabilitation for bone metastasis after surgery or RT

Because of the advances in diagnostic and therapeutic technologies, the overall survival of cancer patients has been prolonged, although the cancer survivors treated with RT has increasing. Patients during/after RT often suffer from the RT-related toxicities including radiation sickness, fatigue, nausea, vomiting, mucous membrane disorder, etc. These symptoms markedly reduce the physical activity level of patients and lead to deconditioning, such as muscular weakness, flexibility deterioration, cardiorespiratory dysfunction and psychological symptoms. Therefore, the rehabilitation intervention which increases the physical activity level and prevents deconditioning is important. Mock et al. reported that the walking exercise program during RT improved the physical functions, fatigue, emotional distress and difficulty sleeping in breast cancer patients during RT [31]. And Segal et al. showed that the resistance/aerobic training improved the QOL, aerobic fitness and strength in prostate cancer patients during RT [32]. Also in the guidelines from American College of Sports Medicine (ACSM) [33], the rehabilitation intervention recommended to improve physical function, aerobic fitness, QOL and fatigue in cancer patients during/after RT.

Furthermore, the number of elderly cancer patients treated with RT has been recently increasing. The elderly patients who have sarcopenia and frailty easily suffer from RT-related toxicities and deconditioning, then, decrease the completion rate of treatment [34], so the rehabilitation should be positively applied to cancer patients during/after RT, especially for elderly patients.

Moreover, the incidence of cancer survivors with bone metastasis has increased. Troublesome bone metastasis develops in 10–20% of patients with cancer. The majority of these patients have an increased risk for skeletal-related events (SREs) including pathologic fractures, spinal cord compression, the need for surgery, the need for RT and hypercalcemia [35]. SREs have been associated with significant morbidity, limited function and a decreased QOL [36–38]. In particular, pathologic fractures and spinal cord compression restrict ADL. Therefore, multidisciplinary team management of SREs (so-called bone management) is paramount in these patients. In these patients, rehabilitation over the course of treatment for the prevention of SREs and improvement of ADL and QOL is a key aspect of "bone management".

5.1. Purpose of rehabilitation for patients with bone metastasis

The essential points of the rehabilitative interventions for patients with bone metastasis are as follows [39]. (1) Rehabilitation aims to prevent patients from becoming bed-bound and helps them to maintain as much independence as possible with regard to ADL. (2) Rehabilitation commonly focuses on training patients to use their residual functions or to develop compensatory techniques by training in the use of assistive equipment or orthoses and educating both patients and their family members to help them adjust to the altered way of life. (3) Rehabilitation has inherent risks such as pathologic fractures and spinal cord compression. Improvements in physical function and physical activity levels due to rehabilitation might lead to an increased risk of pathologic fracture during ADL. However, bed rest, as an alternative, has various complications including muscle contractures, weakness and atrophy, orthostatic hypotension, pressure sores, pneumonia, confusion and disorientation (so-called disuse syndrome). Therefore, rehabilitation with the management of SREs risk would be more beneficial compared with bed rest.

5.2. Rehabilitative intervention paradigms

For patients with bone metastasis, rehabilitation mostly provides the adequate settlement of bed rest angles, training for the use of orthoses, instructions for adequate movements for ADL and exercises to maintain and increase physical function and ADL through discussion at bone metastasis board.

5.2.1. Settlement of bed rest levels: spinal bone metastasis

In cases of pathologic fracture or fragility in the vertebral body (high risk of paralysis), the head end of the Gatch bed should be raised by 30 degrees and patients wear a rigid spinal brace. Patients are moved using the logroll technique without flexion or rotation of the spine. In cases with a low risk of pathologic fracture (bone cortex remains), patients should wear a rigid spinal brace, but there is no restriction on the bed rest angle.

5.2.2. Settlement of bed rest levels: pelvic/lower extremity bone metastasis

In the case of pathologic fracture or fragility in weight-bearing bones or joints, patients are advised to avoid weight-bearing on the affected bone or joint. In patients with remaining bone cortex and an absence of pain, there are no restrictions in ADL.

5.2.2.1. Introduction of orthoses

In patients with bone metastasis, orthoses are applied to decrease bone pain, prevent or treat pathologic fractures and paralysis and to improve physical function. In patients with cervical metastasis, in stable cases, a soft cervical collar is applied to restrict flexion and extend the cervical vertebrae. In unstable cases, a Philadelphia collar and halo vest is applied to inhibit flexion, extension, rotation and lateral bending of the cervical vertebrae. In patients with thoracolumbar metastasis, spinal orthoses are applied to facilitate local rest by restricting the flexion, extension, rotation and lateral bending of the spinal column, which helps to reduce bone pain and inflammation, thereby reducing adverse psychological effects.

In the case of conservative treatment, a functional brace is applied to the humeral diaphyseal fracture and a patellar tendon-bearing orthosis is applied to the weight-bearing bone or joint below the lower leg. It takes a long time to increase bone strength, even after RT and long-term nonweight bearing is necessary. Therefore, surgery should be considered for the bone metastasis in the weight-bearing bones of the lower extremities.

5.2.2.2. Instructions for adequate movements

In the rehabilitation setting, to decrease the risk of the pathologic fractures and pain, patients are instructed on how to move when conducting ADL. The examples are shown in **Table 6**.

Examples	
Daily life behaviors	·For patients with spinal bone metastasis, excess flexion, and rotation of the trunk should be avoided in rolling over and getting up from bed.
	·For patients with bone metastasis of the weight-bearing bones in the lower extremities and pelvis, the transfer of motion with non-weight bearing should be instructed.
	·In getting up from the bed, patients should use the automatic bed Gatch up function.
Assistive device	·A cane, crutch, or walker should be used to decrease pain and weight-bearing.
	·A wheelchair should be used to decrease the physical burden in moving long distances.
	·Self-help devices, such as a Sox aid, should be used to avoid the pain caused by trunk flexion.
Living environment	·Install handrails to decrease pain with ambulation.
adjustment	·Install handrails and higher toilet seats in the restroom to decrease pain and assist with standing up from a seated position.

Table 6. Examples of instructions of movements for activities of daily living.

5.2.2.3. *Bone metastasis board*

Under the concept of "bone management," the multidisciplinary team approach is necessary to achieve the early detection and treatment of bone metastasis and the clinical practice of multidisciplinary therapy. In the treatment of bone metastasis, surgery, radiation therapy, rehabilitation and pain control should be considered, so the multidisciplinary team should discuss and decide the treatment plan in bone metastasis board. The necessity of rehabilitation and orthosis, settlement of bed rest level and risk management are also discussed in bone metastasis board, so the rehabilitation intervention can be safely provided to the bone metastatic patients.

5.3. Efficacy of rehabilitation

Previous studies have reported that rehabilitation during multidisciplinary therapy improved pain, physical function, ADL, QOL and prognosis in patients with bone metastasis (**Table 7**). Ruff et al. [40] showed that patients with spinal epidural metastasis who underwent rehabilitation had less pain, consumed less pain medication, were less depressed and had a greater satisfaction with life, compared with those who did not undergo rehabilitation. Other studies have reported that the rehabilitative intervention in patients with bone metastases improved functional independence measure scores, prognosis, physical function (muscle strength, submaximal aerobic exercise capacity and ambulation), physical activity level and QOL [41–44]. The rehabilitation with risk management by the multidisciplinary team could be effective in preventing SREs and improving pain, ADL, QOL and prognosis in patients with bone metastases. However, reports on the efficacy of rehabilitation in patients with bone metastasis are limited and were usually conducted in small populations. Therefore, further studies in larger populations are needed to validate the efficacy of rehabilitation.

Author	Subjects	Study design	Intervention	Primary outcome	Major results
Ruff [40]	42, spinal epidural metastasis	Controlled retrospective study	Training in transfers, bowel and bladder care, incentive spirometry, nutrition, and skin care	Pain, depression, life satisfaction	Intervention group had less pain, consumed less pain medication, were less depressed, and had greater life satisfaction.
Tang [41]	63, metastatic spinal cord compression	Retrospective descriptive study	Neuro-oncology rehabilitation, tailored to the needs of the patient	Functional independence measure scores, Tokuhashi score	Functional independence measure score improved. Longer survival in patients with high Tokuhashi scores.
Cormie [42]	20, bone metastatic prostate cancer	Randomized controlled study	Aerobic exercise and resistance exercise	Fatigue, physical function, body composition	Physical function, physical activity level, and lean mass improved.
Jane [43]	72, bone metastasis	Randomized controlled study	Massage: 3-month training program	Pain intensity, sleep quality, symptom distress scale	Beneficial effects on pain, mood, muscle relaxation, and sleep quality.
Rief [44]	60, bone metastasis	Randomized controlled study	Isometric resistance training of the muscles along the entire vertebral column	Pain, concurrent medication, oral morphine equivalent dose	Pain relief over a 6-months period and reduced oral morphine equivalent dose, as well as concomitant pain medication.

Table 7. Details of previous reports concerning rehabilitation for bone metastasis patients.

6. Reirradiation for bone metastases

RT is one of the most useful modalities for pain relief in patients with bone metastases. Although the American Society for Therapeutic Radiology and Oncology guidelines recommend 8 Gy in a single fraction as the standard method for palliative RT in uncomplicated painful bone metastases, reirradiation is required in 20–40% of cases [45, 46]. The reirradiation rates are 2.5-fold higher after single fraction RT compared with after multifraction RT [1]. Single fraction RT is commonly used for reirradiation. According to the prospective randomized trial of reirradiation undertaken by the National Cancer Institute of Canada Clinical Trial Group, single fraction RT of 8 Gy seemed to be noninferior and less toxic than multifraction RT of 20 Gy [47]. The pain relief response rate following reirradiation is 60–70%, with complete and partial responses of about 20 and 50%, respectively [46, 48], which are similar to the response rates seen with an initial effective RT. Although initial responders are more likely to respond to reirradiation than initial nonresponders, about half of the nonresponders can be expected to respond to retreatment [48].

Reirradiation is also effective to maintain walking abilities of patients with MSCC. However, the median duration of response is relatively short (about 4–5 months) [49, 50]. The degree of motor function after reirradiation is associated with the walking ability before RT. More than

80% of ambulant patients before RT will be expected to maintain the walking ability, whereas less than 20% of not ambulant patients will recover the function [49, 50]. SBRT is well suited for reirradiation of the spine due to its superiority of dose distribution compared with conventional techniques. SBRT has a major potential to provide superior local control without increasing toxicity (**Table 8**) [51–54]. A care must be taken when SBRT is applied to patients with MSCC, because the existence of tumor too close to the spinal cord is a risk factor for local recurrence due to underdose [51]. Relatively little is known regarding the long-term toxicities of reirradiation. Because reirradiation has the potential to exceed normal tissue tolerance, it might be appropriate to sum the biologically effective doses (BEDs) from the initial and repeat treatment regimens to estimate the safety of treatment. The BED is calculated according to the liner-quadratic model [BED = $D \times (1+ d/\alpha/\beta)$, D: total dose, d: fractional dose] with generally using α/β value of 2 (Gy_2) for the late effects. For example, the BED for 30 Gy in 10 fractions is 75 Gy_2 and 8 Gy in single fraction is 40 Gy_2. Regarding the spinal cord, higher cumulative RT doses (BED > 135.5 Gy_2), higher doses for each RT course (BED > 98 Gy_2) and a short interval between the courses (<6 months) could be associated with a higher probability of developing radiation-induced myelopathy [55]. These dose constraints for the spinal cord seem to be reproducible in SBRT [56].

Author (year)	Patients/ lesions (n)	Previous EBRT dose/Fx	Median dose/Fx (range)	Local control	Overall survival	Neural toxicity
Garg [52]	59/63	NA	30 Gy in 5 fx, 27 Gy in 3 fx	76% at 1 year	76% at 1 year	2 of G3 Radiculopathy
Mahadevan [53]	60/81	30 Gy in 10 fx (median)	24 Gy in 3 fx, 25–30 Gy in 5 fx	93% at last follow-up	11 month (median)	None
Hashmi [54]	215/247	30 Gy in 10 fx (median)	8-22 Gy in 1 fx, 14–50 Gy in 3(2–20) fx	93% at 6 months	64% at 6 months	None

SBRT, Stereotactic body radiotherapy; EBRT, external beam radiotherapy; Fx, fraction; NA, not available; G3, grade3

Table 8. Outcomes of reirradiation by spinal SBRT.

7. Beyond metal implant artifacts

Metallic surgical implants are commonly used in patients who undergo RT for bone metastasis. In computed tomography, metallic hardware can dramatically attenuate the X-ray beam and severe beam hardening effect and lead to faulty or inconsistent projection data [57, 58]. Consequently, so-called metallic artifacts or bright and dark streak artifacts can dramatically degrade the image quality. **Figure 4** illustrates a typical case of a patient who underwent spine-stabilization before adjacent RT. Strong artifacts induced by the titanium-based pedicle screws make it difficult to distinguish target lesions from surrounding normal tissues.

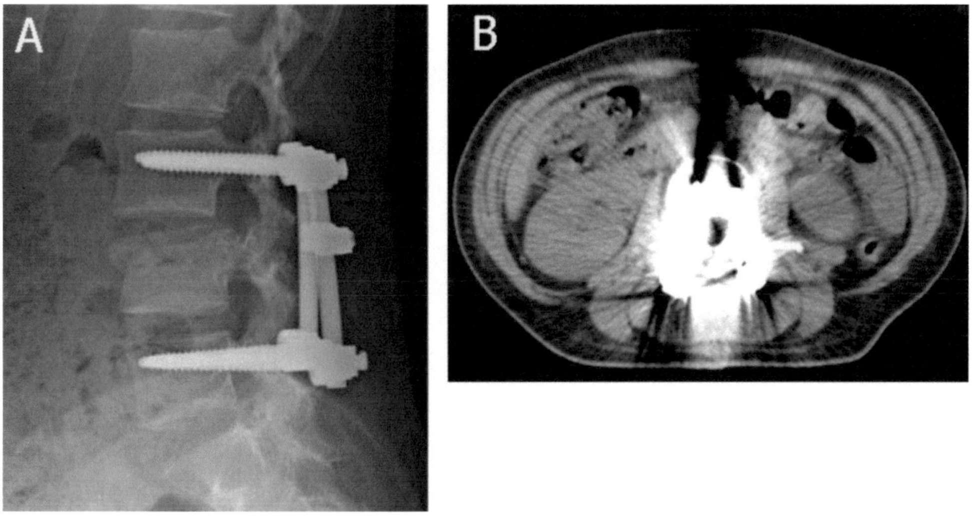

Figure 4. Artifacts of metallic surgical implants. (A) 2D radiography image shows a patient with implanted titanium pedicle screws. (B) Computed tomography image of a patient with titanium pedicle screws. Streak artifacts are present around the metallic implants.

For modern-era RT protocols, target delineation and dose calculation are performed on CT images using treatment-planning systems. Therefore, metallic artifacts, that are commonly located directly adjacent to the target volume and organs-at-risk and that degrade the delineation accuracy and dose calculation might lead to poor local control and a high risk of complications. Several studies have investigated the metallic-implant-related dosimetric impact using Monte Carlo simulations. Spadea et al. [59] reported that low-Z materials such as titanium might not cause relevant dose discrepancies, while high-Z materials including gold and platinum might lead to underestimation of the delivered dose during photon beam irradiation. Verburg et al. [60] investigated the effect of titanium implants on dosimetric errors in photon therapy treatment planning. They revealed dose discrepancies of up to 10% with range differences of up to 10 mm in artifact-contaminated areas. **Figure 5** illustrates examples of dose differences caused by titanium-based artifacts introduced by Verburg [58]. Factors including the beam-implant interaction, radiation beam type and the physical characteristics of the metals differ and eventually lead to dose uncertainties. For bone metastasis, especially in cases of infield recurrence of metastatic spinal lesions, the high dosimetric accuracy for organs-at-risk becomes clinically significant because of the limited spinal cord radiation tolerance. Recently, several promising approaches to reduce metallic artifacts have been proposed, such as metal artifact reduction (MAR) algorithms [61–63] and monoenergetic extrapolations from dual-energy computed tomography (DECT) [64, 65]. **Figure 6** briefly illustrated reduction of metal artifacts using a frequency split MAR method introduced by Meyer et al. Antiartifact approaches have proven useful for improving target delineation and dose calculation in RT, but to date, they have not been widely implicated for routine clinical use.

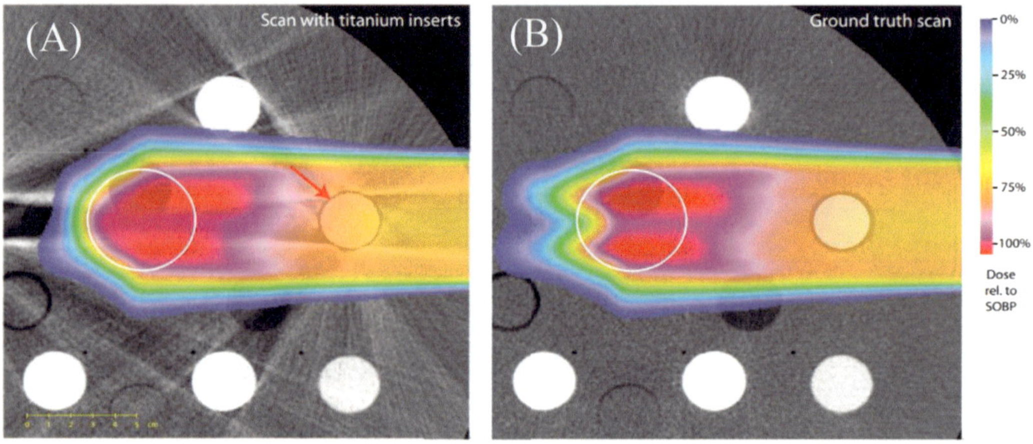

Figure 5. Differences in dose calculation of photon beams passing through the metal artifact region. (A) Dose calculation on the artifact-affected computed tomography image. The arrow indicates the titanium insert. (B) Dose calculation on the ground truth computed tomography image without the artifact.

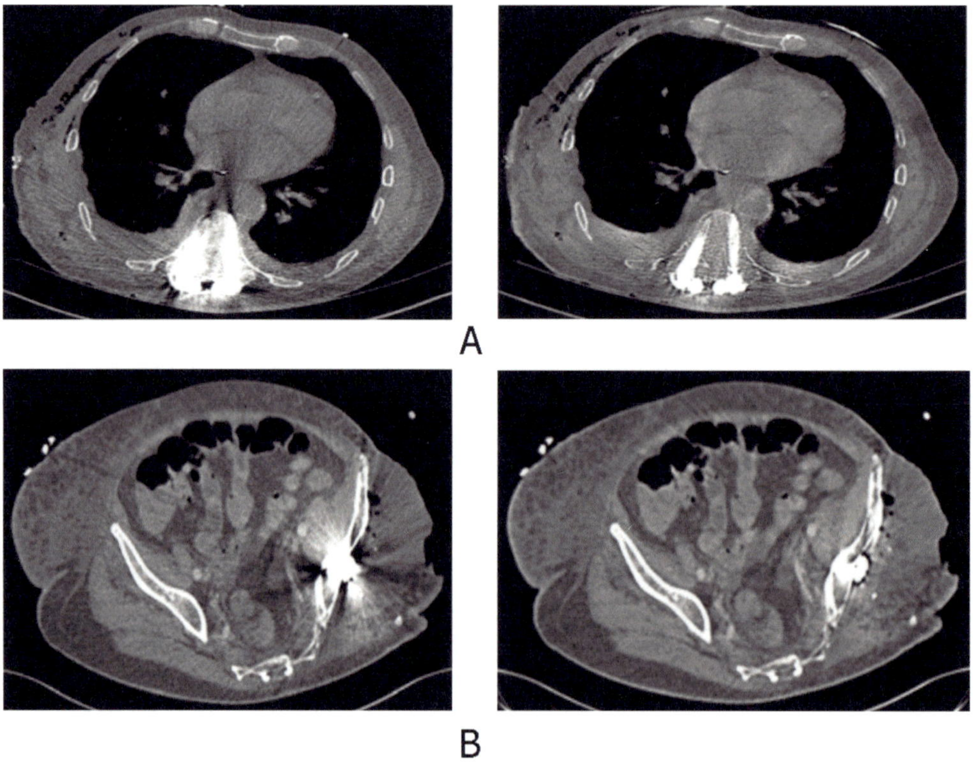

Figure 6. Reduction of metal artifacts using a frequency split MAR method. (A) Patient with implanted pedicle screws. (B) Patient with implanted unilateral hip endoprosthesis, Left: original computed tomography image; right: MAR corrected computed tomography image.

In conclusion, in cases of bone metastases, the impact of dose uncertainties due to metallic implants is critical in modern RT, especially in patients undergoing reirradiation. Promising antiartifact approaches might be useful options to achieve the anticipated magnitude of clinical benefit.

8. Conclusion

RT plays a central role in the management of painful bone metastasis. Compared with conventional RT, IMRT, or SBRT enables the delivery of higher doses to the target tumor while minimizing the dose to adjacent organs. Not only pain relief but also the restoration of spinal stability and preservation of neurologic function are associated with RT in patients with spinal bone metastases. A multidisciplinary team, especially one consisting of a spinal surgeon and rehabilitation physician, is particularly helpful for treating patients with spinal bone metastases characterized by spinal instability. Reirradiation using IMRT or SBRT is a valuable option for the management of bone metastasis. Future developments in surgical procedures and RT will likely improve the management protocols for bone metastases and technology to reduce metal artifacts in radiation planning might improve the efficacy and safety of combination therapy.

Author details

Yasuo Ejima[1], Takeaki Ishihara[1], Daisuke Miyawaki[1], Kenichiro Kakutani[2], Kotaro Nishida[2], Junichiro Inoue[3], Yoshitada Sakai[3], Tianyuan Wang[1] and Ryohei Sasaki[1]*

*Address all correspondence to: rsasaki@med.kobe-u.ac.jp

1 Division of Radiation Oncology, Kobe University Graduate School of Medicine, Kobe City, Hyogo, Japan

2 Department of Orthopaedic Surgery, Kobe University Graduate School of Medicine, Kobe City, Hyogo, Japan

3 Division of Rehabilitation Medicine, Kobe University Hospital, Kobe City, Hyogo, Japan

References

[1] Chow E, Harris K, Fan G, Tsao M, Sze WM. Palliative radiotherapy trials for bone metastases: a systematic review. J Clin Oncol. 2007;**25**:1423–1436. DOI: 10.1016/j.clon.2011.11.004

[2] Bone Pain Trial Working Party. 8 Gy single fraction radiotherapy for the treatment of metastatic skeletal pain: randomized comparison with a multifraction schedule over 12 months of patient follow-up. Radiother Oncol. 1999;**52**:111–121.

[3] Foro A, Fontanals A, Galceran J, Lynd F, Latiesas XS, de Dios NR, Castillejo AR, Bassols ML, Galán JL, Conejo IM, López MA. Randomized clinical trial with two palliative radiotherapy regimens in painful bone metastases: 30 Gy in 10 fractions compared with 8 Gy in single fraction. Radiother Oncol. 2008;**89**:150–155. DOI: 10.1016/j.radonc.2008.05.018

[4] Hartsell W, Scott CB, Bruner DW, Scarantino CW, Ivker RA, Roach M 3rd, Suh JH, Demas WF, Movsas B, Petersen IA, Konski AA, Cleeland CS, Janjan NA, DeSilvio M. Randomized trial of short- versus long-course radiotherapy for palliation of painful bone metastases. J Natl Cancer Inst. 2005;**97**:798–804.

[5] Nielsen O, Bentzen S, Sandberg E, Gadeberg CC, Timothy AR. Randomized trial of single dose versus fractionated palliative radiotherapy of bone metastases. Radiother Oncol. 1998;**47**:233–240.

[6] Roos D, Turner S, O'Brien P, Smith JG, Spry NA, Burmeister BH, Hoskin PJ, Ball DL; Trans-Tasman Radiation Oncology Group, TROG 96.05. Randomized trial of 8 Gy in 1 versus 20 Gy in 5 fractions of radiotherapy for neuropathic pain due to bone metastases (Trans-Tasman Radiation Oncology Group, TROG 96.05). Radiother Oncol. 2005;**75**:54–63.

[7] Steenland E, Leer J, van Houwelingen, Post WJ, van den Hout WB, Kievit J, de Haes H, Martijn H, Oei B, Vonk E, van der Steen-Banasik E, Wiggenraad RG, Hoogenhout J, Wárlám-Rodenhuis C, van Tienhoven G, Wanders R, Pomp J, van Reijn M, van Mierlo I, Rutten E. The effect of a single fraction compared to multiple fractions on painful bone metastases: a global analysis of the Dutch Bone Metastasis Study. Radiother Oncol. 1999;**52**:101–109.

[8] Maranzano E, Trippa F, Casale M, Costantini S, Lupattelli M, Bellavita R, Marafioti L, Pergolizzi S, Santacaterina A, Mignogna M, Silvano G, Fusco V. 8 Gy single-dose radiotherapy is effective in metastatic spinal cord compression: results of a phase III randomized multicenter Italian trial. Radiother Oncol. 2009;**93**:174–179. DOI: 10.1016/j.radonc.2009.05.012

[9] Rades D, Lange M, Veninga T, Stalpers LJ, Bajrovic A, Adamietz IA, Rudat V, Schild SE. Final results of a prospective study comparing the local control of short-course and long-course radiotherapy for metastatic spinal cord compression. Int J Radiat Oncol Biol Phys. 2011;**79**:524–530. DOI: 10.1016/j.ijrobp.2009.10.073

[10] Rades D, Panzner A, Rudat V, Karstens JH, Schild SE. Dose escalation of radiotherapy for metastatic spinal cord compression (MSCC) in patients with relatively favorable survival prognosis. Strahlenther Onkol. 2011;**187**:729–735. DOI: 10.1007/s00066-011-2266-y

[11] Rades D, Freundt K, Meyners T, Bajrovic A, Basic H, Karstens JH, Adamietz IA, Wildfang I, Rudat V, Schild SE, Dunst J. Dose escalation for metastatic spinal cord compression in

patients with relatively radioresistant tumors. Int J Radiat Oncol Biol Phys. 2011;**80**:1492–1497. DOI: 10.1016/j.ijrobp.2010.04.026

[12] Hellmann S, Weichselbaum RR. Oligometastases. J Clin Oncol. 1995;**13**:8–10.

[13] Milano MT, Zhang H, Metcalfe SK, Muhs AG, Okunieff P. Oligometastatic breast cancer treated with curative-intent stereotactic body radiation therapy. Breast Cancer Res Treat. 2009;**115**:601–608. DOI: 10.1007/s10549-008-0157-4

[14] Niibe Y, Hayakawa K. Oligometastases and oligo-recurrence: the new era of cancer therapy. Jpn J Clin Oncol. 2010;**40**:107–111. DOI: 10.1093/jjco/hyp167

[15] Milano MT, Katz AW, Zhang H, Okunieff P. Oligometastases treated with stereotactic body radiotherapy: long-term follow-up of prospective study. Int J Radiat Oncol Biol Phys. 2012;**83**:878–886. DOI: 10.1016/j.ijrobp.2011.08.036

[16] Murai T, Murata R, Manabe Y, Sugie C, Tamura T, Ito H, Miyoshi Y, Shibamoto Y. Intensity modulated stereotactic body radiation therapy for single or multiple vertebral metastases with spinal cord compression. Pract Radiat Oncol. 2014;**4**:e231–237. DOI: 10.1016/j.prro.2014.02.005

[17] Yamada Y, Bilsky MH, Lovelock DM, Venkatraman ES, Toner S, Johnson J, Zatcky J, Zelefsky MJ, Fuks Z. High-dose, single-fraction image-guided intensity-modulated radiotherapy for metastatic spinal lesions. Int J Radiat Oncol Biol Phys. 2008;**71**:484–490. DOI: 10.1016/j.ijrobp.2007.11.046

[18] Guckenberger M, Mantel F, Gerszten PC, Flickinger JC, Sahgal A, Létourneau D, Grills IS, Jawad M, Fahim DK, Shin JH, Winey B, Sheehan J, Kersh R. Safety and efficacy of stereotactic body radiotherapy as primary treatment for vertebral metastases: a multi-institutional analysis. Radiat Oncol. 2014;**9**:226. DOI: 10.1186/s13014-014-0226-2

[19] Degen JW, Gagnon GJ, Voyadzis JM, McRae DA, Lunsden M, Dieterich S, Molzahn I, Henderson FC. CyberKnife stereotactic radiosurgical treatment of spinal tumors for pain control and quality of life. J Neurosurg Spine. 2005;**2**:540–549.

[20] Falicov A, Fisher CG, Sparkes J, Boyd MC, Wing PC, Dvorak MF. Impact of surgical intervention on quality of life in patients with spinal metastases. Spine (Phila Pa 1976). 2006;**31**:2849–2856.

[21] Schick U, Marquardt G, Lorenz R. Intradural and extradural spinal metastases. Neurosurg Rev. 2001;**24**:1–5; discussion 6–7.

[22] Fisher CG, DiPaola CP, Ryken TC, Bilsky MH, Shaffrey CI, Berven SH, Harrop JS, Fehlings MG, Boriani S, Chou D, Schmidt MH, Polly DW, Biagini R, Burch S, Dekutoski MB, Ganju A, Gerszten PC, Gokaslan ZL, Groff MW, Liebsch NJ, Mendel E, Okuno SH, Patel S, Rhines LD, Rose PS, Sciubba DM, Sundaresan N, Tomita K, Varga PP, Vialle LR, Vrionis FD, Yamada Y, Fourney DR. A novel classification system for spinal instability in neoplastic disease: an evidence-based approach and expert consensus from the Spine Oncology Study Group. Spine (Phila Pa 1976). 2010;**35**:E1221–1229. DOI: 10.1097/BRS.0b013e3181e16ae2

[23] Fourney DR, Frangou EM, Ryken TC, Dipaola CP, Shaffrey CI, Berven SH, Bilsky MH, Harrop JS, Fehlings MG, Boriani S, Chou D, Schmidt MH, Polly DW, Biagini R, Burch S, Dekutoski MB, Ganju A, Gerszten PC, Gokaslan ZL, Groff MW, Liebsch NJ, Mendel E, Okuno SH, Patel S, Rhines LD, Rose PS, Sciubba DM, Sundaresan N, Tomita K, Varga PP, Vialle LR, Vrionis FD, Yamada Y, Fisher CG. Spinal instability neoplastic score: an analysis of reliability and validity from the spine oncology study group. J Clin Oncol. 2011;**29**:3072–3077. DOI: 10.1200/JCO.2010.34.3897

[24] Tokuhashi Y, Matsuzaki H, Oda H, Oshima M, Ryu J. A revised scoring system for preoperative evaluation of metastatic spine tumor prognosis. Spine (Phila Pa 1976). 2005;**30**:2186–2191.

[25] Tomita K, Kawahara N, Kobayashi T, Yoshida A, Murakami H, Akamaru T. Surgical strategy for spinal metastases. Spine (Phila Pa 1976). 2001;**26**:298–306.

[26] Katagiri H, Okada R, Takagi T, Takahashi M, Murata H, Harada H, Nishimura T, Asakura H, Ogawa H. New prognostic factors and scoring system for patients with skeletal metastasis. Cancer Med. 2014;**3**:1359–1367. DOI: 10.1002/cam4.292

[27] Kakutani K, Sakai Y, Maeno K, Takada T, Yurube T, Kurakawa T, Miyazaki S, Terashima Y, Ito M, Hara H, Kawamoto T, Ejima Y, Sakashita A, Kiyota N, Kizawa Y, Sasaki R, Akisue T, Minami H, Kuroda R, Kurosaka M, Nishida K. Prospective cohort study of performance status and activities of daily living after surgery for spinal metastasis. Clin Spine Surg. 2016 Oct 19. [Epub ahead of print] DOI: 10.1097/BSD.0000000000000456

[28] Patchell RA, Tibbs PA, Regine WF, Payne R, Saris S, Kryscio RJ, Mohiuddin M, Young B. Direct decompressive surgical resection in the treatment of spinal cord compression caused by metastatic cancer: a randomised trial. Lancet. 2005;**366**:643–648.

[29] Patil CG, Lad SP, Santarelli J, Boakye M. National inpatient complications and outcomes after surgery for spinal metastasis from 1993–2002. Cancer. 2007;**110**:625–630.

[30] Ghogawala Z, Mansfield FL, Borges LF. Spinal radiation before surgical decompression adversely affects outcomes of surgery for symptomatic metastatic spinal cord compression. Spine (Phila Pa 1976). 2001;**26**:818–824.

[31] Mock V, Dow KH, Meares CJ, Grimm PM, Dienemann JA, Haisfield-Wolfe ME, Quitasol W, Mitchell S, Chakravarthy A, Gage I. Effects of exercise on fatigue, physical functioning and emotional distress during radiation therapy for breast cancer. Oncol Nurs Forum. 1997;**24**:991–1000.

[32] Segal RJ, Reid RD, Courneya KS, Sigal RJ, Kenny GP, Prud'Homme DG, Malone SC, Wells GA, Scott CG, Slovinec D'Angelo ME. Randomized controlled trial of resistance or aerobic exercise in men receiving radiation therapy for prostate cancer. J Clin Oncol. 2009;**27**:344–51. DOI: 10.1200/JCO.2007.15.4963.

[33] Schmitz KH, Courneya KS, Matthews C, Demark-Wahnefried W, Galvão DA, Pinto BM, Irwin ML, Wolin KY, Segal RJ, Lucia A, Schneider CM, von Gruenigen VE, Schwartz AL.

American College of Sports Medicine. American College of Sports Medicine roundtable on exercise guidelines for cancer survivors. Med Sci Sports Exerc. 2010;**42(7)**:1409–26. DOI: 10.1249/MSS.0b013e3181e0c112.

[34] Hamaker ME, Vos AG, Smorenburg CH, de Rooij SE, van Munster BC. The value of geriatric assessments in predicting treatment tolerance and all-cause mortality in older patients with cancer. Oncologist. 2012;**17(11)**:1439–49. DOI: 10.1634/theoncologist.2012-0186.

[35] Suva LJ, Washam C, Nicholas RW, Griffin RJ. Bone metastasis: mechanisms and therapeutic opportunities. Nat Rev Endocrinol. 2011;**7**:208–218. DOI: 10.1038/nrendo.2010.227

[36] Fizazi K, Beuzeboc P, Lumbroso J, Haddad V, Massard C, Gross-Goupil M, Di Palma M, Escudier B, Theodore C, Loriot Y, Tournay E, Bouzy J, Laplanche A. Phase II trial of consolidation docetaxel and samarium-153 in patients with bone metastases from castration-resistant prostate cancer. J Clin Oncol. 2009;**27**:2429–2435. DOI: 10.1200/JCO.2008.18.9811

[37] Carlin BI, Andriole GL. The natural history, skeletal complications and management of bone metastases in patients with prostate carcinoma. Cancer. 2000;**88**(12 Suppl):2989–2994.

[38] Saad F, Olsson C, Schulman CC. Skeletal morbidity in men with prostate cancer: quality-of-life considerations throughout the continuum of care. Eur Urol. 2004;**46**:731–739.

[39] Bunting RW, Shea B. Bone metastasis and Rehabilitation. Cancer. 2001;**92**(4 Suppl):1020–1028.

[40] Ruff RL, Ruff SS, Wang X. Persistent benefits of rehabilitation on pain and life quality for nonambulatory patients with spinal epidural metastasis. J Rehabil Res Dev. 2007;**44**:271–278.

[41] Tang V, Harvey D, Park Dorsay J, Jiang S, Rathbone MP. Prognostic indicators in metastatic spinal cord compression: using functional independence measure and Tokuhashi scale to optimize rehabilitation planning. Spinal Cord. 2007;**45**:671–677.

[42] Cormie P, Newton RU, Spry N, Joseph D, Taaffe DR, Galvão DA. Safety and efficacy of resistance exercise in prostate cancer patients with bone metastases. Prostate Cancer Prostatic Dis. 2013;**16**:328–335. DOI: 10.1038/pcan.2013.22

[43] Jane SW, Chen SL, Wilkie DJ, Lin YC, Foreman SW, Beaton RD, Fan JY, Lu MY, Wang YY, Lin YH, Liao MN. Effects of massage on pain, mood status, relaxation and sleep in Taiwanese patients with metastatic bone pain: a randomized clinical trial. Pain. 2011;**152**:2432–2442. DOI: 10.1016/j.pain.2011.06.021

[44] Rief H, Welzel T, Omlor G, Akbar M, Bruckner T, Rieken S, Haefner MF, Schlampp I, Gioules A, Debus J. Pain response of resistance training of the paravertebral musculature under radiotherapy in patients with spinal bone metastases—a randomized trial. BMC Cancer. 2014;**14**:485. DOI: 10.1186/1471-2407-14-485

[45] Lutz S, Berk L, Chow E, Hahn C, Hoskin P, Howell D, Konski A, Kachnic L, Lo S, Sahgal A, Silverman L, von Gunten C, Mendel E, Vassil A, Bruner DW, Hartsell W; American Society for Radiation Oncology (ASTRO). Palliative radiotherapy for bone metastases: an ASTRO evidence-based guideline. Int J Radiat Oncol Biol Phys. 2011;**79**:965–976. DOI: 10.1016/j.ijrobp.2010.11.026

[46] Huisman M, van den Bosch MA, Wijlemans JW, van Vulpen M, van der Linden YM, Verkooijen HM. Effectiveness of reirradiation for painful bone metastases: a systematic review and meta-analysis. Int J Radiat Oncol Biol Phys. 2012;**84**:8–14. DOI: 10.1016/j.ijrobp.2011.10.080

[47] Chow E, van der Linden YM, Roos D, Hartsell WF, Hoskin P, Wu JS, Brundage MD, Nabid A, Tissing-Tan CJ, Oei B, Babington S, Demas WF, Wilson CF, Meyer RM, Chen BE, Wong RK. Single versus multiple fractions of repeat radiation for painful bone metastases: a randomised, controlled, non-inferiority trial. Lancet Oncol. 2014;**15**:164–171. doi: 10.1016/S1470-2045(13)70556-4

[48] Wong E, Hoskin P, Bedard G, Poon M, Zeng L, Lam H, Vulpe H, Tsao M, Pulenzas N, Chow E. Re-irradiation for painful bone metastases—a systematic review. Radiother Oncol. 2014;**110**:61–70. doi: 10.1016/j.radonc.2013.09.004.

[49] Rades D, Rudat V, Veninga T, Stalpers LJ, Hoskin PJ, Schild SE. Prognostic factors for functional outcome and survival after reirradiation for in-field recurrences of metastatic spinal cord compression. Cancer. 2008;**113**:1090–1096. DOI: 10.1002/cncr.23702

[50] Maranzano E, Trippa F, Casale M, Anselmo P, Rossi R. Reirradiation of metastatic spinal cord compression: definitive results of two randomized trials. Radiother Oncol. 2011;98:234–237. doi: 10.1016/j.radonc.2010.12.011.

[51] Garg AK, Wang XS, Shiu AS, Allen P, Yang J, McAleer MF, Azeem S, Rhines LD, Chang EL. Prospective evaluation of spinal reirradiation by using stereotactic body radiation therapy: The University of Texas MD Anderson Cancer Center experience. Cancer. 2011;**117**:3509–3516. DOI: 10.1002/cncr.25918

[52] Mahadevan A, Floyd S, Wong E, Jeyapalan S, Groff M, Kasper E. Stereotactic body radiotherapy reirradiation for recurrent epidural spinal metastases. Int J Radiat Oncol Biol Phys. 2011;**81**:1500–1505. doi: 10.1016/j.ijrobp.2010.08.012

[53] Hashmi A, Guckenberger M, Kersh R, Gerszten PC, Mantel F, Grills IS, Flickinger JC, Shin JH, Fahim DK, Winey B, Oh K, John Cho BC, Létourneau D, Sheehan J, Sahgal A. Re-irradiation stereotactic body radiotherapy for spinal metastases: a multi-institutional outcome analysis. J Neurosurg Spine. 2016;25:646–653.

[54] Ejima Y, Matsuo Y, Sasaki R. The current status and future of radiotherapy for spinal bone metastases. J Orthop Sci. 2015;**20**:585–592. doi: 10.1007/s00776-015-0720-x

[55] Nieder C, Grosu AL, Andratschke NH, Molls M. Proposal of human spinal cord reirradiation dose based on collection of data from 40 patients. Int J Radiat Oncol Biol Phys 2005;**61**:851–855.

[56] Sahgal A, Ma L, Weinberg V, Gibbs IC, Chao S, Chang UK, Werner-Wasik M, Angelov L, Chang EL, Sohn MJ, Soltys SG, Létourneau D, Ryu S, Gerszten PC, Fowler J, Wong CS, Larson DA. Reirradiation human spinal cord tolerance for stereotactic body radiotherapy. Int J Radiat Oncol Biol Phys. 2012;**82**:107–116. DOI: 10.1016/j.ijrobp.2010.08.021

[57] Stradiotti P, Curti A, Castellazzi G, Zerbi A. Metal-related artifacts in instrumented spine. Techniques for reducing artifacts in CT and MRI: state of the art. Eur Spine J. 2009;**18** (Suppl 1):102–108. DOI: 10.1007/s00586-009-0998-5

[58] Yazdia M, Gingras L, Beaulieu L. An adaptive approach to metal artifact reduction in helical computed tomography for radiation therapy treatment planning: experimental and clinical studies. Int J Radiat Oncol Biol Phys. 2005;**62**:1224–1231.

[59] Spadea MF, Verburg JM, Baroni G, Seco J. The impact of low-Z and high-Z metal implants in IMRT: a Monte Carlo study of dose inaccuracies in commercial dose algorithms. Med Phys. 2014;**41**: 011702. DOI: 10.1118/1.4829505

[60] Verburg JM, Seco J. Dosimetric accuracy of proton therapy for chordoma patients with titanium implants. Med Phys. 2013;**40**:071727. DOI: 10.1118/1.4810942

[61] Meyer E, Raupach R, Lell M, Schmidt B, Kachelriess M. Normalized metal artifact reduction (NMAR) in computed tomography. Med Phys. 2010; **10**:5482–5493.

[62] Meyer E, Raupach R, Lell M, et al. Frequency split metal artifact reduction (FSMAR) in computed tomography. Med Phys. 2012;**39(4)**: 1904–1916.

[63] Verburg JM, Seco J. CT metal artifact reduction method correcting for beam hardening and missing projections. Phys Med Biol. 2012;**57**: 2803–2818. doi: 10.1088/0031-9155/57/9/2803

[64] Zhou C, Zhao YE, Luo S, Shi H, Li L, Zheng L, Zhang LJ, Lu G. Monoenergetic imaging of dual-energy CT reduces artifacts from implanted metal orthopedic devices in patients with factures. Acad Radiol. 2011;**18**:1252–1257. doi: 10.1016/j.acra.2011.05.009

[65] Bamberg F, Dierks A, Nikolaou K, Reiser MF, Becker CR, Johnson TR. Metal artifact reduction by dual energy computed tomography using monoenergetic extrapolation. Eur Radiol. 2011;**21**:1424–1429. DOI: 10.1007/s00330-011-2062-1

Chapter 2

Radiotherapy in Lung Cancer

Fiona Lim Mei Ying

Additional information is available at the end of the chapter

http://dx.doi.org/10.5772/67204

Abstract

Lung cancer remains one of the top five cancers worldwide. Around 85% are nonsmall cell lung cancer (NSCLC) and only one-third present with early stage diseases. Radiotherapy had an important role both in radical and palliative treatment. With advancement in technology, newer techniques of stereotactic body radiotherapy allow delivery of much higher biologically effective dose to tumor achieving similar outcomes to radical surgery in early stage diseases. However, the usually large tumor volume together with preexiting poor lung condition makes radiotherapy challenging to deliver a radical dose to tumor while maintaining normal tissue constrains. In this chapter, different indications and techniques used in treating NSCLC will be discussed and reviewed.

Keywords: nonsmall cell lung cancer, external beam radiotherapy, stereotactic body radiotherapy

1. Introduction

According to the World Cancer Report 2014, lung cancer remains the top five most common cancers among both men and women worldwide. And it is also the leading cause of cancer deaths. Majority (around 85%) are nonsmall cell lung carcinomas [1, 2]. Incidence of adenocarcinoma had been rising and now became the most common histological subtypes in both men and women. About one-third of them are presented with early stage localized disease (stage I–II), another one-third with locally advanced disease (stage III), and remaining one-third with metastatic disease (stage IV) at diagnosis [3, 4].

2. Anatomy

Lungs are a paired structure that is separated into left and right by the mediastinum, which contains the tracheal, heart, esophagus, and lymph nodes. The left lung is divided into upper and lower lobe by oblique fissure, while the right lung is divided into three lobes (upper, middle, and lower) by oblique and horizontal fissures.

Lung cancers can arise from mucosa of the tracheobronchial tree or the alveolar lining cells of peripheral lung parenchyma. Tumor can spread locally within lung parenchyma or invading surrounding structures including mediastinum, major vessels, or chest wall (**Figure 1**). They can also spread along major airways causing obstruction, distal collapse, or atelectasis (**Figure 2**).

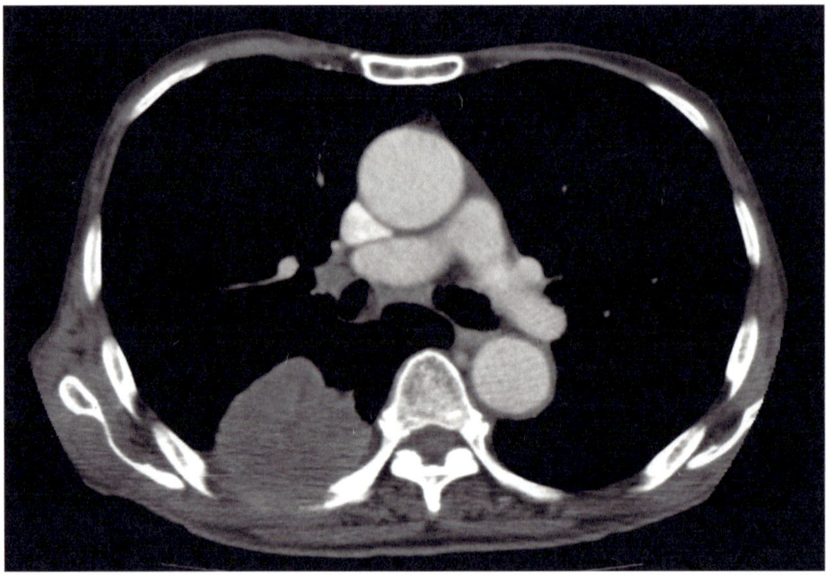

Figure 1. Tumor invasion to chest wall.

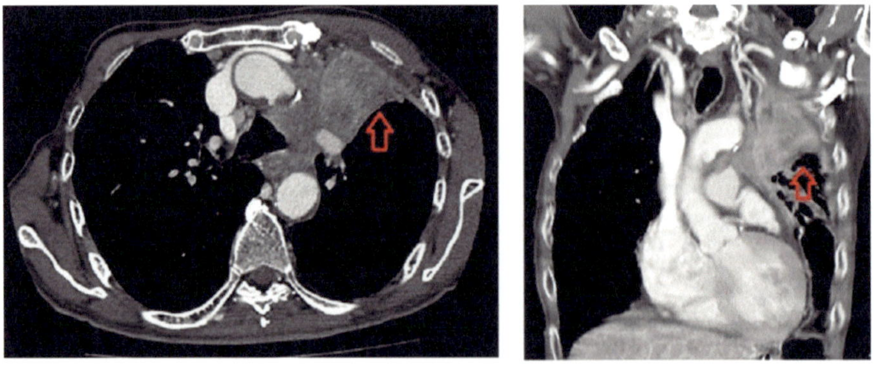

Figure 2. Tumor over left main bronchus causing collapse of left upper lobe (red arrow).

There is rich lymphatic within the respiratory system that accounts for the high rate of nodal metastasis. The lymph node map proposed by the International Association for the Study of Lung Cancer (ISALC) in 2009 divides the lymph nodes into 14 stations and sever zones [5]. It is adopted by the latest seventh edition of AJCC and UICC Manual for N staging, with involvement of ipsilateral hila node as N1, ipsilateral mediastinal nodes as N2, and contralateral mediastinal or supraclavicular nodes as N3. Lymph nodes drainage depends on the location of tumors, with those in left upper lobe drain predominantly into subaortic node and those in right upper lobe drain predominantly into right upper paratracheal node. Middle and lower lobe tumors drain more commonly into subcarinal and lower paratracheal nodes. However, skip metastasis to mediastinal nodes bypassing hilar nodes occur in around 10–25% tumors [6]. Lymph nodes with short axis diameter ≥10 mm is considered suspicious of nodal metastasis (**Figure 3**).

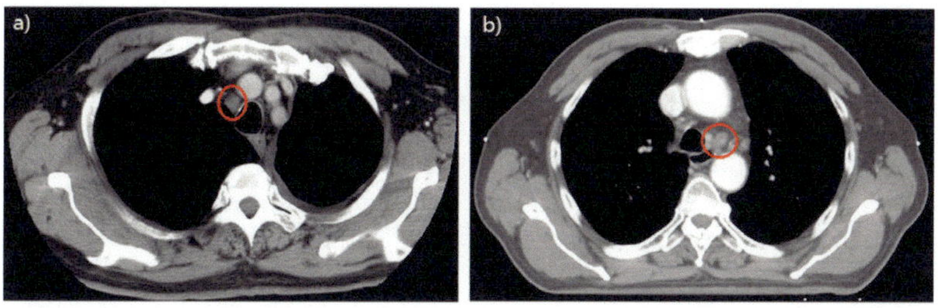

Figure 3. Enlarged mediastinal lymph node over (a) right upper paratracheal node (station 2R) and (b) subaortic node (station 5).

3. Staging and assessment

All patients with suspected lung cancer should have computer tomography (CT) of thorax with intravenous contrast for proper staging. Histological proof from primary tumors can be obtained by bronchoscopy if centrally located or by image-guided approach if peripherally located. For those patients planned for radical treatment, positron emission tomography (PET) scan is recommended to exclude any distant metastasis. Unanticipated metastasis may be detected in up to 10–20% cases. It is also more useful than CT in differentiating collapse or atelectasis from primary tumors (**Figure 4**). Any suspicious lymph nodes based on enlargement on CT or uptake in PET should be confirmed by needle technique (e.g., endoscopic ultrasound) or mediastinoscopy.

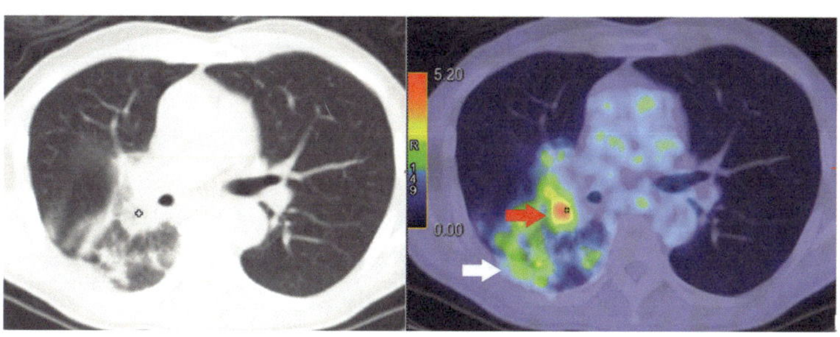

Figure 4. Use of PET in differentiating primary tumor with intense uptake (red arrow) from surrounding collapse or atetactasis (white arrow).

4. Indications of radiotherapy

4.1. Nonsmall cell lung cancer

4.1.1. Early stage I–II disease: curative treatment

Radical surgery remained the preferred treatment in early stage I–II lung cancer with 5-year overall survival rate of around 60–80%. Radical radiotherapy can be an alternative to patients who are medically unfit for surgery due to medical comorbidities or who declined surgery. Currently, there are no phase III trials to directly compare the outcomes after surgery with radiotherapy. Retrospective and historical databases showed that the long-term survival after conventional radiotherapy may be half (or even less) than that after surgery, with 5-year survival of around 20–30% in most series. But this indirect comparison is difficult due to the different population groups with more elderly, comorbidities, or poor lung function in those nonsurgical series. For elderly patients, hypofractionated scheme using 55 Gray (Gy) in 20 daily fractions is as effective as conventional radiotherapy in 2Gy per fraction.

Stereotactic body radiotherapy (SBRT) is now a newly emerging treatment option that allows delivery of a much higher radiation dose to a precise area than conventional radiotherapy. The reported local control rate in early stage lung cancer can be up to 80–90% in 2 years and is well tolerated. Therefore, it becomes the preferred radiotherapy modality for stage I lung cancer patients who are not fit for surgery. But extra care should be given when treating tumors that are centrally located around the major airways due to the potential higher complications with the hypofractionated regime.

4.1.2. Locally advanced stage III disease: curative treatment

This stage of disease was considered locally advanced either due to extensive primary tumor extension to extrathoracic structures nearby (T3 or T4) or mediastinal lymph nodes involvement (N2 or N3). It is a heterogeneous population that requires multimodality treatments. The reported 5-year survival was around 10–30%. A multidisciplinary discussion involving cardiothoracic surgeons, radiologists, and oncologists is needed to individualize and optimize the treatment plan for each patient. Patients with good performance status 0–1, no significant weight loss of >10% in the preceding 3 months and good pulmonary function (forced expiratory volume in 1 second FEV1 > 1.0 L) are candidates for radical combined modality treatment.

For potentially operable N2 disease, induction treatment with either chemotherapy alone or chemoirradiation is recommended over surgery alone. There is no solid evidence to support the superiority of either approach. Addition of preoperative radiotherapy may have the potential effect in downstaging the tumor and achieving a higher pathological complete remission rate of mediastinal disease. Special precaution should be given with its use in candidates before a planned pneumonectomy due to the higher perioperative mortalities. When preoperative radiotherapy is considered, a dose higher than 45–54 Gy in 1.8–2 Gy per fraction had not been shown to give addition survival benefit.

For infiltrative N2 or N3 (contralateral mediastinum) disease, risk of systemic micrometastases is high. Definitive chemoirradation is the commonly used approach. Addition of chemotherapy to radical radiotherapy led to a survival benefit of 5–10% at 5 years. Concomitant use of chemotherapy had a further improvement in survival by 4.5% at 5 years when compared with sequential approach, but with the expense of higher toxicities (mainly esophagitis and/or pneumonitis). Platinum-based doublet chemotherapy is the preferred regime and usually 2–4 cycles are given [7, 8]. Thus, concurrent chemoirradiation is the preferred strategy for fit patients, while sequential approach can be used for less fit patients with disease still within a treatable radical radiotherapy volume. A dose higher than 70 Gy in conventional fractionation is not recommended due to the associated higher toxicities but no added survival benefit. A continuous, hyperfractionated, accelerated radiotherapy (CHART) using 54 Gy in 36 fractions of 1.5 Gy three times per day can be considered for selected patients opting for radiotherapy alone. It had around 20% relative risk reduction in 2-year local progression rate and survival compared with conventional radiotherapy, but implementation can be challenging.

For patients with performance status 3–4, significant comorbidities and poor lung function that preclude a radical treatment approach, palliative radiotherapy may be considered for local symptoms control.

4.1.3. *Metastatic stage IV disease: palliative treatment*

Early radiotherapy to thorax in patients with incurable disease but no or minimal symptoms had not been shown to improve symptom control, survival, or quality of life. Hence, palliative thoracic radiotherapy can be deferred till symptoms emerged. Common indications are cough, hemoptysis, chest pain, and airway obstruction [9]. The optimal radiotherapy dose and fractionation schedule remained unclear. While there is no significant difference in symptom control with different dose schedules, a small survival improvement may be seen with higher dose radiotherapy.

For malignancy-related superior vena cava obstruction, external beam radiotherapy is effective in 60% patients with nonsmall cell lung cancers and 80% patients with small cell lung cancers [10]. Chemotherapy is another treatment option for patients with chemosensitive tumors like lymphoma, germ cell tumors, or small cell tumors. Intravascular stent insertion may be considered for patients that require rapid relief of symptoms, those who fail to response or relapse after radiotherapy.

Palliative radiotherapy can also be given to distant metastatic sites (e.g., bone, skin). Single fraction radiotherapy is as effective as longer course radiotherapy in pain and local symptom control.

4.1.4. *Postoperative treatment*

Adjuvant postoperative radiotherapy (PORT) helps to improve local control in patients with high risk of local recurrence after surgery, including those with pathological N2 disease and incomplete resection either microscopically or macroscopically. A careful evaluation of general conditions and remaining lung reserves is required before the start of treatment. It is not routinely given to early stage I–II disease with clear resection due to the potential detrimental effect on overall survival from previous meta-analyses that include trials using large radiation fields and nonconformal radiation techniques. However, its role with the use of modern radiotherapy machine and conformal radiotherapy are unclear and further research is warranted.

5. Radiotherapy data acquisition

5.1. External beam radiotherapy

5.1.1. Immobilization

Patient will lie supine with arms above head holding a T-bar device and elbow supported laterally (**Figure 5**) to facilitate different beam angle entry for treatment. Knee support can be given to allow a more comfortable position when needed. Vacuum bag can be added to reduce movement if treatment time is long. For palliative setting using AP beams only, patients usually lie supine with arms beside body.

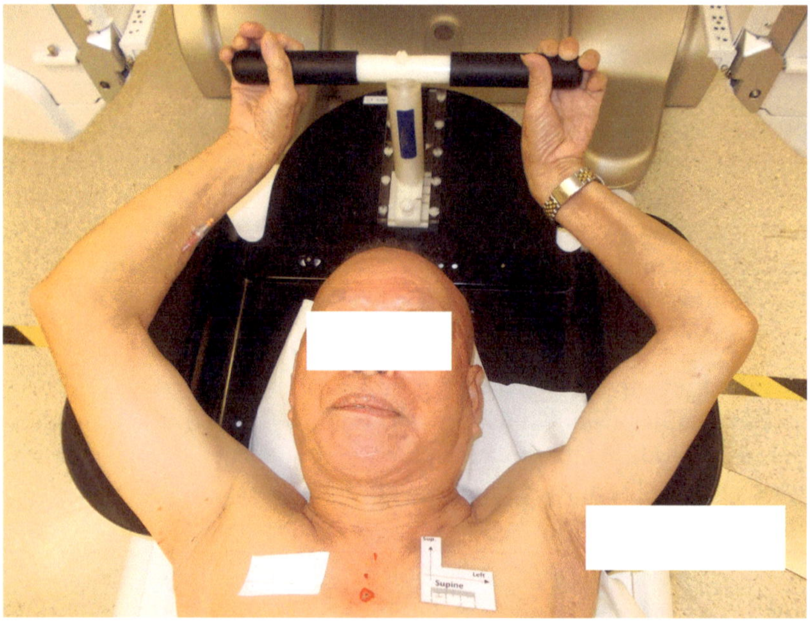

Figure 5. Immobilization for thoracic radiotherapy with T-bar and elbow support.

5.1.2. Simulation

For treatment with radical intent, computer-tomography from cricoid to lower border of L1 is needed to cover the whole lung for calculation of lung dose. Slice thickness of 3–5 mm allows better quality of images for target volume delineation. Intravenous contrast is not essential but is preferred when mediastinal disease is present so as to allow better visualization of the extent.

http://dx.doi.org/10.5772/67204

For treatment of palliative intent, radiation field border can be defined by simple X-ray simulation. Radio-opaque markers (e.g. lead wire) can be used to mark any clinically palpable diseases that are going to be included for radiotherapy (e.g., chest wall mass, supraclavicular lymph nodes).

To aid set-up, tattoos will be marked on beam center or isocenter, together with lateral reference points over left and right side of the body.

5.2. Stereotactic body radiotherapy (SBRT)

5.2.1. Immobilization

Patient should be immobilized in a comfortable position to avoid movement during the longer treatment length of each fraction. In this way, a supine position with arms above head immobilized by wing board and vacuum bag is commonly used (**Figure 6**).

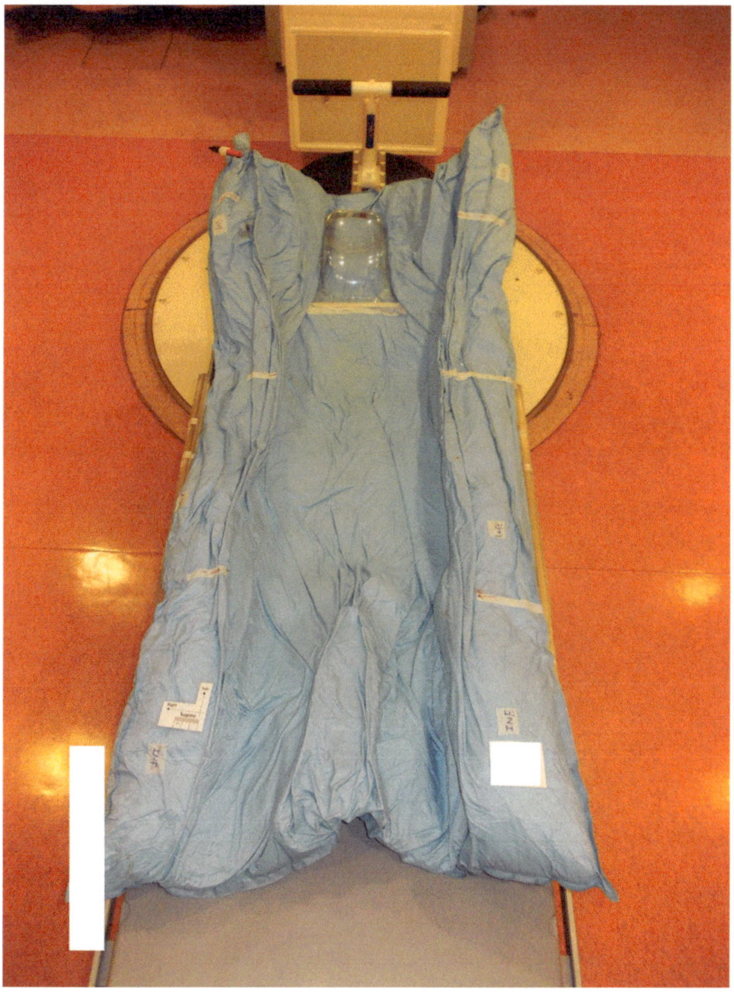

Figure 6. Immobilization with wing board and vacuum bag for SBRT of lung cancer.

5.2.2. Breathing motion assessment and correction

Fluoroscopy can be used to visualize tumor motion. But it only allows tumor motion assessment in two dimensions and can be difficult if with indistinct border of tumors. Noncontrast four-dimensional CT (4D CT) is a better option, which is a fast scanner that acquires multiset of CT images over consecutive phases of breathing cycle. Information about patients' breathing cycle and amplitude can be recorded by infrared reflecting marker and a coupled camera (**Figure 7**). And different CT images set will be sorted according to different phases in the respiratory cycle (**Figure 8**).

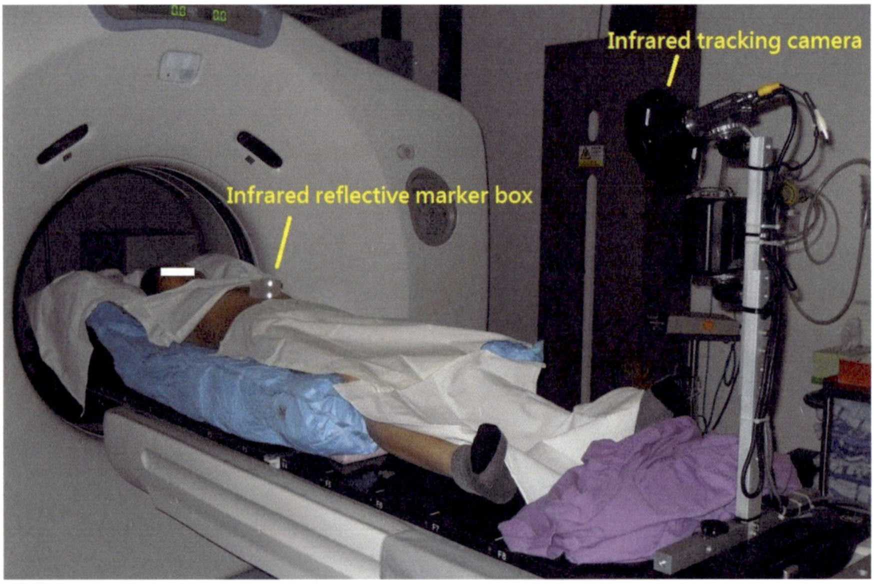

Figure 7. Infrared system including reflecting marker on patient's xiphsternum and coupled camera for tracking breathing cycle.

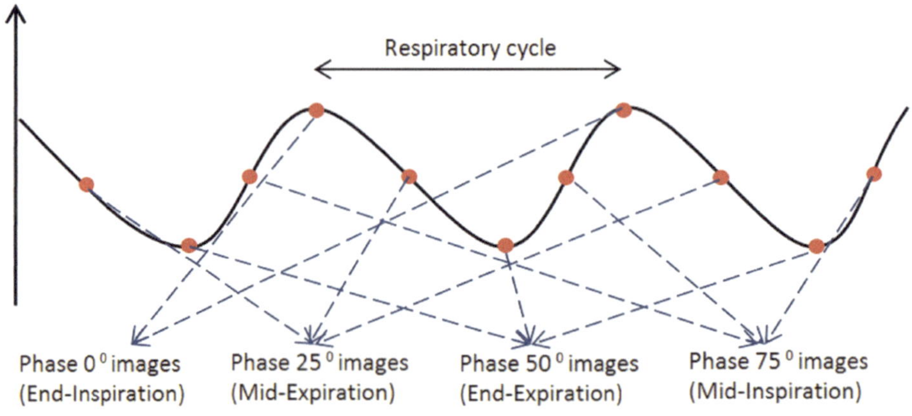

Figure 8. Sorting of 4D CT images by different phases in respiratory cycle.

http://dx.doi.org/10.5772/67204

Additional methods should be considered to reduce the tumor movement when it is ≥1cm, including abdominal compression, breath-hold, respiratory gating, or active breathing control. Both breath-hold and active breathing control require sufficient lung reserve to allow holding each breath for at least 20 seconds, which may be difficult for most of patients with lung cancers. Respiratory gating allows free breathing and beam on in certain phase of respiration. But it requires the use of fiducial markers to track internal tumor motion and is time consuming. Abdominal compression is the most commonly used method but reproducibility can be difficult (**Figure 9**). So the best method to be used depends on the patient's condition, tolerance, and corporation.

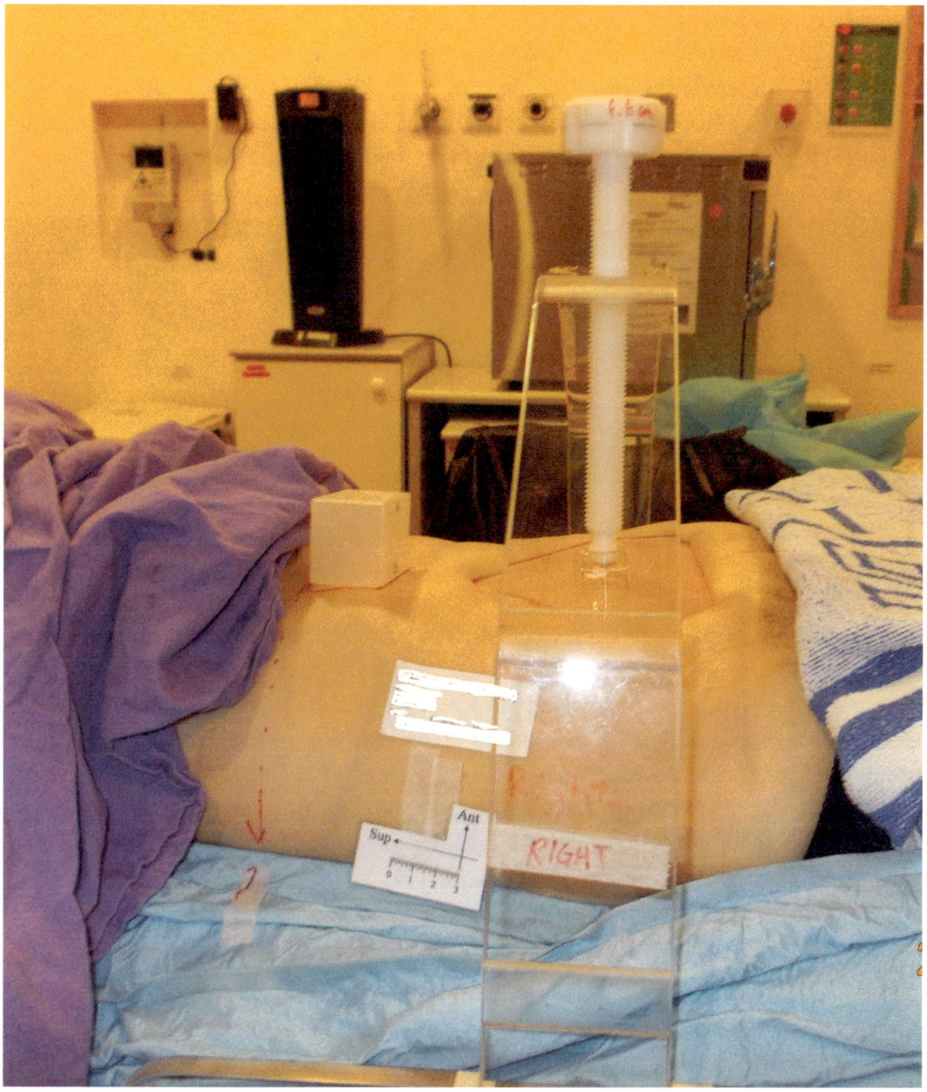

Figure 9. Abdominal compressor on patient's belly to reduce respiratory motion.

6. Target volume delineation

6.1. Conventional radiotherapy

Any clinical information and findings from bronchoscopy and mediastinoscopy should be gathered and correlated with diagnostic images. For postoperative cases, surgical records and pathology reports should be reviewed. And in case with doubt, discussions with surgeons and pathologists are encouraged to identify sites at risk of recurrence. Clips that are placed intraoperatively at sites with incomplete resection are useful for target identification.

An appropriate window setting should be used to delineate different targets on planning CT. Extent of primary lung tumor and mediastinal disease is best visualized by lung setting (window width 1600 and window level -600) and soft tissue setting (window width 400 and window level 20), respectively (**Figure 10**). Diagnostic imaging (e.g., CT or PET) should be coregistered with the planning of CT for contouring. PET images can help delineate area of collapse and atelectasis from tumors, but care should be taken when matching the images due to poor spatial resolution and breathing motion artifact.

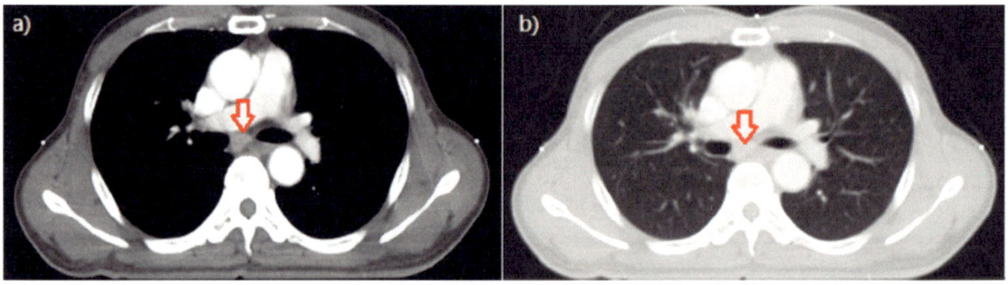

Figure 10. Soft tissue window setting (a) in planning CT to define the mediastinal lymph node (red arrow), which cannot be easily seen in lung window (b).

Gross tumor volume of primary tumor (GTV-P) is best contoured on lung window setting to include any visible tumor within lung parenchyma and the speculated border. Any local invasion to surrounding structures (e.g., chest wall, vertebra) should be included as well based on soft tissue window setting. Areas of collapse or atelectasis were excluded but can be difficult to differentiate. Input from radiologists and PET may be useful. Elective nodal irradiation is not recommended as isolated nodal recurrences are rare. So GTV of lymph node (GTV-N) will only include any pathologically confirmed lymph nodes (fine needle cytology or core biopsy) and any suspicious lymph nodes based on imaging characteristics (including short axis diameter ≥1 cm, necrotic center or PET uptake). If chemotherapy had been used before radiotherapy, all initial sites of tumor involvement should be contoured unless it exceeds a tolerable radiotherapy portal.

An isotropic margin is then added to GTV-P to cover microscopic tumor spread to form the clinical target volume (CTV-P). Usually, a 6 mm margin for adenocarcinoma and an 8 mm margin for squamous cell carcinoma are used as it had been shown to cover around 95% of microscopic tumor extension on pathological specimens [11]. Subsequent CTV-P is edited

http://dx.doi.org/10.5772/67204

according to the presence of natural barriers (e.g., great vessels, bone). For GTV-N, usually no additional margin is needed for CTV.

A margin from CTV to PTV (planning target volume) depends on tumor motion and daily set-up errors (**Figure 11**). Tumor motion can be quite variable from zero in cases using implanted fiducial markers in image-guided radiotherapy to certain centimeters in cases without any breathing motion control. Set-up errors are regularly measured in each department and usually within 5 mm in all directions. In common practice with free breathing treatment, a 1 cm isotropic margin is usually given to form the PTV. But a larger superior-inferior margin of 1.5 cm may be used for tumors with greater movement as long as the lung dose is within the tolerance limit.

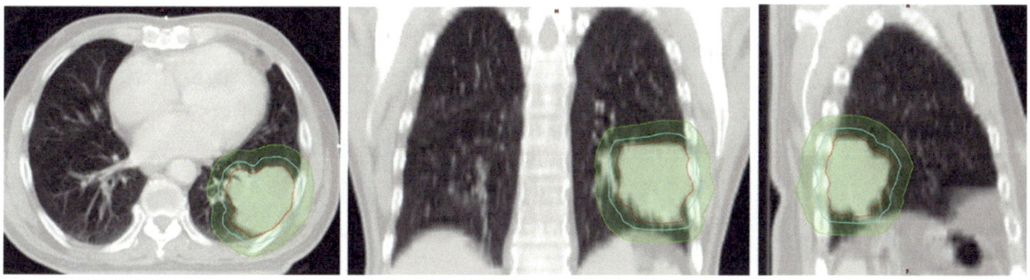

Figure 11. Target volume delineation: primary lung tumor (T) is contoured on lung window as gross tumor volume (GTV; red line); an additional 6 mm is added to form clinical target volume (CTV; blue line) to cover microscopic spread; further 1 cm margin is added to form the planning target volume (PTV; green line) to account for tumor motion and set-up error.

For palliative radiotherapy using AP beams, information about tumor extent from diagnostic imaging can be superimposed on those visible on simulator to form the GTV. And a further 1.5 cm margin from GTV can be used to define the radiotherapy field border.

6.2. Stereotactic body radiotherapy

Internal target volume (ITV) takes into account both GTV and internal tumor motion. It can be generated from the 4D CT using the maximum intensity projection (MIP) scan, maximum inspiratory, and expiratory scans, or all 10 phases of respiratory cycles (**Figure 12**). No CTV is needed. The usual CTV to PTV margin is 3–5mm, but it depends on methods of immobilization, tumor motion assessments, and treatment verification.

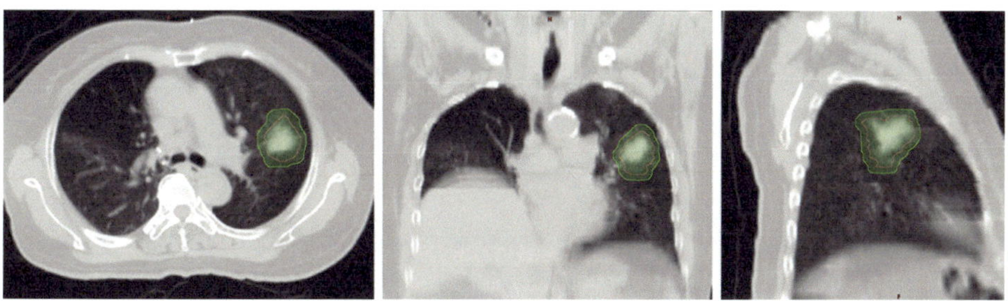

Figure 12. Target delineation on 4D CT: tumor is contoured on MIP images to form the internal target volume (ITV; red line); addition 5 mm margin was used to generate the planning target volume (PTV; green line).

7. Organs at risk delineation

Organs at risk including heart, esophagus, and spinal cord will be contoured using soft tissue window. The heart includes the whole structure within pericardial sac starting from the pulmonary artery to the apex. All layers of esophagus will be included and contoured from the cricoid cartilage to the esophagogastric junction. Spinal cord will be contoured at least 10 cm above and below PTV. For tumors over upper chest, the ipsilateral brachial plexus should also be contoured. Both left and right lungs are also contoured and then used to form a new structure called lung minus PTV after subtraction.

For SBRT, the tracheal and proximal bronchial tree should be contoured as well. Trachea will start from the level of cricoid cartilage to 2 cm above the carina, where it then continuous with the proximal bronchial tree (PBT, **Figure 13**) including the distal 2 cm trachea, main carina, bilateral main bronchi, bilateral upper lobe bronchi, lingular bronchus, intermedia bronchus, right middle lobe bronchus, and bilateral lower lobe bronchi. A 2 cm margin applied around the PTB will then be used to form a PRV (planning organ at risk volume).

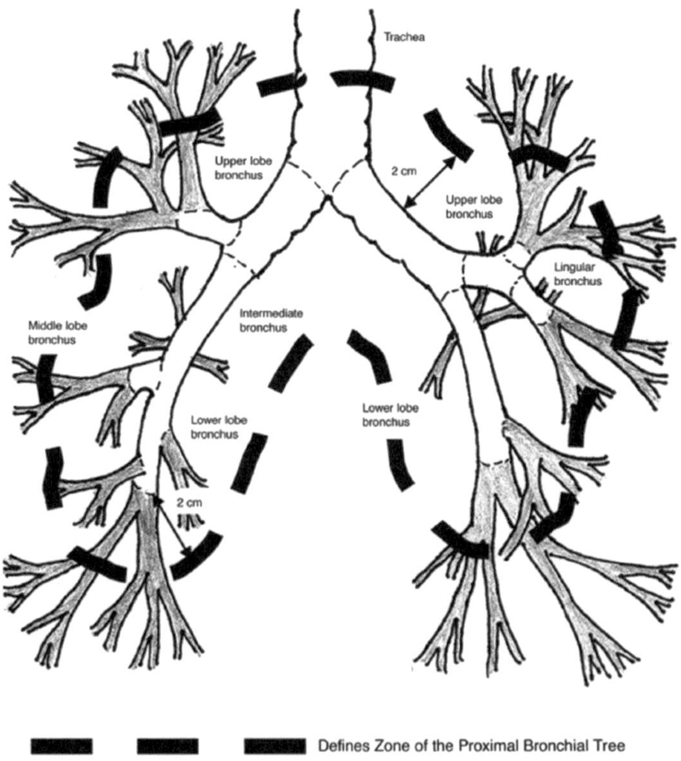

Figure 13. Definition of proximal bronchial tree.

http://dx.doi.org/10.5772/67204

8. Radiotherapy planning

For radical treatment, three-field conformal radiotherapy is most commonly used. The choices of beam numbers and beam angles depend on the location of the tumor and proximity to OARs. For early stage I–II tumors with lateralized target volume, a lateral, anterior, and posterior oblique beams are usually chosen to reduce irradiate contralateral lung (**Figure 14**).

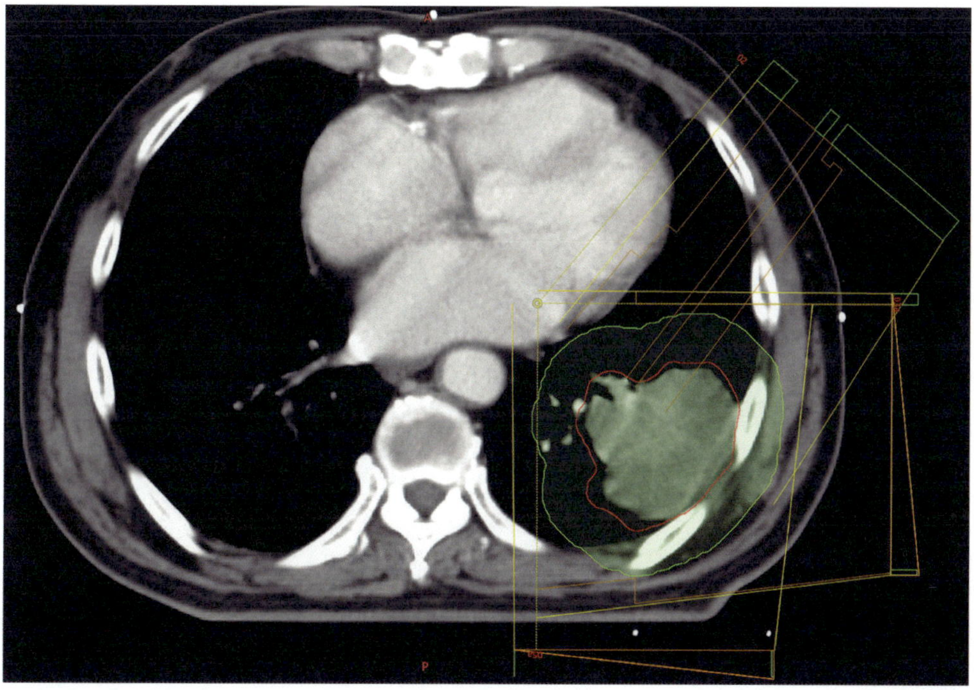

Figure 14. Beam arrangement in a three-field conformal radiotherapy for early stage lung cancer (red line = GTV; green line = PTV).

For more advanced stage disease with tumor involvement to mediastinum or across midline, the above three-field technique using ipsilateral beams only may not give good dose coverage to target, and addition of contralateral beam will increase total lung dose. In such case, two phases treatment should be considered. First phase will treat the mediastinum using AP beams shaped by multileaf collimator (MLC), while the second phase will use conformal technique to give adequate coverage to all the target volume. With this approach, total lung dose can be reduced but OARs near midline (e.g., esophagus, spinal cord) will receive higher dose.

For palliative radiotherapy, anterior and posterior fields modified by MLC are usually used with dose prescribed to midplane. Energy of photon beam used will depend on separation at the center of the field.

Radiotherapy plans should be carefully evaluated using dose-volume histogram (DVH). Optimal plan should aim at 95% PTV receiving at least 100% of the prescribed dose and 99% PTV receiving a minimum of 90% of the prescribed dose. For OARs, commonly used dose constrains for lung minus PTV is V20 (volume receiving >20 Gy) below 35%, preferably below 30%. However, a tighter constrain to reduce the risk of radiation pneumonitis should be considered when there is presence of other risk factors including preexiting lung disease and concurrent use of chemotherapy. Another frequently used limit is the mean lung dose below 20 Gy. The dose constrains for other OARs are maximum dose to spinal cord less than 45 Gy and heart V20 less than 40 Gy. Care should be given to avoid irradiation of more than 10 cm length of the esophagus due to higher long-term risk of stricture.

For SBRT, either intensity-modulated radiotherapy using 6–8 fields (IMRT) or rapidarc therapy is recommended to deliver a high and conformal dose to a precise area (**Figure 15**). Dose to skin should be minimized to avoid cutaneous and subcutaneous toxicities. Recommendations to other OARs can be made reference to that published by ROSEL study and RTOG 0813 study.

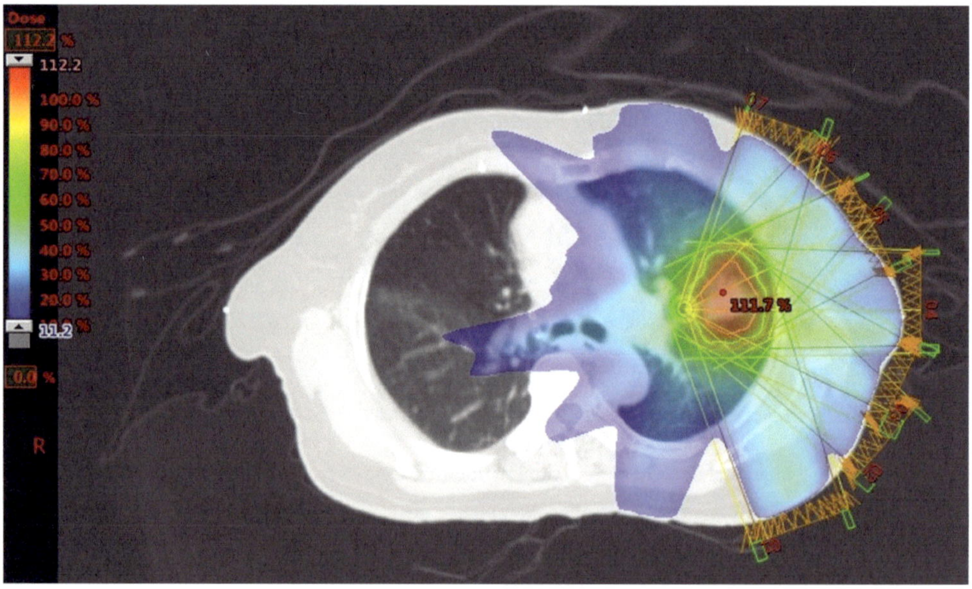

Figure 15. Beam arrangement and dose color wash from SBRT for lung cancer using IMRT technique.

9. Radiotherapy dose and fractionation

9.1. Radical treatment

9.1.1. Early stage T1-3N0 disease and fit patients: use SBRT

- For peripherally located tumor: 54 Gy in three fractions or 60 Gy in five fractions, alternate day treatment over 1–2 weeks (more conservative schedule is recommended if PTV is in contact with chest wall to avoid rib toxicities).

- For centrally located tumor (defined as GTV within 2 cm from proximal bronchial tree): 50 Gy in 10 fractions, alternate day treatment over 2 weeks.

9.1.2. Other early stage I–II disease: use conventional radiotherapy

- 60–70 Gy in 30–35 daily fractions over 6–6.5 weeks.
- Consider hypofractionated regime of 55 Gy in 20 daily fractions over 4 weeks if elderly.

9.1.3. Locally advanced stage III disease: use conventional radiotherapy

- For preoperative treatment (with or without chemotherapy): 45–54 Gy in 1.8–2 Gy per fraction over 5–6 weeks.
- For definitive treatment with concurrent chemotherapy: 60–66 Gy in 30–33 daily fractions over 6–6.5 weeks (consider treat up to 70 Gy in 35 daily fractions over 7 weeks if no chemotherapy given and within lung dose tolerance).

9.2. Adjuvant treatment

- For complete resection: 50 Gy in 25 daily fractions over 5 weeks.
- For incomplete resection: 60 Gy in 30 daily fractions over 6 weeks (consider boost up to 66 Gy in 33 daily fractions if gross residual disease).

9.3. Palliative treatment

- For PS 0–1 and life expectancy >6 months: 30 Gy in 10 daily fractions over 2 weeks (consider 39 Gy in 13 daily fractions over 2.5 weeks if spinal cord not within treated volume).
- For PS ≥ 2: 20 Gy in five daily fractions over 1 week or 10 Gy single fraction.

10. Treatment verification and delivery

Portal images by electronic portal imaging device on treatment machines are taken on first 3 days on treatment and then weekly afterwards. These are compared and registered with digitally reconstructed radiography (DRR) from CT simulations to allow offline corrections. For SBRT, cone beam CT by onboard imaging on treatment machine is done daily to allow online correction before delivery of each fraction of treatment.

During treatment period, patients should be reviewed at least once by radiation oncologists for assessment of any acute radiation side effects. Mild chest symptoms like cough or dyspnea are common but concomitant chest infection should be excluded if symptoms worsened. Dysphagia can occur due to esophagitis which usually start at around third week. Adequate analgesics and diet advice should be given to minimize severity and the impact on nutrition or weight loss.

11. Follow-up

After radical treatment, CT of thorax and upper abdomen should be done 3 monthly in the first 2 years, then half yearly till 5 years, and then annually to evaluate disease status. Long-term toxicities especially on lung function and esophageal stricture should be regularly reviewed and managed accordingly.

Author details

Fiona Lim Mei Ying

Address all correspondence to: fionalimmy@gmail.com

Department of Oncology, Princess Margaret Hospital, Hong Kong

References

[1] International Agency for Research on Cancer. 2014. Available from: http://publications.iarc.fr/Non-Series-Publications/World-Cancer-Reports/World-Cancer-Report-2014

[2] Lortet-Tieulent J, Soerjomataram I, Ferlay J, Rutherford M, Weiderpass E, Bray F. International trends in lung cancer incidence by histological subtype: Adenocarcinoma stabilizing in men but still increasing in women. Lung Cancer. 2014;**84**(1):13–22. DOI: http://dx.doi.org/10.1016/j.lungcan.2014.01.009

[3] Govindan R, Page N, Morgensztern D, et al. Changing epidemiology of small-cell lung cancer in the United States over the last 30 years: Analysis of the surveillance, epidemiologic, and end results database. Journal of Clinical Oncology. 2006;**24**:4539–4544.

[4] Morgensztern D, Ng SH, Gao F, Govindan R. Trends in stage distribution for patients with non-small cell lung cancer. A National Cancer Database Survey. Journal of Thoracic Oncology. 2010;**5**:29–33.

[5] Rusch VW, Asamura H, Watanabe H, Giroux DJ, Rami-Porta R, Goldstraw P. The IASLC Lung Cancer Staging Project. A proposal for a new international lymph node map in the forthcoming seventh edition of the TNM classification for lung cancer. Journal of Thoracic Oncology. 2009;**4**:568–577.

[6] Riquet M, Hidden G, Debesse B. Direct lymphatic drainage of lung segments to the mediastinal nodes. An anatomic study on 260 adults. The Journal of Thoracic and Cardiovascular Surgery. 1989;**97**:623–632.

[7] O'Rourke N, Roque i Figuls M, Farre Bernado N, Macbeth F. Concurrent chemoradiotherapy in non-small cell lung cancer. Cochrane Database of Systematic Reviews. 2010;6:CD002140. DOI: 10.1022/14651858.CD002140.pub3.

[8] Auperin A, Pechoux CL, Rolland E, Curran WJ, Furuse K et al. Meta-analysis of concomitant versus sequential radiochemotherapy in locally advanced non-small-cell lung cancer. Journal of Clinical Oncology. 2010;**28**:2181–2190. DOI: 10.1200/JCO.2009.26.2543

[9] Fairchild A, Harris K, Barnes E, Wong R, Lutz S, Bezjak A, et al. Palliative thoracic radiotherapy for lung cancer: a systematic review. Journal of Clinical Oncology. 2008;**26**:4001–4011. DOI: 10,1200/JCO.2007,15,3312

[10] Rowell NP, Gleeson FV. Steroids, radiotherapy, chemotherapy and stents for superior vena caval obstruction in carcinoma of the bronchus. Cochrane Database Systemic Review. 2001;**4**(4):CD001316.

[11] Giraud P, Antoine M, Larrouy A, Milleron B, Callard P, De Rycke Y, et al. Evaluation of microscopic tumor extension in non-small-cell lung cancer for three-dimensional conformal radiotherapy planning. International Journal of Radiation Oncology Biology Physics. 2000;**48**(4):1015–1024.

Chapter 3

Adaptive Radiotherapy for Lung Cancer Using Uniform Scanning Proton Beams

Yuanshui Zheng

Additional information is available at the end of the chapter

http://dx.doi.org/10.5772/67445

Abstract

Lung cancer remains the leading cause of cancer death in North America and is one of the major indications for proton therapy. Proton beams provide a superior dose distribution due to their finite ranges, but where they stop in the tissue is very sensitive to anatomical change. To ensure optimal target coverage and normal tissue sparing in the presence of geometrical variations, such as tumor shrinkage and other anatomical changes, adaptive planning is necessary in proton therapy of lung cancer. The objective of the chapter is to illustrate the rationale, process, and strategies in adaptive lung cancer treatment using uniform scanning proton beams. In addition, practical considerations for adaptive proton planning are discussed, such as software limitations, the associated costs and risks, and the criteria on whether and how to adapt a plan.

Keywords: uniform scanning, proton therapy, lung cancer, adaptive radiotherapy

1. Introduction

Lung cancer continues to be the leading cause of cancer death in the United States, and over 158,000 lung cancer deaths were estimated in 2015 [1]. Radiation is one of the major treatment modalities for lung cancer treatment. Because of proton beams' finite range, proton beam therapy (PBT) has been increasingly used for lung cancer. Compared to 3D conformal or intensity modulated photon radiation (IMRT), proton beams can better spare the lung, esophagus, heart, cord, and other normal tissues while delivering the same or higher dose to the treatment target [2–4]. The dosimetric advantage of proton therapy could lead to potential better tumor control and less toxicity. Proton beams provide a superior dose distribution due to their finite ranges, but where they stop in the tissue is very sensitive to anatomical change. To ensure optimal target coverage and normal tissue sparing in the presence of geometrical variations, such as tumor shrinkage and other anatomical changes, plan adaptation is often needed in proton therapy of lung cancer.

The chapter aims at illustrating the rationale and process in adaptive proton treatment of lung cancers, as well as the strategies and practical considerations in plan adaptation, with a focus on the use of uniform scanning proton beams.

2. Proton therapy system

Depending on how proton beams are spread out laterally and in depth, there are mainly three proton delivery systems in clinical use: passive scattering proton therapy (PSPT), uniform scanning proton therapy (USPT), and pencil beam scanning (PBS). In PSPT, the proton beam is spread out laterally by a static scatterer (or double scatterers) located in the beam axis, and the beam modulation in depth is typically achieved by using a rotating range modulation wheel, which is composed of multiple steps of various thicknesses. Both USPT and PBS proton therapy use scanning magnets to sweep proton beams laterally and deliver the dose to a target volume layer by layer at various depths using proton beams of various energies. The main difference between USPT and PBS is that proton beams are scanned continuously with a uniform intensity in a zigzag pattern at a fixed frequency for each energy layer in USPT, while delivered with various beam intensities from one spot to another or continuously for each layer in PBS. PBS can be further divided into single field uniform dose (SFUD) delivery, which delivers a uniform dose to the target for each field, and multiple field uniform dose (MFUD), which delivers a heterogeneous dose to the target for each field but achieves a homogeneous combined dose from all fields. MFUD is also called intensity modulated proton therapy (IMPT).

Since our main focus for this chapter is USPT, a detailed description of a USPT system at our center is described below. The proton therapy center is equipped with an IBA Cyclotron (IBA, Louvain-la-Neuve, Belgium), which accelerates proton beams to approximately 230 MeV before they are extracted to treatment rooms through a beam transportation system. The proton beam passes through an energy degrader, which can lower the energy when necessary, and an energy selection system (ESS) is then transported to a nozzle in the treatment room. After entering the nozzle, the proton beam will first pass through a first scatterer, which broadens the beam laterally to achieve the desired spot size at isocenter. The beam then passes through a range modulator wheel, which does not rotate continuously for uniform scanning beam delivery and mainly serves as an energy degrader. Together with the first scatterer, the modulator wheel lowers the proton energy to deliver a peak dose layer by layer in depth. The beam is scanned laterally with a constant frequency by two scanning magnets in a zigzag pattern to deliver a uniform dose for a near rectangular scanning area. It then passes through the main and backup ionization chambers that monitor the proton dose. At the end of the nozzle is a snout that holds an aperture and a compensator and can translate along the beam axis to achieve variable snout to isocenter positions. An aperture is used to collimate the beam to the treatment target laterally, and a range compensator is used to conform the proton penetration to the distal boundary of the treatment target. More details on this system were described by Zheng *et al.* [5]. **Figure 1** shows a schematic diagram of the uniform scanning nozzle at our proton therapy center.

http://dx.doi.org/10.5772/67445

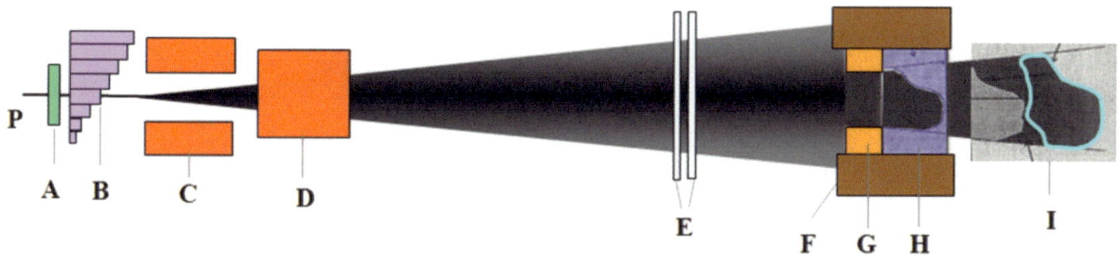

Figure 1. A schematic diagram of the uniform scanning nozzle at the ProCure Proton Therapy Center in Oklahoma City. Proton beams (P) go through a first scatterer (A), a range modulator wheel (B), two scanning magnets (C and D), the main and backup monitor unit ionization chambers (E), a snout (F), an aperture (G), a range compensator (H), and stop at the patient (I). The nozzle has a distance of about 290 cm between the first scatterer and the isocenter, and 211 cm between the effective source and the isocenter. (From Zheng *et al.* [5]).

3. Treatment techniques

3.1. Treatment simulation

Patient immobilization and simulation for lung cancer patients under proton therapy are similar to those under photon therapy. However, since proton beams are very sensitive to setup uncertainty and patient motion, the reproducibility of immobilization and proper motion management are critical in proton therapy. At our center, patients typically lie supine, are immobilized with a vacuum bag, which is on top of an index fixed framing device (wing board), and with their arms up and hands holding the pegs on the wing board, as shown in **Figure 2**. The patient is scanned at 2.5 mm slice thickness. If contrast is used, one computerized tomography (CT) scan should be taken before the contrast is injected in addition to one after the injection. The CT data with intravenous contrast will be used primarily for target delineation, and the CT data set without contrast will be used for dose calculation.

Four dimensional (4D) computerized tomography (CT) scanning is typically used for lung cancer patients in proton therapy to evaluate patient motion. The motion can be monitored by a belt system or a Varian RPM system during the 4D CT scan. The magnitude of tumor motion is typically evaluated for each 4D CT scan and used to determine the strategies in motion management. Depending on facility and beam delivery system, a limit of motion magnitude is set, beyond which the patient will need additional motion management or be excluded from proton treatment. For example, at our center, we generally treat patients using USPT with a maximum motion of 10–15 mm, while at the MD Anderson Proton Therapy Center, 5 mm maximum motion was used for patients under PBS proton treatment [6]. While respiratory gating or breath holding could reduce the tumor motion, currently, it is only used clinically in a very few proton centers due to challenges such as relatively low proton dose rate that leads to long treatment time for gated treatment, lack of connection between the respiratory device and the proton beam delivery machine, and difficulty of holding breath for lung cancer patients.

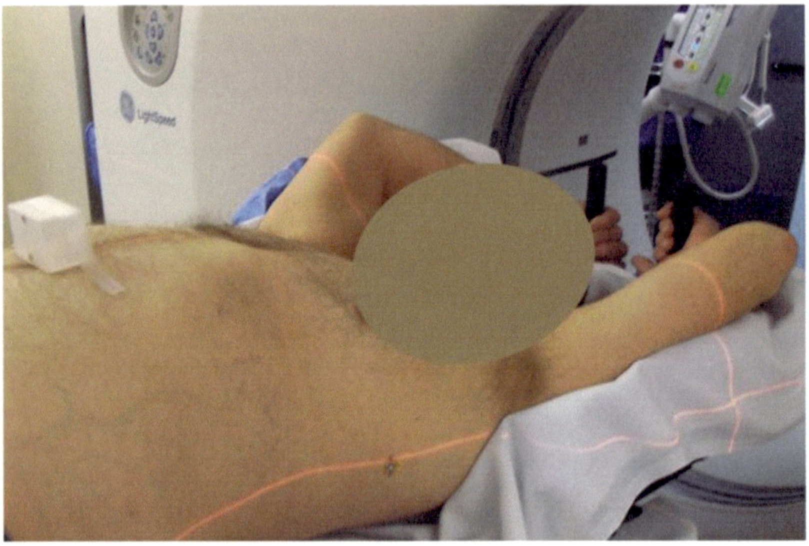

Figure 2. Typical CT simulation and immobilization technique for lung cancer treatment using uniform scanning proton therapy.

3.2. Treatment planning

Treatment planning can be performed on the average CT based on the 4D CT scan, or at a certain respiratory phase when gating or breast holding is used. At our center, we use the average CT and an Internal target volume (ITV) approach to account for motion effect during treatment, which is similar to what used at MD Anderson Cancer Center for lung treatment using passive scattering proton beams [7]. The internal gross target volume (IGTV) is contoured on the maximum intensity pixel (MIP) images and expanded 7–10 mm to generate the clinical target volume (CTV), which is expanded further by 5 mm to obtain the planning target volume (PTV). The average CT will be used for treatment planning and dose calculation. The magnitude of motion will be evaluated by a physicist, and the treatment of lung patient with uniform scanning proton beams is often limited to those who have a motion magnitude of 10 mm or less. To be conservative, a smearing of 10 mm is used in compensator calculation for all lung cancer treatment planning. To ensure adequate coverage of the target at the presence of tumor motion, the stopping power ratio of IGTV is overridden with the average stopping power ratio of the tumor tissue, which is about 1.01 based on sampling of over 10 lung patients treated at our center. Each patient is treated with uniform scanning proton beams typically using 2–4 fields. The prescription is typically 74 Cobalt Gray-equivalent (CGE) at 2 CGE per fraction for 37 fractions.

3.3. Dosimetric advantages

Proton beams provide a superior dose distribution for lung cancer treatment compared to photon beams. Chang *et al.* reported that PSPT significantly reduced dose to normal tissues

http://dx.doi.org/10.5772/67445

and the integral dose to patients with non-small cell lung cancer (NSCLC) compared to three-dimensional conformal radiation therapy (3D-CRT) and intensity modulated radiation therapy (IMRT) [2]. Kadoya *et al.* reported that using proton beam significantly reduced Lung dose compared to stereotactic body radiation therapy (SBRT) for Stage I non-small-cell lung cancer [8]. The mean dose, V5, V10, V15, and V20 were 4.6 Gy, 13.2%, 11.4%, 10.1%, and 9.1% for proton therapy compared to 7.8 Gy, 32%, 21.8%, 15.3%, and 11.4%, respectively, for SBRT with a prescribed dose for 66 Gy. In a similar study, Hoppe *et al.* reported that in addition to better dose sparing to the lung, PSPT delivered less dose ($D_{0.1cm}{}^3$ and $D_{5cm}{}^3$) to the heart, esophagus and bronchus compared to SBRT [9]. For locally advanced Stage III NSCLC patients, Wu *et al.* found that proton beam therapy was feasible and superior to three-dimensional conformal radiotherapy for several dosimetric parameters such as the mean dose for lung, heart, and spinal cord [3]. Using IMPT, doses to normal tissues, such as the lung, spinal cord, heart, and esophagus, can be further reduced compared to passive scattering proton therapy and IMRT for extensive Stage IIIB NSCLC, as reported by Zhang *et al.* [10]. The dosimetric advantage of IMPT would allow further dose escalation from 74 to 84.4 Gy while keeping normal tissue sparing at a lower or similar lever. IMPT proved also advantageous in terms of lung sparing compared to both Tomotherapy and IMRT in a study by Stuschke *et al.* [11]. A brief summary of literature on plan comparison between proton and photon therapy discussed here is listed in **Table 1**.

When uniform scanning proton therapy is used, similar normal tissue sparing to passive scattering proton therapy can be achieved. **Figure 3** shows the dose comparison of USPT versus IMRT for a lung case. The patient was a 72-year-old female with severe chronic obstructive pulmonary disease (COPD) and Stage IIIA (cT1aN2MpG2) squamous cell carcinoma of the right upper lung.

References	Year	Institution	Tumor stage (patient no)	Proton vs. photon	Normal tissues receiving less dose from proton therapy
Chang *et al.* [2]	2006	MDACC	Stage I (10) and III (15)	PSPT vs. 3DCRT	Lung, spinal cord, heart, esophagus, integral dose
Kadoya *et al.* [8]	2011	STPTC	Stage I (21)	PSPT vs. SBRT	Lung
Hoppe *et al.* [9]	2010	UFPTI	Stage I (8)	PSPT vs. SBRT	Lung, heart, esophagus, bronchus
Zhang *et al.* [10]	2010	MDACC	Stage IIIB (10)	IMPT vs. IMRT	Lung, spinal cord, heart, esophagus
Stuschke *et al.* [11]	2012	UHE	NA (6)	IMPT vs. IMRT/ tomotherapy	Lung
Wu *et al.* [12]	2016	NCCHE	Stage III (33)	PSPT vs. 3DCRT	Lung, heart, cord

Abbreviations: MDACC: M. D. Anderson Cancer Center; STPTC: Southern Tohoku Proton Therapy Center; UFTPI: University of Florida Proton Therapy Institute; NCCHE: National Cancer Center Hospital East; UHE: University Hospital Essen. Others see above.

Note: Reports from the literature.

Table 1. Comparison studies between proton and photon therapy for NSCLC patients.

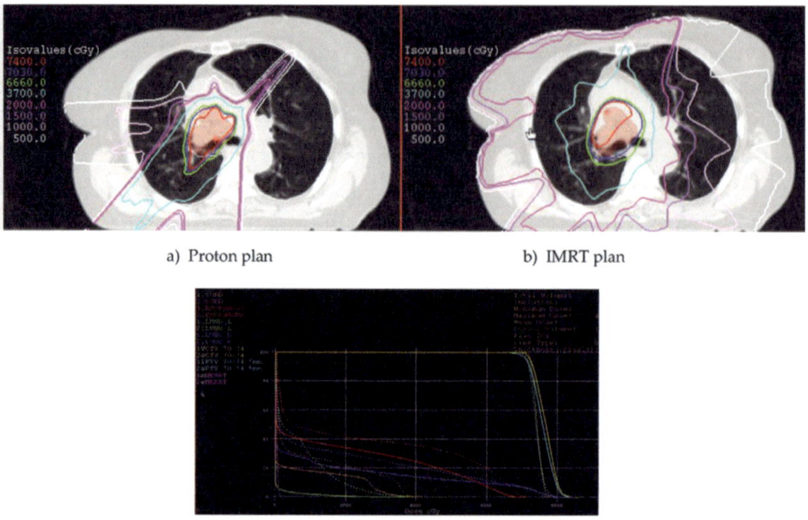

a) Proton plan b) IMRT plan

c) DVH comparison

Figure 3. Dose comparison of Uniform Scanning proton plan and IMRT plan. (a) Proton plan, (b) IMRT plan, and (c) DVH comparison (solid line—proton, dashed line—IMRT). The prescribed dose was 74 cobalt gray equivalent (CGE) at 2 CGE per fraction for 37 fractions.

4. Adaptive proton therapy of lung cancers

4.1. Rationale

Adaptive radiation therapy (ART) is a closed-loop process where the treatment plan will be re-optimized for treatment variations such as patient anatomy change using a systematic feedback of measurements. [13]. Thanks to the advancement of imaging modalities available for treatment planning and delivery, such as 4D CT and onboard imaging, ART has been feasible and clinically implemented at many cancer centers. The main goal of plan adaptation is to adjust the treatment plan to the change of patient anatomy, tumor motion, or setup, so that the target coverage and normal tissue sparing remain optimal for each individual patient during the whole course of treatment. For lung cancer patients, anatomy change is often inevitable due to tumor regression, pleural and pericardial effusions, or atelectasis. Adaptive photon therapy has been shown to be beneficial in lung cancer treatment, resulted in a mean reduction of 21% for the volume of ipsilateral lung receiving 20 Gy (V20) [14], and an average of 65 cGy reduction in mean lung dose and reductions in cord max dose, mean esophageal dose, and heart dose [15]. It was reported that ART has the potential to improve the accuracy of radiation treatments, thus reducing the exposure of organs at risk and facilitating safe dose escalation, leading to potentially better local control and overall survival [16–19].

Because a proton beam has a finite range and sharp distal dose fall off, the dose distribution of a proton plan is very sensitive to anatomy change; therefore, the need for lung cancer treatment adaption in proton therapy is even greater than photon therapy. Hui *et al.* found that the effects of inter-fractional motion and anatomic change could lead to a result of up to 8% reduction of the CTV coverage, a mean 4% dose increase of the volume of the contralateral lung receiving at least 5 CGE, and a mean 4.4 CGE increase in spinal cord maximum dose [20]. Koey *et al.* reported that without adaptive planning, target coverage could be dropped to below 60% compared with adaptive planning for some lung cancer case undergoing proton therapy [21]. The potential considerable dose change in proton therapy due to anatomy variation indicates that plan adaptation is essential in proton therapy of lung cancer.

4.2. Process for adaptive proton planning

A typical adaptive planning process includes measuring the treatment variations such as anatomic change, evaluating their dosimetric and clinical impact, and adapting the radiation treatment to the updated information as necessary. In proton therapy of lung cancer, anatomic change is of main concern. Repeated CT scans are commonly used to measure the anatomic change during the treatment course. Ideally, the repeated CT scans should be performed frequently with a 4D CT scan so that patient anatomy and motion can be accurately evaluated. However, depending on facility resources and patient compliance, in room CBCT or slow CT scans can also be used. The repeated CT will be registered to the initial CT, and a QA plan will be generated by applying the same beam configuration from the initial plan to the registered repeated CT data, which will be evaluated on dosimetric change and potential clinical impact. The physicist and physician will then determine whether and how the plan will be adapted. If plan adaptation is determined necessary, plan change will be made according to the physician/physicist instruction, and the new plan will be changed and go through the process of plan review, QA, and approval before beam delivery similar to the initial plan. In addition to deciding whether a plan adaptation is needed, one should also decide whether any other change is needed for the patient. For example, if the patient anatomy is likely to change significantly before the next scheduled CT scan, we may want to increase the imaging frequency for the patient.

A clinical workflow of the adaptive planning for lung cancer treatment at our center is shown in **Figure 4**. After initial 4D CT imaging, treat planning, and beam delivery, QA CT (i.e., repetitive CT) will be performed after a patient receives 14, 30, and 50 CGE of proton dose, that is, after the 7th, 15th, and 25th fraction for most patients treated with 2 CGE per fraction. The repeated average CT was fused to the original average CT based on bony anatomy by a dosimetrist using the VelocityAI software system (Version 3.1.0, Varian Medical Systems, Palo Alto, CA). A quality assurance (QA) plan was generated after each CT scan by applying the same proton beams and hardware (apertures and compensators) in the original plan to the registered new CT dataset using the XiO TPS (Version 5.0, Elekta Inc., St. Louis, MO). A physicist will first review the CT fusion to evaluate the anatomic change and check the correctness of the fusion. The physicist will then review the QA plan to evaluate the dosimetric change and the correlation between the dosimetric change and the anatomy variation. Together with the attending physician, the physicist will make a recommendation on whether plan adaption is needed. If plan adaptation is determined to be necessary, a dosimetrist will make the plan change, and treatment with the new plan will start as soon as possible. The process of treatment, QA CT, QA planning, and plan adaptation will be repeated until the patient complete the treatment course.

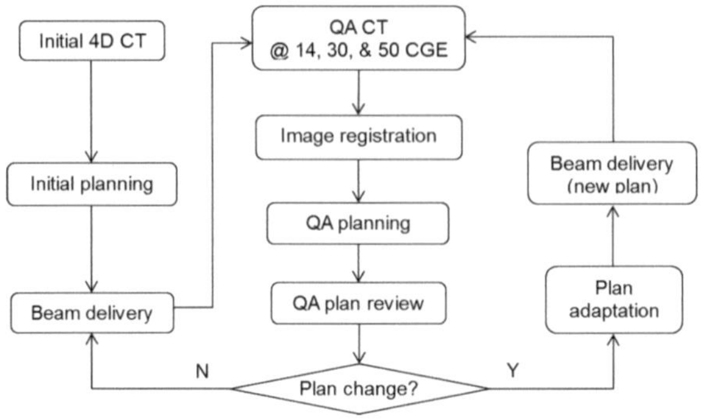

Figure 4. A clinical workflow of adaptive planning for lung cancer treatment using uniform scanning proton therapy.

4.3. Strategies for plan adaptation

One straightforward way of plan adaptation is to re-plan based on the newly obtained CT, repeating the same process as how the initial plan is created. Re-planning has been used for most adaptive treatment in both photon therapy and proton therapy and generally includes target contouring, beam placement, dose optimization, plan review and approval, documentation and billing, calendar adjustment, QA, and so on. For adaptive proton therapy where PSPT and USPT are used, new patient specific devices such as apertures and compensators are also needed during re-planning, which can lead to added cost and long turnaround time due to the manufacturing process. Substantial effort is needed from the dosimetrists, physicist, and machinists, and it can take several days to make the new plan available for treatment. Before the new plan becomes available, the patient can either continue to be treated with the initial plan or have a treatment break, depending on the extent of anatomy change and its impact on dose distribution and potential clinical effect. On the other hand, re-planning can fully adapt a plan and achieve the best optimization of dose distribution based on the new CT data set. **Figure 5** shows an example of re-planning with new patient specific hardware. Substantial tumor shrinkage was observed on the repeated CT scan, which led to a large increase in lung and cord dose (**Figure 5b**). A new plan was created based on the new 4D CT (**Figure 5c**), with an improved normal tissue sparing while maintaining target coverage similar to the initial plan.

Another way of plan adaptation is to make some simple changes in beam parameters, such as range, modulation, or beam weight of any combination. Because a uniform scanning or passive scattering proton beam delivers a uniform dose to patients, it is possible to adjust the range and/or modulation for a proton beam to shift the depth of the spread out Bragg peak (SOBP) region so that the adjusted beam would conform to the target after the water equivalent thickness (WET) changes due to anatomy change. For uniform scanning proton beams, such parameter change is very easy and can be made for the TPS and R&V in minutes plus some additional work on documentation. **Figure 6** shows an example of such case that patient developed pleural effusion at the 25th fraction. After simply increasing the proton

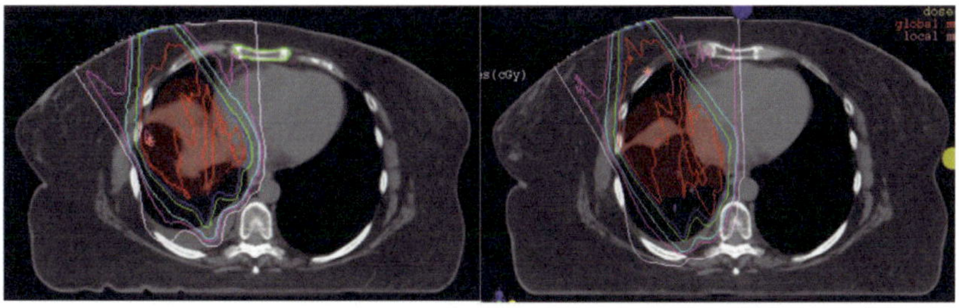

a) Original plan b) QA plan

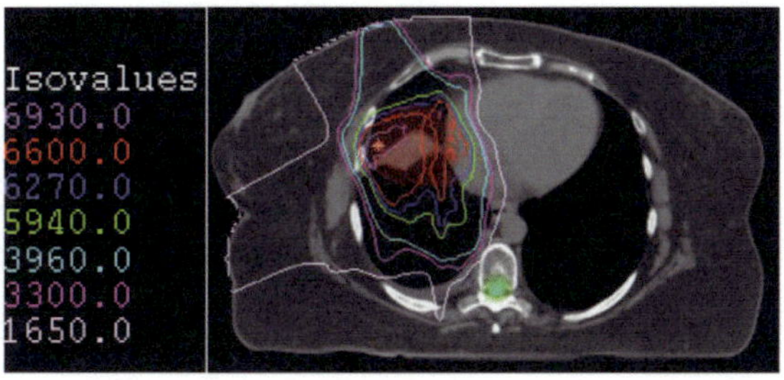

c) Adapted plan

Figure 5. An example case of re-planning with new patient specific device. The patient has small cell Stage IIIA lung cancer with COPD. A 66 CGE was delivered at 33 fractions using uniform scanning proton beams. (a) Original plan; (b) QA plan; (c) adapted plan based on the new CT data.

range by 2.2 cm, the target became fully covered while the normal tissues of lung and heart were still well protected. This simple approach can be highly desirable for certain anatomy changes such as patient weight change which pulls back or increase the range relatively uniform, and/or a quick plan adaptation is needed due to concern on treatment breaks. Please note that such approach is unique in uniform scanning and may not be available in PBS or passive scattering PT.

Other strategies of plan change for USPT could be beam weight change, for example, decrease the weight of beam(s) that is adversely affected by the anatomy change, and increase the weight of beam(s) that is least affected. In addition, a hybrid approach, such as re-planning for one beam and range adjustment for another, can also be used as appropriate.

The strategy used for plan adaptation depends largely on the institutional practice and the beam delivery technique used for lung cancer treatment. For lung cancer treatment with PSPT, Koay *et al.* reported that 20.5% of patients underwent adaptive planning using re-planning with new patient-specific hardware [21]. For USPT, Zheng *et al.* reported that 18.8% of lung cancer patients underwent adaptive planning, using various strategies including range change only (10.9%), range and modulation change (1.8%), range, modulation, and beam weight change (1.2%), and re-planning with new hardware (5.5%) [22]. For PBS or IMPT, Chang *et al.* reported that 26.5% patients were re-planed [6]. A brief summary of adaptive proton therapy literature discussed here is listed in **Table 2**.

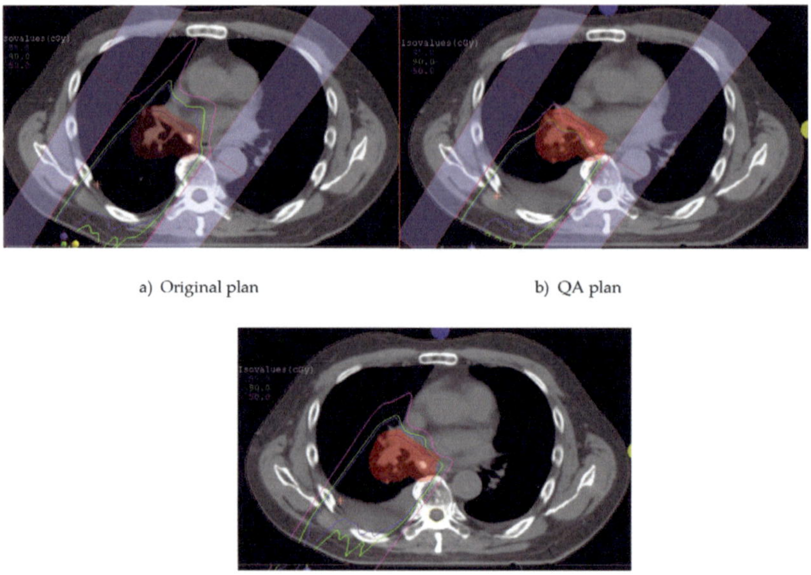

a) Original plan b) QA plan

c) Adapted plan

Figure 6. The dose distribution from the right posterior oblique beam normalized at the isocenter for a lung cancer patient undergoing adaptive proton therapy using parameter adjustment. (a) Initial plan; (b) QA plan; (c) adapted plan with a 2.2 cm range increase. The patient had a right hilar mass and was treated with three proton beams for a total dose of 74 CGE. Fluid buildup was observed on a repeated CT scan after the 25th fraction.

References	**Year**	**Institution**	**Treatment technique**	**No. of patients**	**Adaptation percentage**	**Repeated CT scanning**	**Median time for plan change**
Koay *et al.* [21]	2012	MDACC	PSPT	44	20.5%	At week 3 or 4	At 24 fractions
Chang *et al.* [6]	2014	MDACC	PBS/IMPT	34	26.5%	Every 2 weeks	After 10 fractions
Zheng *et al.* [22]	2015	ProCure	USPT	165	18.8%	After 7, 15, and 25 fractions	After 18 fractions

Abbreviations: MDACC: M. D. Anderson Cancer Center; STPTC: Southern Tohoku Proton Therapy Center; UFTPI: University of Florida Proton Therapy Institute; NCCHE: National Cancer Center Hospital East; UHE: University Hospital Essen.

Note: Reports from the literature.

Table 2. Adaptive proton therapy.

5. Practical considerations

While adaptive planning can potentially improve the dose distribution and clinical outcome, there are also many pitfalls and limitations in the current adaptive planning process. An optimal adaptive planning process should be developed based on both practical considerations and theoretical dosimetric and clinical gains.

5.1. Frequency of repeated CT scanning and QA planning

The frequency of repeated CT scans depends on facility-specific protocol or individual patient need. Chang reported that 4D CT scans were repeated during week 3 or 4 of treatment or as clinically indicated by the treating physician for lung cancer patients undergoing PSPT [23], and weekly or every 2 to 3 weeks for those receiving intensity modulated proton therapy at MD Anderson Cancer Center [6]. At our center, 4D CT is generally repeated after 7, 15, and 25 fractions of treatment. However, for special cases, more repeated CT scans may be needed such as when patients have a pleural effusion or large weight change. In addition, if hypo-fractionated or hyper-fractionated treatment is used, more frequent monitoring should be considered. Daily imaging has becoming available with the introduction of in room CT like CBCT into proton therapy; however, its clinical implementation may be limited due to the extra treatment time and human effort as well as concerns on the increased imaging dose to patients.

5.2. Limitations of image registration and QA planning

One key component of adaptive planning is the image registration. Accurate imaging registration can be challenging, especially for lung adaptive planning where considerable anatomy change may be observed due to disease progression, tumor response to therapy and respiratory motion [24, 25]. It is important to setup and immobilize the patient for repeated CT as close as possible to the initial CT scan that is used for the treatment planning as large patient setup variation could lead to difficulty on image registration and anatomy change evaluation. The accuracy of image registration needs to be carefully evaluated. In addition, there can be limitation on how a QA plan is generated. For example, our treatment plan system does not account for the patient pitch and roll when a QA plan is applied to the new CT data, although our image registration software does. Another issue is that there could be human errors associated with the image registration and QA plan process, such as beams may be placed with an incorrect isocenter in a QA plan. Limitations or errors in the image registration and QA plan process could result in artificial dose deviation unrelated to anatomy change and potential errors in decision-making of plan adaptation. Therefore, it is critical to understand these limitations and evaluate the accuracy of image registration and QA planning to avoid errors in decision-making that may lead to unnecessary plan change and potential mistreatment. Our guideline is, in addition to review the QA plan and dose distribution beam by beam, we also analyze the anatomy change and the correlation between the dose change and anatomy change. Any noticeable dose change in the QA plan should be correlated to either patient anatomy/motion change or setup variation; otherwise, the dose change may be artificial as a result of software limitations or human errors, and further investigation should be warranted.

5.3. Correlation between dose change and anatomy variation

The penetration depth of a proton beam is a function of the proton energy and the WET of the materials it passes through. Therefore, for a proton beam of given energy, the depth of the dose falloff is directly correlated to the WET associated with the anatomy in the beam path. Common changes in anatomy that could lead to plan adaptation include patient weight gain or loss, tumor shrinkage or growth, pleural effusion, atelectasis, and so on. For example, when a patient gains weight, the WET in beam path will increase, leading to a range pull back. The effect of patient weight change typically is more noticeable for anterior proton beams, and may be addressed by simply adjusting the range and/or modulation as the WET change is relatively uniform within the field. Similarly, tumor shrinkage will result in a decrease in WET and beam overshoot, which could lead to more dose to normal tissues such as lung and cord. Target coverage is generally not an issue when a tumor shrinks but can be severely compromised when a tumor progresses and increases in volume. Tumor shrinkage or progression will have an effect on the dose distribution from all beams and is likely to lead a re-planning if the tumor volume change is considerable. About half of cancer patients develop a plural effusion, which is a buildup of extra fluid in space between lung and chest cavity. Clearly, any change in pleural effusion would lead to change in WET and dose deviation from the beam passing through the fluid buildup. If the tumor is far away from the fluid buildup and no beam passes through it, the effect of pleural effusion could be negligible on the dose distribution and no plan adaptation is needed. In most cases, one would only need to make adjustments for the beam(s) that passes the fluid, by either changing the range and/or modulation or re-planning the beam with a new compensator.

Please note that for the composite dose distribution from several proton beams, the correlation to the anatomy may not be straightforward. Anatomy and WET changes will lead to visible dose change for one beam; their effect may not show up well on the overall dose distribution and the DVH. For example, the volume of the target receiving at least 95% of the prescription dose (V95) may show minimal change, while there is a clear under coverage due to a range pullback from a certain beam and plan adaptation should be used. Therefore, beam-by-beam analysis is strongly recommended to evaluate the dose correlation due to the anatomy change.

5.4. Patient motion and motion management

Given the sensitivity of proton beam to anatomy variation, accurate evaluation and appropriate management of motion are very important in lung cancer therapy. For PSPT and USPT, the patient motion is typically accounted for during the initial treatment planning using techniques such as target expansion (ITV), range smearing, and stopping power ratio override [7, 26]. In addition, motion can be managed using respiratory gated system [27]. From our experience, the effect of motion variation in the QA plan based on repeated 4D CT scan seems to be relatively low, and the original plan is typically robust enough to adequately cover the target as long as no anatomy change is present. For PBS, the interplay of patient motion and dynamic beam delivery could result in dose heterogeneity in target and potential under coverage. To mitigate the interplay effect, the motion magnitude for patients treated with PBS is often restricted, such as at a maximum of 5 mm. In addition, several techniques have been used or proposed to mitigate the interplay effect, such as layer repainting, large beam spot, respiratory gated beam delivery, robust planning optimization accounting for the motion, and tumor tracking [6, 12, 28–31]. It has also been reported that the interplay effect may be averaged out during fractionated treatment [32]. However, to fully achieve the potential of IMPT, it may be necessary to routinely evaluate motion change and adapt treatment accordingly.

5.5. Resource constraints and potential risk associated with plan change

When re-planning is used in plan adaptation, new patient specific apertures and compensators may need to be manufactured for both PSPT and USPT. The manufacturing process usually takes hours or more to complete, depending on field size and shape as well as the queuing status of other hardware. If no machine shop is available onsite, the hardware needs to be manufactured by other contracting companies which may take 1–2 days to become available. Furthermore, additional time is needed for the following QA process for the hardware and output measurement. While no hardware is needed for PBS, the robust treatment planning and optimization and the consequent QA process can be very time and effort consuming. In addition, the plan change can lead to unexpected consequences and increased risk of treatment errors, especially when it is not communicated well. Therefore, we have to take the associated cost and risk into account in addition to the dosimetric and clinical gain when deciding whether plan change is necessary.

5.6. Treatment volume with tumor shrinkage

It is still unclear on whether the clinical target volume should be reduced accordingly when a tumor shrinks during the treatment course. Siker *et al.* cautioned field reductions for tumor shrinkage during radiotherapy, questioning the significance of tumor regression because histologic tumor clearance was hard to document [33]. However, Guckenberger *et al.* believed that adaptation of radiotherapy to the shrinking GTV did not compromise the dose coverage of volumes of subclinical microscopic disease [34]. In adaptive proton therapy for both USPT and PSPT, the treatment target volume is commonly kept the same as the initial plan and the same apertures are used, while the beam penetration is adjusted, that is, the range is adjusted or the compensator is recalculated, to account for the WET change associated with the tumor shrinkage. Exceptions can be made per physicians' discretion for cases that normal tissue sparing is critical, such as for patients with a very large initial tumor volume and normal dose can be close or exceed the tolerance with the initial plan. One proposal is to treat the initial target volume for at least 50 Gy, the standard dose for microscopic disease, and then treat the reduced volume to the full dose with a boost [35].

5.7. Dose accumulation

Accurate accounting doses at the presence of anatomy change and plan adaptation is important to make informed decision on whether and how to adapt a plan. However, this can be challenging due to limitation of image registration when large anatomic change or setup variation exist. In addition, CT scans are often repeated on a non-daily basis, and the exact patient anatomy between CT scans is unknown. To estimate the actual dose delivered between two image scans when daily patient anatomy information is not available, one may use a weighted summation of the doses calculated on the two CT data sets, or interpolate patient anatomy between the two scans and calculate doses based on the interpolated data sets. The latter can be more realistic, but a good software tool for interpolation is needed.

5.8. Criteria on plan change

The criteria on when and how to adapt a plan can differ from institution to institution and depend on the attending physician and/or individual patient. There are several considerations during QA plan evaluations including: (1) Is there noticeable anatomic change? How will the anatomy change affect the dose? (2) How much does the PTV coverage change compared to the initial plan? Is the target coverage still acceptable? (3) How much does the normal tissue dose change? Is the normal tissue dose within tolerance? (4) How much is the dose deviation from the original plan? Will a re-planning improve the dose distribution significantly? (5) How long does it take to have the revised plan ready for treatment? Will a treatment break be needed before the new plan becomes available? (6) How much are the cost and effort for a plan adaptation (e.g., whether new hardware fabrication was involved, or just some parameter change)? How many fractions are left? Is it worthwhile to make a plan change for the remainder of treatment? (8) Are there any special consideration for the patients, for example, does the patient need more sparing in lung due to pre-existing lung function such as COPD?

Change *et al.* reported that the main criteria for plan adaptation was whether CTV or GTV receives <95% of dose and whether doses for normal tissues such as heart and cord dose were out of tolerance [6]. At our center, in addition to looking into dosimetric effect such as the target coverage and normal tissue dose, we take into account the potential clinical gain as well as the cost and time associated with plan adaptation to decide on whether and how to adapt a plan. For example, if the patient is close to the end of treatment and the clinical impact of plan adaptation is low, we may use a simple adaptation strategy like range adjustment or no adaptation at all for the rest of treatment.

6. Future directions

The technology of proton therapy is evolving very quickly, and many progresses are being made toward more accurate and efficient adaptive planning. Currently, only offline adaption has been reported in proton therapy due to the lack of accurate in-room imaging system and long turnaround of manufacturing patient specific hardware for both PSPT and USPT. However, PBS has been increasingly used for lung cancer treatment, and CBCT and other in-room CT have become available. The advancement of both PBS and in-room CT makes online adaptive planning possible in proton therapy in the future. Before online proton adaptive planning becomes a reality, many challenges need to be addressed. Better tools are needed for automatic image registration and dose accumulation, the dose calculation accuracy of in-room CT such as CBCT needs to be improved, and automatic and fast robust re-planning and QA with IMPT should be developed. In addition, criteria on plan adaptation based on both dosimetric parameters and clinic outcome should be developed for quick and accurate decision-making.

While adaptive planning is needed for proton therapy of lung cancer, it is time and effort consuming, and not every patient can benefit from this process. It would be helpful to be able to predict when adaptive planning is needed and for which patients. This would allow personalized adaptive planning process for patients, improve treatment efficiency, save costs, reduce risks of treatment errors from the plan adaptation process, and eliminate unnecessary imaging dose to patients with the repeated CT scanning. Berkovic *et al.* used volume and dosimetric data to construct lookup tables in attempt to predict whether and when ART could be useful based on the timing of the radiation treatment, the tumor volume, and whether it was a concurrent or sequential chemo-radiotherapy [36]. Based on our experience with USPT, it is found that patients with noticeable weight change (e.g., 3% or more), pleural effusion, and pneumonitis in addition to the tumor volume change are indicatives of plan adaptation.

7. Summary

Adaptive planning is necessary for proton therapy treatment of lung cancer to maintain optimal dosimetric distribution when patient anatomy changes. To achieve optimal adaptive planning process and clinical outcome, we need to consider not only the benefits from the improved dosimetric distribution and potential clinical outcome with plan adaptation but also its cost and limitations, available resources, and potential risks associated with plan change. Better tools for image registration, dose accumulation, and plan automation are desired to make the plan adaption process more efficient and accurate. The plan adaptation process, for instances, the frequency of repeated CT scanning and the criteria for plan adaptation, needs to be adapted with institutional resource and experience. Online adaption in proton therapy can be feasible with the advancement of pencil beam scanning and in-room CT, but many challenges, such as the limitation of the in room CT image quality, efficient robust proton re-planning and quality assurance, need to be addressed before its clinical use.

Author details

Yuanshui Zheng

Address all correspondence to: yuanshuizheng@yahoo.com

Atlantic Health System, Morristown, NJ, USA

Oklahoma State University, Still Water, OK, USA

References

[1] Siegel, R.L., K.D. Miller, and A. Jemal, Cancer statistics, 2015. CA Cancer J Clin, 2015. **65**(1): 5–29.

[2] Chang, J.Y., et al., Significant reduction of normal tissue dose by proton radiotherapy compared with three-dimensional conformal or intensity-modulated radiation therapy in Stage I or Stage III non-small-cell lung cancer. Int J Radiat Oncol Biol Phys, 2006. **65**(4): 1087–96.

[3] Wu, C.T., et al., Dosimetric comparison between proton beam therapy and photon radiation therapy for locally advanced non-small cell lung cancer. Jpn J Clin Oncol, 2016. **46**(11): 1008–1014.

[4] Wang, C., et al., Comparisons of dose-volume histograms for proton-beam versus 3-D conformal x-ray therapy in patients with stage I non-small cell lung cancer. Strahlenther Onkol, 2009. **185**(4): 231–4.

[5] Zheng, Y., et al., Commissioning of output factors for uniform scanning proton beams. Med Phys, 2011. **38**(4): 2299–306.

[6] Chang, J.Y., et al., Clinical implementation of intensity modulated proton therapy for thoracic malignancies. Int J Radiat Oncol Biol Phys, 2014. **90**(4): 809–18.

[7] Kang, Y., et al., 4D Proton treatment planning strategy for mobile lung tumors. Int J Radiat Oncol Biol Phys, 2007. **67**(3): 906–14.

[8] Kadoya, N., et al., Dose-volume comparison of proton radiotherapy and stereotactic body radiotherapy for non-small-cell lung cancer. Int J Radiat Oncol Biol Phys, 2011. **79**(4): 1225–31.

[9] Hoppe, B.S., et al., Double-scattered proton-based stereotactic body radiotherapy for stage I lung cancer: A dosimetric comparison with photon-based stereotactic body radiotherapy. Radiother Oncol, 2010. **97**(3): 425–30.

[10] Zhang, X., et al., Intensity-modulated proton therapy reduces the dose to normal tissue compared with intensity-modulated radiation therapy or passive scattering proton therapy and enables individualized radical radiotherapy for extensive stage IIIB non-small-cell lung cancer: A virtual clinical study. Int J Radiat Oncol Biol Phys, 2010. **77**(2): 357–66.

[11] Stuschke, M., et al., Potentials of robust intensity modulated scanning proton plans for locally advanced lung cancer in comparison to intensity modulated photon plans. Radiother Oncol, 2012. **104**(1): 45–51.

[12] Casares-Magaz, O., et al., A method for selection of beam angles robust to intra-fractional motion in proton therapy of lung cancer. Acta Oncol, 2014. **53**(8): 1058–63.

[13] Yan, D., et al., Adaptive radiation therapy. Phys Med Biol, 1997. **42**(1): 123–32.

[14] Ramsey, C.R., et al., A technique for adaptive image-guided helical tomotherapy for lung cancer. Int J Radiat Oncol Biol Phys, 2006. **64**(4): 1237–44.

[15] Dial, C., et al., Benefits of adaptive radiation therapy in lung cancer as a function of replanning frequency. Med Phys, 2016. **43**(4): 1787.

[16] Sonke, J.J. and J. Belderbos, Adaptive radiotherapy for lung cancer. Semin Radiat Oncol, 2010. **20**(2): 94–106.

[17] Tvilum, M., et al., Clinical outcome of image-guided adaptive radiotherapy in the treatment of lung cancer patients. Acta Oncol, 2015. **54**(9): 1430–7.

[18] Kataria, T., et al., Adaptive radiotherapy in lung cancer: Dosimetric benefits and clinical outcome. Br J Radiol, 2014. **87**(1038): 20130643.

[19] Persoon, L.C., et al., First clinical results of adaptive radiotherapy based on 3D portal dosimetry for lung cancer patients with atelectasis treated with volumetric-modulated arc therapy (VMAT). Acta Oncol, 2013. **52**(7): 1484–9.

[20] Hui, Z., et al., Effects of interfractional motion and anatomic changes on proton therapy dose distribution in lung cancer. Int J Radiat Oncol Biol Phys, 2008. **72**(5): 1385–95.

[21] Koay, E.J., et al., Adaptive/nonadaptive proton radiation planning and outcomes in a phase II trial for locally advanced non-small cell lung cancer. Int J Radiat Oncol Biol Phys, 2012. **84**(5): 1093–100.

[22] Zheng, Y., et al., Adaptive radiation therapy for lung cancer using uniform scanning proton beams: Adaptation strategies, practical considerations, and clinical outcomes. Int J Radiat Oncol Biol Phys, 2015. **93**(3): S29.

[23] Chang, J.Y., et al., Toxicity and patterns of failure of adaptive/ablative proton therapy for early-stage, medically inoperable non-small cell lung cancer. Int J Radiat Oncol Biol Phys, 2011. **80**(5): 1350–7.

[24] Hardcastle, N., et al., Accuracy of deformable image registration for contour propagation in adaptive lung radiotherapy. Radiat Oncol, 2013. **8**: 243.

[25] Balik, S., et al., Evaluation of 4-dimensional computed tomography to 4-dimensional cone-beam computed tomography deformable image registration for lung cancer adaptive radiation therapy. Int J Radiat Oncol Biol Phys, 2013. **86**(2): 372–9.

[26] Moyers, M.F., et al., Methodologies and tools for proton beam design for lung tumors. Int J Radiat Oncol Biol Phys, 2001. **49**(5): 1429–38.

[27] Lu, H.M., et al., A respiratory-gated treatment system for proton therapy. Med Phys, 2007. **34**(8): 3273–8.

[28] Grassberger, C., et al., Motion mitigation for lung cancer patients treated with active scanning proton therapy. Med Phys, 2015. **42**(5): 2462–9.

[29] Liu, W., et al., Impact of respiratory motion on worst-case scenario optimized intensity modulated proton therapy for lung cancers. Pract Radiat Oncol, 2015. **5**(2): e77–86.

[30] Kardar, L., et al., Evaluation and mitigation of the interplay effects of intensity modulated proton therapy for lung cancer in a clinical setting. Pract Radiat Oncol, 2014. **4**(6): e259–68.

[31] Schatti, A., et al., Experimental verification of motion mitigation of discrete proton spot scanning by re-scanning. Phys Med Biol, 2013. **58**(23): 8555–72.

[32] Li, H., et al., Dynamically accumulated dose and 4D accumulated dose for moving tumors. Med Phys, 2012. **39**(12): 7359–67.

[33] Siker, M.L., W.A. Tome, and M.P. Mehta, Tumor volume changes on serial imaging with megavoltage CT for non-small-cell lung cancer during intensity-modulated radiotherapy: How reliable, consistent, and meaningful is the effect? Int J Radiat Oncol Biol Phys, 2006. **66**(1): 135–41.

[34] Guckenberger, M., et al., Adaptive radiotherapy for locally advanced non-small-cell lung cancer does not underdose the microscopic disease and has the potential to increase tumor control. Int J Radiat Oncol Biol Phys, 2011. **81**(4): e275–82.

[35] Hindawi Publishing Corporation Journal of Oncology. 2011, Article ID 898391;10 doi: 10.1155/2011/898391

[36] Berkovic, P., et al., Adaptive radiotherapy for locally advanced non-small cell lung cancer, can we predict when and for whom? Acta Oncol, 2015. **54**(9): 1438–44.

Chapter 4

Radiation for Gynaecological Malignancies

Papa Dasari, Singhavajhala Vivekanandam and
Kandepadu Srinagesh Abhishek Raghava

Additional information is available at the end of the chapter

http://dx.doi.org/10.5772/67202

Abstract

Gynaecological malignancies are the most common cancers of women and they contribute to the significant amount of mortality. Women in developing countries are diagnosed in late stages and hence radiation is the common modality of therapy. Radiation is required in managing 80–90% of women with carcinoma cervix, 60% of women with endometrial cancer and 50% of women with carcinoma vulva. The stage of the disease is the most important factor in survival and counselling is essential to ensure complete therapy. Radiation is used as a primary therapy, adjuvant therapy, neo-adjuvant therapy and as palliation. The techniques include external beam radiation and brachytherapy or the combination of both. The newer techniques include IMRT-, IGRT- and PET-CT-guided therapies. Side effects/complications occur as acute during therapy, subacute within 3 months and chronic after 6 months. Management of these side effects is essential for increasing compliance of the patient so as to achieve high cure rates. Management of recurrent disease is a challenge and requires multidisciplinary approach involving Gynaecological Oncologist, Radiation Oncologist and Surgical Oncologist.

Keywords: radiotherapy, counselling, gynaecological malignancies, side effects, survival rates

1. Introduction

Radiation therapy in gynaecological malignancies is an essential component in achieving cure as well as palliation. Radiotherapy is required up to 80–90% of women with carcinoma cervix, 60% of women with endometrial carcinoma, 50% of women with carcinoma vulva, all women with vaginal cancer and 5% of women with ovarian cancer. The aim of radiotherapy is to kill the tumour cells without damaging the neighbouring normal tissues. The side effects of radiation can be severe and need to be recognized early to be treated effectively. Counselling of women suffering from gynaecological malignancies who receive radiation is of great importance as adherence to treatment is one of the factors that influences survival rates. The most important part is the selection and categorization of women for radiation. The aim of this chapter is to appraise the readers about the burden of the gynaecological malignancies in a tertiary-care set up, counselling and selection criteria for radiation, methods of radiation and the side effects and the outcome.

1.1. Burden of gynaecological malignancies in tertiary care set up

Cancer is the first and foremost cause of death in developing countries and the second most common cause in developed countries. Genital tract malignancies are the most common cancers in women and the most common site affected is cervix followed by ovary and Uterine corpus [1]. The incidence of carcinoma cervix is 9 per 100,000 in developed countries as against 17.8 per 100,000 in developing countries. The mortality attributed to carcinoma cervix is 3.2 per 100,000 in developed regions when compared to 9.8 per 100,000 women in developing regions [2]. The cancer registry of our hospital recorded carcinoma cervix to be occurring in 70%, ovarian cancer in 20%, endometrial cancer in 9% and other cancers in 1% of cases in women. In India, every year 122,844 women were reported to be diagnosed with carcinoma cervix and 67,477 died of the disease and at present the trend of this malignancy is decreasing in incidence [3]. The incidence of carcinoma cervix has declined by 75% in developed countries [1].

2. Selection criteria for radiation

Staging of the malignant disease is the most important factor in determining therapy and while planning contraindications to radiation to be looked for and histopathological examination report is mandatory.

Contraindications for radiation: (1) Severe acute sepsis or febrile illness, (2) severe cancer cachexia, (3) myocardial infarction and (4) unequivocal histopathological report. Though there are no absolute contraindications, radiation is not the preferred therapy for radio-insensitive tumours like fibrosarcoma, leiomyosarcoma and melanoma.

Carcinoma cervix: The most common histopathological type is squamous cell carcinoma. The incidence of adenocarcinoma is on the rise contributing to as much as 25% [4]. In spite of the availability of screening tests in the modern era, as high as 85% are still presenting in late stage. Adherence to therapy is poor as it was reported that only 38.8% complete radiotherapy [5]. Pre-therapy staging is based on clinical examination and imaging findings. Recently, imaging techniques are playing a great role in planning therapy even though traditionally staging is done by clinical examination.

Role of imaging in staging:

- The accuracy of CT in staging carcinoma cervix is 63–88%. The sensitivity and specificity of CT in detecting pelvic lymph node involvement is shown in (**Table 1**)
- MRI distinguishes early from advanced disease, thereby stratifying patients for surgery and chemoradiation.

- MRI is used to assess cervical stromal invasion and extra-uterine extension and for assessing proximal extension of cervical tumour in young women with early-stage disease for the feasibility of fertility-preserving surgery [6].
- PET has sensitivity of 75% and specificity of 96% for the detection of pelvic lymphadenopathy and sensitivity of 100% and specificity of 99% for the detection of para-aortic lymphadenopathy. Its use has been increased, combined with CT, in the detection of nodal disease for locally advanced disease (>IB) [3, 5]. For early stage disease, the sensitivity and specificity of PET CT were about 73% and 97%, respectively.
- Grigsby et al. compared CT and FDG-PET scanning for lymph node staging in 101 patients with carcinoma of the cervix. CT detected enlarged pelvic lymph nodes and para-aortic lymph nodes in 20 and 7 patients, respectively, whereas PET detected abnormal FDG uptake in pelvic lymph nodes in 67, in para-aortic lymph nodes in 21 and in supraclavicular lymph nodes in 8. Based on para-aortic lymph node status, the 2-year progression-free survival rate was 64% in CT-negative and PET-negative patients, 18% in CT-negative and PET-positive patients and 14% in CT-positive and PET-positive patients [7].

Survival rates are shown in **Table 2**.

CT	Sensitivity (%)	Specificity (%)
Pelvic + para-aortic lymph nodes	44	93
Para-aortic lymph nodes	67	100

Table 1. Sensitivity and specificity of CT.

Radiotherapy is advocated in the following situations:

(1) All stages especially when the woman is not fit for surgery or refuses surgery

(2) Following radical hysterectomy with positive pelvic lymph nodes

(3) Stages IIB to IV B

(4) Fertility sparing surgery which revealed a focus of positive lymph nodal metastasis

(5) Advanced stage carcinoma cervix following termination of pregnancy

(6) Persistent or recurrent disease

2.1. Carcinoma endometrium/Uterine Corpus

Carcinoma endometrium is the most common cancer of the uterus and its incidence is increasing. The median age is 63 years and more than 90% belong to 50 years of age or more and 25% occur before pre-menopause. More than 75% are diagnosed in Stage I as the most common symptom is abnormal or postmenopausal bleeding. Survival rates are more than 75%. Adenocarcinoma is the most common type with good prognosis, but it is relatively radioresistant.

S. no.	Stage (FIGO)	TNM (AJCC)	Survival rates (5-year observed rates)
	Stage 0		93%
1	Stage I A1	**(T1a1, N0, M0**	**93%**
2	Stage I A1	**(T1a2, N0, M0)**	
3	Stage I B	**(T1b, N0, M0)**	**80%**
4	Stage B 1	**(T1b1, N0, M0)**	
5	Stagve I B2	**(T1b2, N0, M0)**	
	Stage II	**(T2, N0, M0)**	**63%**
6	Stage II A	**(T2a, N0, M0)**	
7	Stage II A1	**(T2a1, N0, M0)**	
8	Stage II A2	**(T2a2, N0, M0)**	
9	Stage 2 B	**(T2b, N0, M0)**	**58%**
	Stage III	**(T3, N0, M0)**	
10	Stage III A	**(T3a, N0, M0**	**35%**
11	Stage III B	**T3b, N0, M0; OR T1-T3, N1, M0) Hydronephrosis**	**32%**
	Stage IV		
12	Stage IV A	**(T4, N0, M0)**	**16%**
13	Stage IV B	**(any T, any N, M1)**	**15%**

Table 2. Staging grouping of carcinoma cervix.

HPE grading:

Gx = Grade cannot be assessed

Grade 1 = Tumour cells are well-differentiated

Grade2 = Tumour cells are moderately differentiated

Grade 3 = Tumour cells are poorly differentiated

The histopathological types are as follows:

1. Endometroid adenocarcinoma (secretory, ciliated, papillary)
2. Adenocarcinoma with squamous differentiation
3. Adenoacanthoma (benign squamous component)
4. Adenosquamous carcinoma (malignant squamous component)
5. Papillary serous carcinoma
6. Clear cell adenocarcinoma
7. Carcinosarcoma/malignant mixed mullerian tumour
8. Uterine sarcomas

9. Mucinous tumours

10. Undifferentiated.

Staging of endometrial carcinoma with survival rates is shown in **Table 3**. Radiotherapy is also indicated in Stage I as per risk stratification.

TNM	FIGO stages	Surgico-pathological findings	Endometrial adenocarcinoma; 5-year survival	Endometrial carcinosarcoma; 5-year survival
Tx		Primary tumour cannot be assessed		
T0		No evidence of primary tumour		
Tis		Carcinoma *in situ* (Pre-invasive carcinoma)		
T1	**I**	**Tumour confined to Corpus**	88–75%	70%
T1 a	IA	Tumour limited to endometrium or Less than a half of endometrium is involved		
T1 b	IB	Tumour invasion of half or more than half of myometrium	f	
T2	**II**	**Tumour invades stroma of cervix and confined to uterus**	69%	45%
T3 a	**III A**	**Tumour involvement of serosa and/or adnexa (direct extension or metastasis)**	58–47%	30%
T3 b	III B	Vaginal involvement or parametrial involvement (direct extension or metastasis)		
	III C	Metastasis to pelvic and/or para-aortic lymph nodes		
	III C1	Pelvic lymph node metastasis		
	III C2	Para-aortic lymph node metastasis		
	IV	**Tumour invades bladder mucosa and/or bowel mucosa and/or distant metastasis**	17–15%	15%
T4	IV A	Bladder mucosa and Bowel mucosa are involved by tumour but no distant metastasis Bullous oedema is not considered as involvement		
	IV B	Distant metastasis; Lymph nodes, Lungs, bones Upper abdomen omentum; liver		

Note: T = denotes extent of the tumour; N = designates whether cancer has spread to the lymph nodes; M = denotes distant metastasis.

Nx = Spread to nearby lymph nodes cannot be assessed; N0 = no spread to nearby lymph nodes; N1 = spread to pelvic lymph nodes; N2 = spread to para-aortic lymph nodes.

Lymph node involvement: Stage I A-5%, Stage I B-10%; Stage I C-15%; Stage II-20% and Stage III-55%.

Distant spread: M0 = there is no spread to distant lymph nodes, organs and tissues; M1 = spread to distant lymph nodes, upper abdomen, omentum, other organs, liver, lung.

Table 3. TNM classification and FIGO staging [8].

Stage I low risk includes Stage I A grade 1 and 2 endometroid adenocarcinoma without or with minimal myometrial invasion.

Stage I intermediate-risk group includes Stage I with grade 1 or 2 adenocarcinoma with >50% myometrial invasion or grade 3 adenocarcinoma with superficial invasion and with extensive lymphovascular involvement

High-risk endometrial cancer includes Stage II with deep cervical stromal involvement and Stage III and IV disease.

2.2. Picture of USG and gross specimen of endometrial carcinoma (Figure 1)

Vulval and vaginal cancer:

A. Vulval carcinoma: Most common after 65 years of age but recently the incidence of carcinoma vulva in the age group between 40 and 49 years is reported to have been doubled. Its incidence is 1.3/100,000 women. Pathological types: Squamous cell carcinoma—90%; others include malignant melanoma, Paget's disease, Bartholin gland tumours, adenocarcinoma and basal cell carcinoma. Local recurrence is common when there is lymphovascular involvement, when the growth is of infiltrative type and when prominent fibromyxoid tumour is present at the edge of resected margins [9]. Gross picture of carcinoma vulva is shown in **Figure 2**.

Primary modality of therapy is surgical excision and groin lymph node dissection. Survival rates with staging are shown in **Table 4**.

Selection criteria for radiation:

Primary radiotherapy is suggested in women:

- When optimal surgical therapy is not possible.
- When Ulcerated groin nodes. Radiotherapy is followed by surgery or surgery followed by radiotherapy. However, surgery following radiation is associated with high morbidity.

Adjuvant radiotherapy is advised to groin and pelvic nodes in the following situations

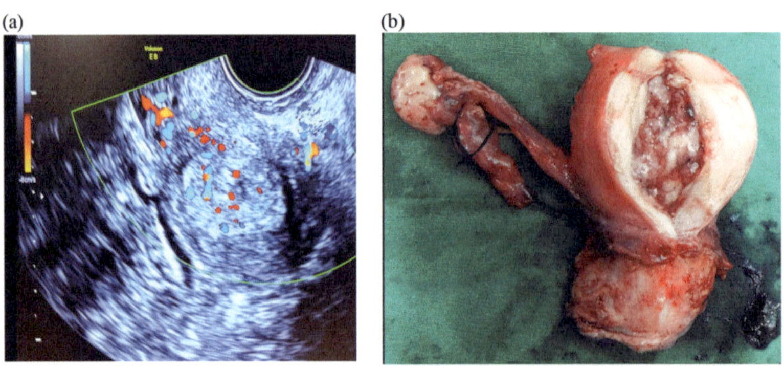

Figure 1. (**A**) USG (TVS) picture of endometrial carcinoma showing increased endometrial thickness and increased vascularity and (**B**) picture of same uterus (panel A) as gross specimen showing endometrial carcinoma in the cavity.

http://dx.doi.org/10.5772/67202

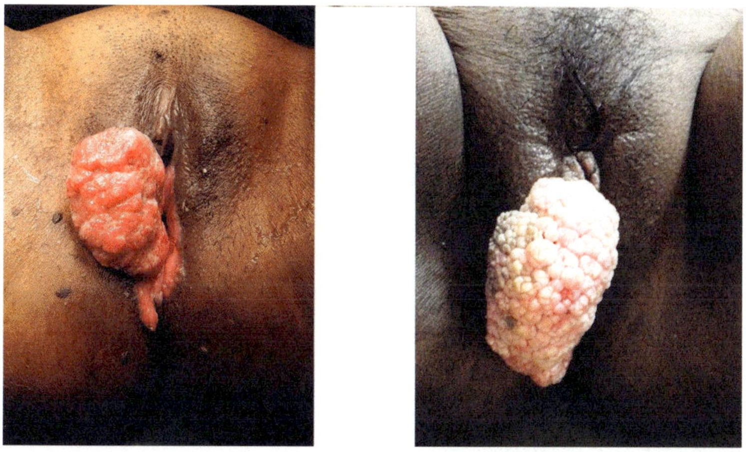

Figure 2. Cauliflower type of growth on the vulva.

(1) When one or two nodes show the spread either microscopic or extra capsular.

(2) When the resected margins are involved.

Pre-operative radiotherapy is advocated to preserve anal sphincter function when the tumour is close to the anal sphincter. Radiotherapy may also be combined with chemotherapy. Chemo-RT may increase the morbidity, especially skin toxicity.

Recurrence is very common in vulvar cancer and it varies from 15 to 33%. The sites of recurrence can be vulva itself (69.5%), groin nodes (24.3%) and distant sites (18.5%).

Stage grouping	Explanation	Survival rates (%)
Stage 0 (Tis,N0, M0)	Carcinoma *in situ*(only vaginal epithelium is involved)	84
Stage I (T1, N0, M0)	Cancer-confined vagina; no spread to lymph nodes/ distant sites	
Stage II (T2, No,M0)	Cancer invades the connective tissue below vagina No spread to lymph nodes and distant sites	
Stage III (T3, N0/1,M0) or (T1,/T2,N1, M0)	Spread of cancer to pelvic wall but not to lymph nodes or distant sites Or spread to lateral pelvic wall and/to lymph nodes pelvic or inguinal Not spread to distant sites	75
Stage IVA (T4, N0/N1,M0)	Cancer spread to rectum/bladder Lymph nodes may or may not have been involved No distant metastasis	57
Stage IV B (Any T, Any N, M1)	Cancer involves pelvic organs and spread to distant sites like lungs and liver, bone, etc.	

Note: Five-year survival rates for all stages together are reported as 50%; for squamous cell carcinoma 50%;for adenocarcinoma 60% and malignant melanoma 30%.

Table 4. FIGO and AJCC stage grouping and survival; carcinoma vulva.

B Vaginal carcinoma: Vaginal cancer is rarely encountered and its incidence is reported to be 1 in 11,000 and ocxcurs in women more than 70 years of age and only 15% occur in women less than 40 years. Presenting symptoms are usually abnormal discharge, bleeding per vaginum, post-coital bleeding and mass per vaginum. Symptoms during late stages include constipation, pelvic pain and difficulty in micturition. Confirmation of diagnosis is by speculum examination demonstrating a cervix free of disease and growth in the vagina. Biopsy determines the type of cancer. If the growth involves cervix and vagina, it is classified under cervical cancer. If it involves vagina and vulva, it is classified as vulvar cancer. The most common pathological type is squamous cell carcinoma (70%); and others include adenocarcinoma (15%), melanoma (9%), sarcoma (4%) and miscellaneous [10].

3. Counselling for radiation

Counselling prior to radiotherapy is of utmost importance because of three reasons:

(1) To make the patient understand the process through which she would be going, i.e. the technique, the duration of therapy and the possible side effects and their significance and management.

(2) To make her compliant and complete the therapy for curative purposes or palliative purposes and follow-up for further therapy like surgery or chemotherapy and also the possibility or chances of recurrence.

(3) To help the patient to make informed decision and consent for the process.

Informed consent: [11]

Informed consent is to be taken by the radiotherapy counsellor/radiotherapy physician and it should include the diagnosis and stage of the disease, name of the procedure or treatment like external radiotherapy or brachytherapy or radio-isotope treatment, site of the body where radiation would be delivered and Whether the procedure is done under sedation, local/regional/general anaesthesia. The duration of therapy and the proposed sessions of therapy and whether it is for curative purpose or for palliative purpose is to be stated and signed by the concerned health professional involved in the care of the woman. The most common acute side effects and late side effects should be mentioned in the document signed by the health professional. An information leaflet to the patient in the language known to her or relatives would be desirable and is of great benefit.

The second part of the consent form should include statement that the patient has understood the benefits of the therapy, the short-term and long-term side effects that can occur and has the opportunity to ask questions and read the management protocol. The statement should also include the liberty of the patient to ask to stop the treatment at any time during the therapy after understanding the consequences of the same. A separate statement to be obtained from the reproductive aged women that she is not pregnant at this time of initiating the therapy and would not plan to become pregnant during the course of therapy and she would inform the treating physician in case of such occurrence.

A statement for storing the data of the patient and its usage for the future purpose like research also can be included in this consent form.

Written consent would be obtained once prior to the procedure and at each session of treatment a verbal consent would be taken and this statement also to be included in the written consent form and to be signed and dated by the individual concerned.

In case of mental disease incapacitating the patient, a responsible attendant should be involved in the counselling process and in consenting in a similar way.

3.1. Survival rates

It is important to appraise the women and the relatives regarding prognosis and survival in addition to side effects whenever therapy is instituted. Though survival depends on many factors like age at the development of the malignancy, type of the tissue involved for example, cervix or endometrium or adnexa, histopathological type, modality of therapy, complications of therapy, compliance to therapy, associated co-morbidities and the chance for recurrence, the most important factor is found to be the stage of the disease. In other words, spread of the cancerous tissue is the most important factor that is used to prognosticate and explain the modality of therapy and its outcomes like overall survival. Survival rates are expressed variously and the standard way is to express in terms of 5-year survival. The survival rates for carcinoma cervix, endometrium and vulva are shown in **Tables 2–4**, respectively, and these should guide the clinician to explain the patient while undertaking counselling.

For carcinoma cervix, the survival rates reported in India include 47.7% in Mumbai-based registry in North India and 38% in Bangalore-based registry from South India. The 5-year survival rate for recurrent disease is reported to be between 30–60% and the main modality of treatment for recurrence being surgery. The prognosis is better if the recurrence occurs after 6 months of initial cure and the size of the recurrence is less than 3 cm [12].

4. Radiation therapy

Radiation therapy can be delivered as

(1) Primary radiotherapy

(2) Adjuvant radiotherapy

(3) Neoadjuvant radiotherapy

(4) Palliative radiotherapy

Primary radiotherapy: Primary radiotherapy involves the use of radiation therapy as the only modality of treatment either alone or in combination with chemotherapy which is used as a radiation sensitizer. Primary radiotherapy is used in the following situations: (1) women with unresectable, locally advanced disease; (2) women with resectable disease in whom the risk of surgical morbidity is unacceptably high and (3) women with medical risk factors that contraindicate primary surgical therapy.

Adjuvant radiotherapy: Early stage lesions of the lower genitourinary tract can be treated surgically if resection can be accomplished with adequate negative margins and acceptable morbidity. Post-operative radiotherapy/adjuvant radiotherapy is reserved for cases in which histopathologic analysis of the removed specimen reveals features suggesting a high risk of local recurrence.

Neoadjuvant radiotherapy: In advanced stage disease, sometimes neoadjuvant radiation is used before surgery to render an inoperable tumour operable and for preserving the organ.

Palliative radiotherapy: For women with distant metastatic disease at presentation, cure is unlikely and the aim of the treatment is to improve the quality of life. However, palliative radiotherapy is frequently used to palliate the symptoms of a painful bone metastasis, relieve features of raised intracranial tension in brain metastasis and relieve dyspnoea in superior vena cava obstruction.

4.1. Techniques of radiation

The two main modalities of irradiation are teletherapy (external beam radiation) and brachytherapy. External beam irradiation is used to treat the whole pelvis including the uterus, cervix fallopian tubes and ovaries, parametria and the regional nodes. A linear accelerator is used to deliver mega voltage photons to treat the whole pelvis. Gamma rays from a cobalt-60 machine are also used to deliver radiation.

Brachytherapy: In this modality, source of radiation is placed inside the body as close to the tumour as possible. It usually consists of the placement of intrauterine and vaginal applicators. These are then loaded with the source of radiation. Cesium-137 (^{137}Cs) is the most popular low-dose rate (LDR) source and Iridium-192 (^{192}Ir) is the most common high-dose rate source (HDR). Treatment with HDR is usually completed in a few minutes, whereas an LDR source takes 1 or 2 days to complete the treatment.

4.2. Technique of external beam radiation

External beam radiation in the treatment of carcinoma cervix aims at treating the whole pelvis. Whole pelvis involves treating the pelvic organs uterus, adnexa and upper third of vagina, parametrial tissues (cardinal, uterosacral and pubo-cervical ligaments) and pelvic lymph nodes (internal and external iliac, obturator and pre-sacral lymph nodes). Traditionally, the whole pelvis is treated with four fields—anterior-posterior portals and two lateral fields (**Figure 3A** and **B**)]. Upper border is placed at L4-L5 interspace to adequately cover the external iliac and lower common iliacs. The lower border is kept 3 cm below the lower extent of the tumour or lower border of obturator foramen if the vagina is not involved by the tumour.

http://dx.doi.org/10.5772/67202

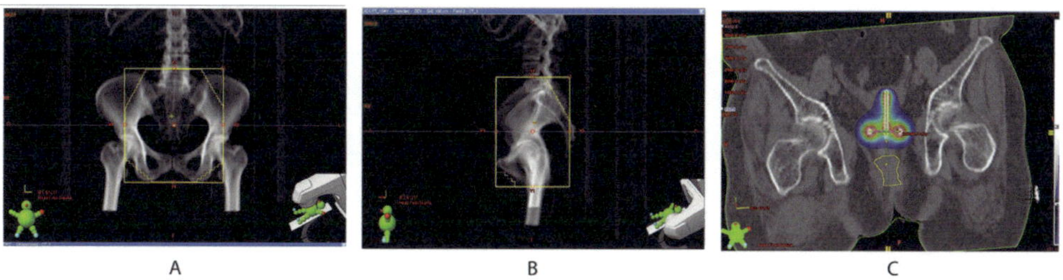

Figure 3. (A) Anterior field borders, (B) lateral field borders, and (C) HDR brachytherapy dose distribution [pear-shaped].

The lateral borders are kept 2 cm lateral to the pelvic brim in order to adequately cover the iliac nodes. The upper and lower borders of the lateral fields correspond with those of the AP-PA fields. The anterior border is kept at the anterior border of the pubic symphysis and the posterior border is placed to cover the entire sacrum. High-energy beams of the range of 6–15MV are used to deliver radiation. Dose of external beam radiation is 46 Gy in 23 fractions, 200 cGy per fraction and one fraction a day 5 days a week. The dose distribution of four field box plan is shown in **Figure 4A** and bladder and rectum contours are shown in **Figure 4B**.

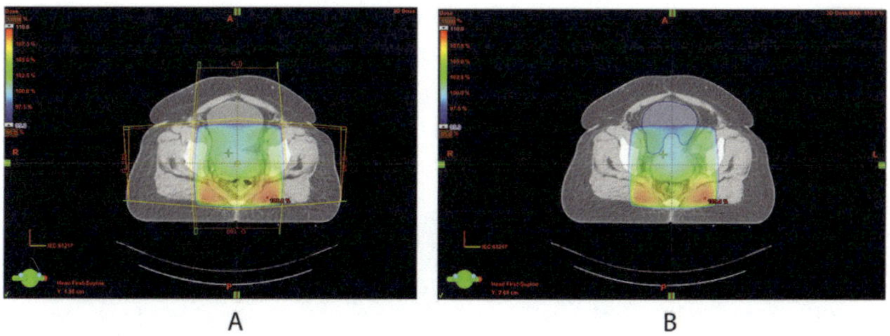

Figure 4. (**A**) 3DCRT plan showing 95% coverage with four fields and (**B**) dose distribution of four field box plan showing 95% coverage with bladder and rectal contours.

4.3. 3D planning techniques

- CT scan is taken with patient supine with arms on the chest, knees and lower legs immobilized, and anterior and lateral tattoos marked with radio-opaque material aligned with lasers to prevent lateral rotation.
- Clinical examination is made in the treatment position and inferior extent of tumour in the vagina marked with radio-opaque material.
- Patients will be instructed to maintain a constant bladder filling—'comfortably full'—and instructions will be given to empty the bladder two hours before simulation and to drink one litre of water mixed with 60 ml of Gastrovideo oral contrast. Ondansetron 8 mg or domperidone 10 mg will be given if needed. To delineate large bowel, instructions will be given to drink one litre

of water mixed with 60 ml of Gastrovideo oral contrast within 1 hour, 24 hours prior to simulation. Only liquid diet will be allowed after that, till simulation. Domperidone 10 mg will be given.

- CT Scan is taken from the first lumbar vertebra to 5 cm beyond the vaginal introitus. Intravenous contrast is used to outline pelvic blood vessels to be used as surrogates for pelvic nodes in CTV delineation.
- *Target volume definition*

  While defining clinical target volume (CTV), gross tumour volume (GTV) along with cervix, uterine volume is added. Entire uterus is delineated including the fundus. CTV-T includes the primary GTV-T with potential microscopic spread to cervix, uterus, parametrial tissues, upper vagina, and broad and proximal utero-sacral ligaments. If posterior extension of cervical tumour is present, the entire utero-sacral ligaments and upper pre-sacral nodes are included. CTV-N includes the pelvic lymph nodes, i.e. obturator, internal, external and common iliac, and upper pre-sacral nodes. These are delineated by identifying contrast-enhanced pelvic blood vessels on each CT scan and using a 7 mm margin to create a 3D CTV.A typical CTV to PTV margin of 10 mm is used around the CTV-T to allow for organ motion of cervix and uterus and measured set-up uncertainties. For CTV-N, organ motion occurs to a lesser extent and a 7–10 mm CTV to PTV margin is typically sufficient for set-up variations. The contours of GTV, bladder and rectum are shown in (**Figure 5**).

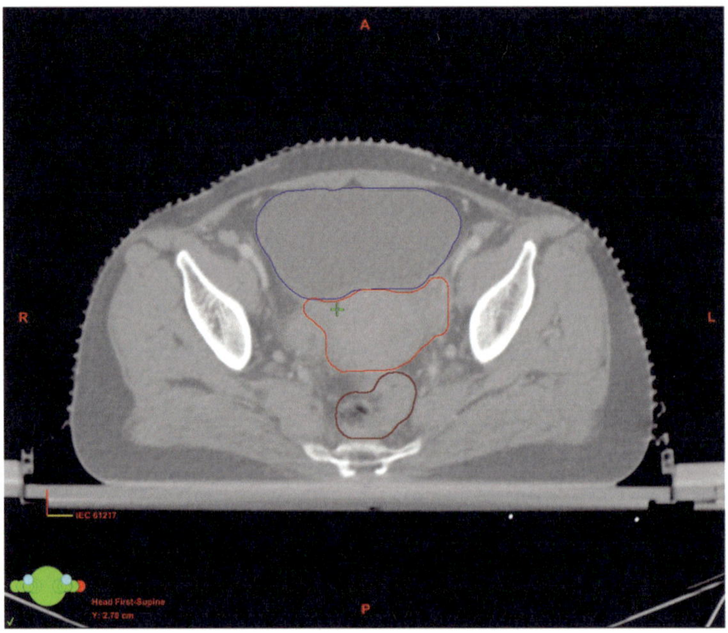

Figure 5. Planning CT showing contours of GTV, bladder and rectum.

4.4. Technique of brachytherapy

The high tolerance of the uterus and vagina make it ideally suited for brachytherapy. In brachytherapy, sealed radioactive sources are used to deliver radiation at short distances. It is possible to deliver a high dose locally to the tumour with a rapid dose fall-off from the surrounding normal tissues. The commonly used isotope for high-dose rate brachytherapy includes Iridium 192 and Cobalt 60. Caesium 137 is used for low-dose rate brachytherapy. Uterine tandem is inserted into the length of which depends on the length of the uterus. Two ovoids are placed in the fornices and the vagina is packed with gauze. This decreases the dose to the rectum and bladder. Using an after loading technique, the source is introduced into the ovoids and tandem. The dwell time and dwell position is calculated so that the desired dose to Point A is achieved. In JIPMER, the dose prescribed to Point A is 8.5 Gy × 3 using Iridium 192. The classical isodose for intra-cavitary brachytherapy of carcinoma cervix is pear-shaped (**Figure 3C**).

4.5. JIPMER radiotherapy protocol for carcinoma cervix—summary (Table 5)

The standard treatment for women with FIGO IB2, IIA, IIB, IIIA, IIIB and IVA disease is concurrent chemo-radiation. Surgery is not preferred because of the increased risk of positive margins and positive nodes. Concurrent chemo-radiotherapy is preferred to radiation alone since the addition of concurrent chemotherapy confers an overall survival advantage [RR risk reduction is 29%] [13]. Platinum-based chemotherapy is preferred over non-platinum-based chemotherapy since there is more benefit with platinum-based compounds (5FU). The hazard ratio (HR) for platinum is 0.70 (95% confidence interval, CI 0.61–0.80; $p< 0.0001$) compared to 0.81 (95% CI 0.56–1.16; $p=0.20$) for non-platinum-based chemotherapy. 118 chemoradiation with cisplatin alone is comparable to chemo-radiation with cisplatin/5-fluorouracil. However, concurrent chemo-radiation for treatment of cervical cancer is associated with increased acute toxicities specifically haematological and gastrointestinal toxicity [13].

4.6. RT for carcinoma cervix in special situations

(1) Acute haemorrhage

Women presenting with acute episode of hemorrhage need to be hospitalised and stabilised with blood transfusion and vaginal packing

Broad spectrum antibiotics and antifibrinolytics are to be started.

Haemostatic RT—Whole Pelvis EBRT-2 Gy/# standard fractionation as per stage-wise treatment protocol. If bleeding persists, brachytherapy with ovoids will be considered.

(2) Pregnancy: First and second trimester pregnant women are managed by medical termination of pregnancy as appropriate for gestational age by medical methods .This is followed by stage-wise treatment after 2 weeks

Third trimester—Pregnancy is continued till 34 weeks with fetal monitoring and institution of steroids for fetal lung maturity followed by elective caesarean section. Stage-wise treatment is undertaken after 4 to 6 weeks of caesarean section.

(3) Utero-vaginal prolapse: Manual reduction during RT if possible; procedentia—prolapse reduction under anaesthesia and labial stitching followed by RT.

(4) HIV:HAART—Highly active anti-retroviral treatment

CD4 > 200 cells/ml—Stage-wise treatment with radiotherapy + chemotherapy

CD4 50–200 cells/ml—Stage-wise treatment with radiotherapy

CD4 < 50 cells/ml—palliation of symptoms

Use of universal aseptic precautions during P/V examination.

Stage	EBRT	ICBT-HDR	BED	LQED at 2 Gy/#	Recommended dose to point A
IA1	0	7 Gy× 6# Ovoid &tandem	71.4	59.5	70–80 Gy
IA2, IB1, IIA1, IB2, IIA2	46 Gy/23# WP	8.5 Gy× 3# Ovoid &tandem or ring &tandem	102.4	85.3	80–85 Gy
IIB	45 Gy/20# WP or 46 Gy/23# WP	8.5 Gy× 3# Ring &tandem or ovoid &tandem	102.3 102.4	85.2 85.3	>85 Gy
IIIA	46 Gy/23# WP 4 Gy/2#PM boost 6 Gy/3# PO	6 Gy× 3# linear applicator	96	80	85–90 Gy
IIIB <2/3 of upper vaginal involvement	45 Gy/20# WP 4.5 Gy/2# PM-Boost Or 46 Gy/23# WP 4 Gy/2# PM-Boost	8.5 Gy× 3# Ring &tandem or Ovoid &tandem	109.8 107.2	89.8 89.3	85–90 Gy
IIIB >2/3 of upper vaginal involvement	46 Gy/23# WP 4 Gy/2#PM boost 6 Gy/3# PO	6 Gy× 3# Linear applicator	96	80	85–90 Gy
IVA (Poor performance status),	30–39 Gy/10–13# (Palliative RT to gross disease)	No brachytherapy	39–50.7	32.5–42.25	
Post-op	46 Gy/23# WP	8 Gy× 2# Vault brachytherapy	84	70	

Table 5. JIPMER radiotherapy protocol for carcinoma cervix—summary.

4.7. Incidentally diagnosed carcinoma cervix after simple hysterectomy/Stump carcinoma after subtotal hysterectomy for benign disease

- Pathological review—no LVSI—Stage I A1— follow-up
- Stage IA1 with LVSI (or) > Stage IA2 Negative margins, negative imaging—pelvic RT + brachytherapy + chemotherapy

  (or)

  Complete parametrectomy + upper vaginectomy + pelvic lymph node dissection + PA LN sampling followed by adjuvant RT or chemo RT as per the above indications

- Positive margins, gross residual disease—if imaging negative for nodal disease—chemo RT, if imaging positive for nodal disease—consider for surgical debulking of grossly enlarged nodes followed by chemo RT.

4.8. Carcinoma of the endometrium protocol at JIPMER

History and physical examination; biopsy report confirmation of carcinoma and type of carcinoma:

- Haemogram
- Kidney function tests—blood urea, serum creatinine, serum electrolytes, creatinine clearance
- Liver function tests
- Random blood sugar
- Chest X-ray
- Ultrasonography—abdomen and pelvis
- HBs antigen
- HIV serology
- CECT/MRI abdomen and pelvis
- Cystoscopy and sigmoidoscopy as clinically indicated

4.9. The evidence present in treating endometrial cancer with radiotherapy

In women with Stage I intermediate-risk external beam pelvic radiotherapy reduces the local as well as vaginal recurrences. Vaginal brachytherapy alone also can achieve similar recurrence rates in this group of women. In women with intermediate- to high-risk group, the overall survival is also similar with external pelvic beam radiation and vaginal brachytherapy. The role of chemotherapy combined with radiation not well established.

5. Evidence-based recommendation ESMO-ESGO-ESTRO consensus [14] (Table 6)

5.1. Normal tissue tolerance

Organs at risk (OAR) in radiation therapy of endometrial cancer include the bladder, rectum, small intestine and the femoral heads.

Radiation therapy for endometrial cancer and tissue tolerance (**Table 7**).

EBRT for endometrial cancer: The technique almost similar as that of carcinoma cervix planning except that the AP/PA field upper border is placed at L5-S1 junction. The pelvis is treated with EBRT to 45–50 Gy in 25–28 daily fractions using 6–18 MV photon beams. The target volume is defined by GTV of the entire uterus in inoperable cases. CTV includes vaginal cuff, obturator nodes, external, internal and common iliac nodes. Planning target volume (PTV) is calculated as CTV plus 0.5–1 cm or ITV (internal target volume) plus 0.5 cm.

Brachytherapy delivers high dose to the vagina while minimizing dose to organs at risk. A vaginal cylinder of largest feasible diameter is the most common applicator used. The radiation is delivered with low-dose rate (LDR) or high-dose rate (HDR) radiotherapy. 50–60 Gy is the LDR prescription to the surface over 60–70 h when used alone. When combined with EBRT, the prescription dose is reduced to 25–30 Gy. The HDR dose prescriptions recommended by the American Brachytherapy Society (ABS) for adjuvant endometrial cancer is as follows. Suggested doses of HDR alone (**Table 8A**) and suggested doses of HDR to be used with 45 Gy EBRT for adjuvant endometrial cancer (**Table 8B**).

5.2. Carcinoma of the vulva

In patients with early stage vulval cancer with high risk features, radiation is commonly delivered following surgery. In patients with locally advanced tumours, surgery will result in unacceptable morbidity and poor cosmetic outcome. Radiotherapy in combination with concurrent chemotherapy is used for 'organ preservation' and cure. Apart from biopsy confirmation of vulval lesion, FNAC of clinically positive inguinal nodes is mandatory and all other investigations prior to RT as per other malignancies are undertaken.

Normal tissue tolerance: Organs at risk (OAR) in radiation therapy of vulvar cancer include the bladder, rectum, small intestine and the femoral head similar to that of endometrial cancer and the tolerance of vagina is <75–80 Gy.

5.3. RT planning techniques: simulation and field arrangements

- Photon energy of more than 6 MV is required for treatment. CT is required for measuring the depth of inguinal nodes. Patients are simulated with custom immobilizations. Supine, frog-leg positions are preferred to reduce the bolus effect from skin folds, with full bladders to reduce dose to small bowel.
- Radio-opaque markers should be used to delineate vulva tumour, scars, palpable lymph nodes, extent of vaginal involvement if present and anal verge.

http://dx.doi.org/10.5772/67202

- Borders of AP field should include superiorly from mid-sacroiliac joint to cover external and internal iliac nodes or L4-L5 level to cover the common iliac nodes if internal or external iliac nodes appear suspicious or positive.
- Inferiorly it should include the entire vulva or lower margin of the tumour (whichever is more caudal).
- Lateral border should include greater trochanter to cover the inguinal nodes in the AP field and 2 cm beyond the outermost point of the pelvic inlet on the PA field.
- *Narrow PA field*: Superior and inferior extent to same as that of wide AP field but lateral extent is farther off from femur-matching supplemental electron fields.
- Anterior electron fields to the lateral inguinal region matched with the exit PA field. Energy of the beam is selected depending on the CT depth of femoral vessels
- *Conedown: After 45 Gy to the pelvis, fields have to be reduced to include the* primary tumour and involved inguinal lymph nodes with 2–3 cm margin.

Risk group	Description	Recommended management
Low	Stage I endometroid, grade 1–2, <50% myometrial invasion, LVSI negative	The risk of recurrence after surgery alone is less than 5% No adjuvant treatment is recommended
Intermediate	Stage I endometroid, grade 1–2, >50% myometrial invasion, LVSI negative	Vaginal brachytherapy (PORTEC-2)
High-intermediate	Stage I endometroid, grade 3, <50% myometrial invasion, regardless of LVSI status Stage I endometroid, grade 1–2, LVSI unequivocally positive, regardless of depth of invasion	Node negative-brachytherapy **No surgical nodal staging:** Adjuvant EBRT recommended for LVSI unequivocally positive to decrease pelvic recurrence Adjuvant brachytherapy alone is recommended for grade 3 and LVSI negative to decrease vaginal recurrence
High	Stage I endometroid, grade 3, >50% myometrial invasion, regardless of LVSI status	**Surgical nodal staging performed, node negative:** Adjuvant EBRT with limited fields should be considered to decrease locoregional recurrence Adjuvant brachytherapy may be considered as an alternative Adjuvant systemic therapy is under investigation **No surgical nodal staging:** Adjuvant EBRT is recommended for pelvic control and relapse free survival Sequential adjuvant chemotherapy may be considered to improve PFS and CSS There is more evidence to support giving chemotherapy and EBRT in combination rather than either treatment modality alone
High	Stage II	**Surgical nodal staging performed, node negative:** Grade 1–2, LVSI negative: recommend vaginal brachytherapy to improve local control Grade 3 or LVSI unequivocally positive: Recommend limited field EBRT Consider brachytherapy boost Chemotherapy is under investigation **No surgical nodal staging:** EBRT is recommended Consider brachytherapy boost Grade 3 or LVSI unequivocally positive: sequential adjuvant chemotherapy should be considered

Risk group	Description	Recommended management
High	Stage III endometroid, no residual disease	EBRT is recommended IIIA: Chemotherapy and EBRT to be considered IIIB: Chemotherapy and EBRT to be considered IIIC1: Chemotherapy and EBRT to be considered IIIC2: Chemotherapy and extended field EBRT to be considered
High	Non-endometroid (serous or clear cell or undifferentiated carcinoma or carcinosarcoma	**Serous and clear cell after comprehensive staging:** Consider chemotherapy; clinical trials are encouraged Stage IA, LVSI negative: Consider vaginal brachytherapy only without chemotherapy – Stage ≥IB: EBRT may be considered in addition to chemotherapy, especially for node-positive disease **Carcinosarcoma and undifferentiated tumours:** Chemotherapy is recommended Consider EBRT; clinical trials are encouraged
Advanced	Stage III residual disease, Stage IVA	Palliative RT/Chemotherapy
Metastatic	Stage IVB	Palliative chemotherapy/RT/best supportive care

Note: The 5-year risk of recurrence is 2–10, 20–25 and 30 % for low risk, intermediate risk and high risk, respectively [15].

Table 6. Evidence-based recommendation ESMO-ESGO-ESTRO consensus [14].

OAR	Dose limitations
Bladder	V80 < 15%, V75 < 25%, V65 < 50%
Rectum	V50 < 50%, V60 < 35%, V65 < 25%, V75 <15%
Small intestine	V15 <120 cc, V45 < 195 cc
Femoral heads	Dmax < 40 Gy

Note: V = volume of tissue receiving *n*% of Gy.

Table 7. Radiation therapy for endometrial cancer and tissue tolerance.

Number of HDR fractions	Dose/fraction	Dose-specific point
3	7	0.5 cm depth
4	5.5	0.5 cm depth
5	4.7	0.5 cm depth
3	10.5	Vaginal surface
4	8.8	Vaginal surface
5	7.5	Vaginal surface

Table 8A. Suggested doses of HDR alone.

5.4. Intensity-modulated radiation therapy

Intensity-modulated radiation therapy (IMRT) improves conformality and eliminates matching problem between electrons and photons over 3DCRT (3D conformal radiation) for vulvar cancer.

Number of HDR fractions	Dose/fraction	Dose-specific point
2	5.5	0.5 cm depth
3	4	0.5 cm depth
2	8	Vaginal surface
3	6	Vaginal surface

Table 8B. Suggested doses of HDR to be used with 45 Gy EBRT for adjuvant endometrial cancer.

IMRT reduces the dose to bladder, rectum, small bowel and head of femur. Definitions of CTV and PTV in 3DCRT and IMRT are as follows: CTV should include 1-cm margin including the entire vulvar region and the bilateral external iliac, internal iliac and inguinofemoral nodes. PTV should include 1 cm margin around CTV.

5.5. Dose prescriptions (Table 9)

Carcinoma of the vagina: Colposcopy-directed biopsy of the cervix and vulva to rule out primary cervical and/or vulvar cancer is undertaken apart from other investigations prior to radiotherapy. In women with early and locally advanced vaginal cancer, radiation is often the sole treatment either alone or in combination with concurrent chemotherapy which is used as a radiation sensitizer. RT comprising both external beam irradiation and brachytherapy is the treatment of choice. Brachytherapy can be intra-cavitary or interstitial depending on the depth of invasion. Intra-cavitary brachytherapy is used to treat superficial lesions <5mm in depth from the vaginal surface. Interstitial brachytherapy is used to treat lesions involving >5mm of depth from the vaginal surface.

5.6. Radiotherapy for vaginal cancer (Table 10)

5.6.1. RT planning techniques simulation and field arrangements

- Patients are simulated in supine, frog-leg positions (to minimize the bolus effect from skin folds) with full bladders (to minimize the volume of small bowel in the radiation field), with custom immobilizations.
- CT scan will be taken from the first lumbar vertebra to 5 cm beyond the vaginal introitus, and anterior and lateral tattoos marked with radio-opaque material aligned with lasers to prevent lateral rotation.

5.6.2. AP/PA field

Superior border will be placed at L5-S1 and inferior border at 3–4 cm below the vaginal marker and lateral borders at 1.5–2cm of the true pelvic rim. If inguinal lymph nodes are to be treated, wide AP fields will be planned to cover inguinal regions with narrow posterior fields with 2:1 weighting.

Setting	Scenario	Dose (Gy)
Preoperative		45–50
Post-operative	Microscopic residual	50
	Extracapsular extension or node positive	55–60
	Gross residual	65–70
Definitive	Concurrent chemoradiation	60–65

Table 9. Dose prescriptions.

Stage	Therapy
Stage I	Brachytherapy alone or combined with EBRT
Stage II	EBRT to the primary and pelvic lymph nodes along with brachytherapy boost is recommended. If the parametria are involved, treatment should include parametrial boost
Stage III–IV A	EBRT to the primary and pelvic lymph nodes along with parametrial boost and brachytherapy boost, with concurrent chemotherapy is recommended

Table 10. Radiotherapy for vaginal cancer.

5.6.3. Dose prescriptions

EBRT dose of 46 Gy with brachytherapy dose of 25–30 Gy is recommended. EBRT boost to 64–70 Gy is used instead of brachytherapy for extensive lesions and those involving recto-vaginal septum.

5.6.4. Normal tissue tolerance

Organs at risk (OAR) in radiation therapy of vaginal cancer include the bladder, rectum, small intestine and the femoral heads **Table 11**.

5.7. Carcinoma of the ovary

The role of radiation is limited in carcinoma ovary. Whole-abdomen radiation has been used, but its popularity has waned because of the favourable toxicity profiles of the current chemo-therapeutic regimens.

6. Newer modalities

Newer external radiation techniques, such as intensity-modulated radiation therapy (IMRT), image-guided radiation therapy (IGRT), stereotactic body radiotherapy (SBRT), proton therapy and PET-CT-guided radiation, have been tried in gynaecological cancers, but these require further validation.

http://dx.doi.org/10.5772/67202

OAR	Dose limitations
Bladder	V45 < 35%
Rectum	V30 < 60%
Small intestine	V15 <120 cc, V45 < 195 cc
Femoral heads	V30 < 15%

Note: Vn% = volume of tissue receiving *n*% of Gy.

Table 11. Tissue tolerance for vaginal RT.

6.1. Intensity-modulated radiation therapy (IMRT)

The technique of IMRT was developed using inverse planning. Intensity of the beam will be modulated spatially with the help of multileaf collimators. The advantage of IMRT lies in the reduction of amount of radiation dose received by small bowel and bone marrow. The use of IMRT is still under evaluation for intact cervix cases, but has been validated in the post-operative setting. Gandhi et al. reported the toxicities of pelvic radiotherapy in 44 patients, of which 22 received 3DCRT and 22 received IMRT. IMRT resulted in significant reduction of gastrointestinal toxicities with comparable clinical outcome. Patients who received IMRT had fewer grade 2 and grade 3 gastrointestinal toxicities as compared with 3DCRT [16]. Du et al. evaluated the dosimetry, efficacy and toxicity of IMRT in advanced cervical cancer. IMRT provided better target dose conformity and better sparing of small bowel, bladder and rectum. They concluded that IMRT resulted in improved dose distributions with significantly lower toxicities with comparable clinical outcome [17]. The dose distribution of IMRT is shown in **Figure 6**.

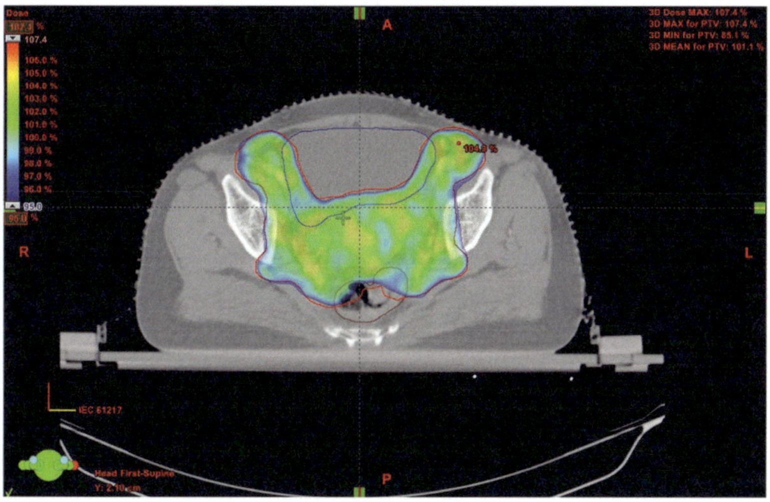

Figure 6. Dose distribution of IMRT showing 95% coverage.

6.2. Image-guided radiation therapy (IGRT)

The definition of IGRT, as given by the American College of Radiology and American Society of Radiation Oncology practice guidelines, is a procedure that refines the delivery of therapeutic radiation by applying image-based target relocalization to allow proper patient repositioning for the purpose of ensuring accurate treatment and minimizing the volume of normal tissue exposed to ionizing radiation [18]. It is particularly useful in cases with a large mobile uterus as seen in young women and with a concern regarding the position of the uterus in the planned radiation field.

6.3. Stereotactic body radiotherapy (SBRT)

SBRT delivers radiation with large fraction sizes using highly conformal treatment techniques. In isolated para-aortic node cases, it has been considered for a nodal boost. It should not be used as replacement for brachytherapy due to the significant increase in normal tissue doses with SBRT as compared with brachytherapy.

6.4. Proton therapy

The rationale for proton therapy lies in the improvement of therapeutic ratio by reducing the radiation dose to non-targeted tissues, thereby reducing toxicity and facilitating dose escalation to achieve increased tumour control. Proton therapy can offer the best way of sparing the small bowel and rectum and can contribute to significant decrease in acute and chronic toxicities in cervical cancer treatment.

6.5. Image-guided brachytherapy

Currently, image-guided adaptive brachytherapy in gynaecological malignancies is based on CT and MRI. Ultrasonography (USG) as an imaging modality for guidance is also being explored. Advantages of USG include easier availability, cost-effectiveness and small learning curve which makes it highly useful in developing countries. Limited availability and accessibility to CT and MRI prevented the early adoption of these promising techniques. Potter et al. reported the clinical outcome of 156 patients treated with image-guided brachytherapy. Ninety-seven percent of patients achieved complete remission with 3-year overall local control rates of 95%, 3-year overall cancer-specific survival rates of 74% and 3-year overall survival rates of 68%. They concluded that there is reduction in major morbidity and pelvic recurrence with the use of image-guided brachytherapy [19].

Side effects of pelvic radiation:

Radiation-induced side effects depend on the type of tissue, dosage and methods of delivery of radiation, and the manifestations can be acute and chronic. Acute side effects usually occur during or within the first 3 months of completing radiation. These include fatigue, skin irritation or redness of the skin and loose bowel movements discomfort when urinating.

Chronic side effects occur 3 months after completion of radiation. It includes skin changes like thinning of skin, radiation enteritis which manifest as loose stools and bleeding per rectum, cystitis, vaginal stenosis and intestinal obstruction and perforation are other uncommon side effects. Common late toxicities include vaginal stenosis/shortening, dryness, fibrosis, telangiectasia, atrophy of skin. Fracture of femoral neck has been implicated with osteoporosis and smoking. Avascular necrosis of the femoral head, though extremely rare, may also occur. Infection, lymphocyst formation and lymphoedema have been associated with groin radiation. Psychosocial consequences which are related to sexual function and body image may occur. With 200 Gy, the rate of tissue necrosis is less than 1% for cervical tissue and vagina is more sensitive with a tolerance of 100–140 Gy, beyond which necrosis is common. The complication of vesicovaginal fistula may result beyond a threshold of 150 Gy and rectovaginal fistula at 80 Gy [5].

Nutrition is important and should contain high protein. Plenty of oral fluids intake of more than 3 litre is necessary to avoid dehydration. When EBRT is employed, skin is the most commonly affected tissue. Avoiding soap and other irritants is important to avoid ulceration.

7. Follow-up and management of side effects

- Two months for the first year, 3 months for the next 2 years, 6 months for the next 2 years and then annually from 5 years.
- History of side effects and physical examination including pelvic and rectal examination and biopsy if recurrent growth.
- CT/MRI for all patients during the first year of follow-up. If cervix cannot be assessed, imaging will be done annually.
- Patient education regarding sexual health, vaginal dilator use, vaginal lubricants/moisturizers (oestrogen creams) is undertaken at each follow-up visit.
- Patients with fistula, who had complete response on follow-up, will be referred for fistula repair.

8. Treatment of recurrent carcinoma of cervix

- *After previous surgery*

Approximately 50% of patients with localized recurrences after surgery alone may be salvaged with radiation. EBRT (45–50 Gy) with concurrent chemotherapy followed by brachytherapy is recommended. If the tumour is inaccessible for brachytherapy, dose escalation with IMRT with at least 65–70 Gy may be attempted.

- *After definitive irradiation*

Important factors to be considered for re-irradiation are the time period between the two treatments, beam energy, volume and doses delivered in the initial treatment. EBRT for recurrent tumour is given to limited volumes (40–45 Gy, 1.8 Gy/fraction).

8.1. Treatment of recurrent carcinoma of endometrium

Radiation therapy can be used to treat small vaginal recurrences in patients who have not received prior radiation. EBRT (45–50 Gy) and brachytherapy are often combined.

8.2. Treatment of recurrent carcinoma of vagina

Lesions that recur after limited surgical procedures can be treated using radiation or more extensive surgery. Most patients have received prior EBRT and, thus, have options limited to surgery.

8.3. Treatment of recurrent carcinoma of vulva

If there is clinical local recurrence confined to vulva or clinical nodal recurrence, no prior RT, then EBRT with concurrent chemotherapy can be delivered. Doses range from 50.4 Gy in 1.8 Gy/# for adjuvant therapy to 59.4–64.8 Gy in 1.8 Gy/# for unresectable disease. Large nodes may be boosted to a dose of 70 Gy.

9. Conclusion

Radiation therapy in gynaecological malignancies involves multidisciplinary approach, careful planning and execution. Counselling is an essential part to increase compliance and to achieve high cure rates.

Author details

Papa Dasari[1,*], Singhavajhala Vivekanandam[2] and Kandepadu Srinagesh Abhishek Raghava[2]

*Address all correspondence to: dasaripapa@gmail.com

1 Department of Obstetrics and Gynaecology, JIPMER, Puducherry, India

2 Department of Radiotherapy, Regional Cancer Centre, JIPMER, Puducherry, India

References

[1] Ramesh N, Anjana A, Kusum N, Kiran A, Ashok A, Somdutt S. Overview of benign and malignant tumours of the genital tract. J Appl Pharm Sci. 2013;3:140–149.

[2] WHO ; International Agency for Research on cancer. American Cancer Society. Global Cancer. Facts and Figures. 2nd edition. Globacon; 2008.

[3] Sridevi A, Javed R, Dinesh A. Epidemiology of cervical cancer with special focus on India. Int J Women's Health 2015;7:405–414.

[4] Schorge JO, Knowles LM, Lea JS. Adenocarcinoma of the cervix. Current treatment options. Curr Treat Options Oncol. 2004;5:119. doi:10.1007/s11864–004–0044–0.

[5] Shrivatsva SK, Mahantshetty U, Narayan K. Principles of radiation therapy in low resource and well developed settings with particular reference to cervical cancer. IJGO. 2012;116S2:S155–S159.

[6] Sethi TK, Bhalla NK, Jena AN et al. Magnetic resonance imaging in carcinoma cervix–does it have a prognostic relevance. J Cancer Res Ther.2005;1:103–107.

[7] Loft A, Berthelsen AK, Roed H et al. The diagnostic value of PET/CT scanning in patients with cervical cancer: a prospective study. Gynecol Oncol. 2007;106:29–34.

[8] American Joint Committee on Cancer. Cervix uteri cancer staging. American Cancer Society. http://www.cancer.org/cancer/cervicalcancer/detailedguide/cervical-cancer-staged.

[9] Plataniotis G, Castiglione M. Endometrial cancer: ESMO clinical practice guidelines for diagnosis, treatment and follow-up. Ann Oncol. 2010;21: 41–45.

[10] Vaginal Cancer-American Cancer Society. www.cancer.org/vaginal-cancer-pdf

[11] Consent for Radiotherapy. NHS Foundation Trust. www.nhs.uk/Conditions/Consent-to-treatment/Pages/Introduction.aspx

[12] Nandakumar A, Ramnath T, Chaturvedi M. The magnitude of cancer cervix in India. Indian J Med Res. 2009;130(3):219–221.

[13] Green J, Kirwan J, Tierney J, Vale C, Symonds P, Fresco L, et al. Concomitant chemotherapy and radiation therapy for cancer of the uterine cervix. Cochrane Database Syst Rev. 2005;(3):CD002225.

[14] Colombo N, Creutzberg C, Amant F et al. ESMO,ESGO-ESTRO Consensus Conference on Endometrial Cancer. Int J Gynecol Oncol. 2016;26:1;1–30.

[15] Kuppets R, ON T, Le T, ON O. The role of adjuvant therapy in endometrial cancer. Joint SOGC-GOC-SCC Clinical Practice guideline. J Obstet Gynaecol Can. 2013;35(4 eSuppl B):S1–S9

[16] Gandhi AK, Sharma DN, Rath GK, Julka PK, Subramani V, Sharma S, Manigandan D, Laviraj MA, Kumar S, Thulkar S. Early clinical outcomes and toxicity of intensity modulated versus conventional pelvic radiation therapy for locally advanced cervix carcinoma: a prospective randomized study. Int J Radiat Oncol Biol Phys. 2013;87(3):542–548.

[17] Du XL, Tao J, Sheng XG, Lu CH, Yu H, Wang C, Song QQ, Li QS, Pan CX. Intensity-modulated radiation therapy for advanced cervical cancer: a comparison of

dosimetric and clinical outcomes with conventional radiotherapy. Gynecol Oncol. 2012;125(1):151–157.

[18] ACR–ASTRO practice guideline for image-guided radiation therapy (IGRT). American College of Radiology. http://www.acr.org/SecondaryMainMenuCategories/quality_safety/guidelines/ro/IGRT.aspx.

[19] Potter R, Georg P, Dimopoulos JC, Grimm M, Berger D, Nesvacil N, et al. Clinical outcome of protocol based image (MRI) guided adaptive brachytherapy combined with 3D conformal radiotherapy with or without chemotherapy in patients with locally advanced cervical cancer. Radiother Oncol 2011;100(1):116–123.

Chapter 5

Image-Guided Adaptive Brachytherapy for Cervical Cancer Using Magnetic Resonance Imaging: Overview and Experience

Kenji Yoshida, Ryo Nishikawa, Daisuke Miyawaki,
Yasuhiko Ebina and Ryohei Sasaki

Additional information is available at the end of the chapter

http://dx.doi.org/10.5772/67382

Abstract

Image-guided adaptive brachytherapy (IGABT) using magnetic resonance imaging (MRI) has been accepted as a novel treatment technique for cervical cancer. During the development of MRI-based IGABT, a very important concept called "High-risk clinical target volume (HR-CTV)" was introduced. However, computed tomography (CT)-based IGABT is the most common modality in Japan.

MRI-based IGABT was initiated in September 2014 at Kobe University Hospital and 50 patients were treated through March 2016. Although a total HR-CTV D90 ranging from 80 to 85 Gy equivalent dose in 2 Gy fractions in combination with 45 Gy of external beam radiotherapy (EBRT) and 7 Gy×4 fractions of IGABT is the most standard treatment aim in European institutions, our aim for a total HR-CTV D90 was a 70–80 Gy because of the use of the central shielding technique for the protection of organs at risk in the late phase of EBRT.

The mean total HR-CTV D90 for our 50 patients was 77 Gy. Although our aim was achieved, it was relatively low because Japanese radiotherapy protocols for cervical cancer still differ from those in European institutions. Therefore, a new treatment protocol, which is closer to the global standard, should be established.

Keywords: image-guided adaptive brachytherapy, high-risk clinical target volume, D90, D2cc, magnetic resonance imaging

1. Introduction

Image-guided adaptive brachytherapy (IGABT) using magnetic resonance imaging (MRI) has been widely accepted as a novel treatment technique for gynecologic malignancies, especially for cervical cancer. In 2005, the primary concept of IGABT, which is high-risk clinical target volume (HR-CTV), was described by the Gynaeacologic (GYN) GEO-ESTRO working group [1]. Around the same time, the first clinical report on the effectiveness of MRI-based IGABT was published by Pötter et al. [2]. In that study, 44 of 48 patients had stage IIB to IVA disease. Overall survival at 3 years was 61%, progression-free survival was 51%, and continuous complete remission for true pelvis was 85% with a median follow up of 33 months.

By using MRI or computed tomography (CT), three-dimensional (3D) description of the HR-CTV and the organs at risk (OAR), such as the bladder, rectum, sigmoid colon, and small bowel, can be achieved. Therefore, dosimetric evaluation for both the HR-CTV and OAR using dose volume histograms (DVH) can be performed with greater accuracy than that with traditional point A treatment planning using the definition of the ICRU report 38 for the OAR doses [3]. The GYN GEO-EATRO working group also published recommendations regarding the 3D dosimetric parameters [4]. Although various dosimetric parameters were described by GYN GEO-EATRO, HR-CTV D90 and OAR D2cc have been emphasized in clinical brachytherapy (BT). The working group also published recommendations for the acquisition protocols of MRI sequences [5].

Implementation of IGABT made it possible to use interstitial needles more safely. This is one of the most important points in performing IGABT, because the use of interstitial needles can change the dose distribution dramatically, especially in large tumors. In European institutions, MRI-based IGABT is a common technique and interstitial needles are frequently used. However, CT-based IGABT is most common in Japanese institutions and interstitial needles are less frequently used than in European institutions. In addition, 3D-conformal radiotherapy (3D-CRT) with a central shielding (CS) technique for the protection of OAR from higher doses has been applied as the standard external beam radiotherapy (EBRT) for many years at most Japanese institutions, even after the introduction of intensity-modulated radiotherapy (IMRT), which is performed without a CS technique at many European institutions. Therefore, radiotherapy (RT) for cervical cancer in Japan is somewhat different from that in institutions in other countries.

MRI-based IGABT for cervical cancer was initiated at Kobe University Hospital in September 2014 and 50 patients were treated with definitive IGABT through March 2016. Similar to other institutions in Japan, for EBRT, a 3D-CRT with a CS technique is still performed. Interstitial needles are applied for some patients with large tumors. The purpose of this chapter is to provide an overview of MRI-based IGABT and the introduction of the experience at Kobe University Hospital along with a comparison with European representative institutions.

http://dx.doi.org/10.5772/67382

2. Applicators for IGABT

Applicators compatible with MRI must be used for MRI-based IGABT. Even if CT-based IGABT is performed, traditional stainless steel applicators should not be used because severe metal artifacts may occur when CT images are acquired. Tandem and ovoid applicators are used most frequently in Japanese institutions.

The Medical University of Vienna, the most representative institution in Europe, and a lot of other institutions in other countries have used Vienna applicators compatible with MRI that were developed for combined intracavitary (IC) and interstitial (IS) BT [6]. This applicator has a tandem and a ring part. The ring part includes the source pathway and it also has a templated function for titanium interstitial needle implantation. By setting the dwell point in the ring, a dose distribution the same as when using a tandem and ovoid applicator can be developed. Therefore, both MRI-based IC-BT alone and combined with IC- and IS-BT can be performed by using the Vienna applicator. Unfortunately, this applicator is not allowed to be used in Japan. In addition, only plastic or stainless steel needles are available for IGABT. When using stainless steel needles, MRI cannot be performed after needle implantation. CT-based IGABT, or acquisition of MR images before needle implantation and fusion of the MRI images to the CT images acquired after needle implantation, is one of the ways to deal with this problem. Plastic needles are also compatible with MRI; however, these are not suitable for hard tumors because of the dull edge. Metal stainless needles may help to create a pathway for plastic needles. After pathway preparation with metal stainless needles, implantation may be easier and acquisition of MR images can be achieved.

Jürgenliemk-Schulz et al. investigated the potential benefit of newly designed tandem and ovoid applicators compatible with IC- and IS-BT using plastic needles [7]. They performed MRI-based IGABT using the applicators in six patients and reported that additional improvement was achieved with a combined IC/IS approach. The results are encouraging because the newly developed applicators for both IC/IS approaches may be used in many countries including Japan, resulting in significant progress in IGABT.

3. Definition of high risk clinical target volume (HR-CTV)

The most important target volume in IGABT, the HR-CTV, can be defined at the time of first BT. In the recommendations from the GYN GEO-ESTRO working group, a brief definition of HR-CTV in 3D image-based 3D treatment is described as follows (1) carrying a high tumor load, includes the gross tumor volume (GTV) and always includes the whole cervix and presumed extracervical tumor extension at the time of BT. Limited disease is defined as a tumor less than 4 cm and/or limited to the cervix at the time of diagnosis. Therefore, in such cases, the whole cervix including the GTV at BT corresponds to the HR-CTV. For extensive disease, presumed tumor extension is defined by clinical examination (visualization and palpation) and imaging (MRI). Interstitial needles are usually required in such extensive cases. Examples of HR-CTVs of both limited and extensive cases treated at Kobe University are shown in **Figures 1** and **2**.

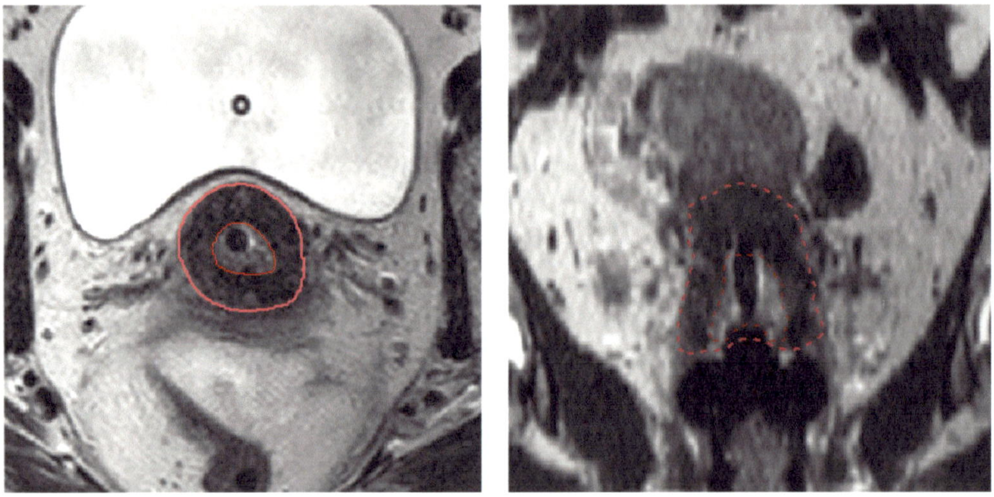

Figure 1. HR-CTV (pink and outer line) and GTV (red and inner line) of limited disease delineated on axial image (original) and coronal image (reconstructed).

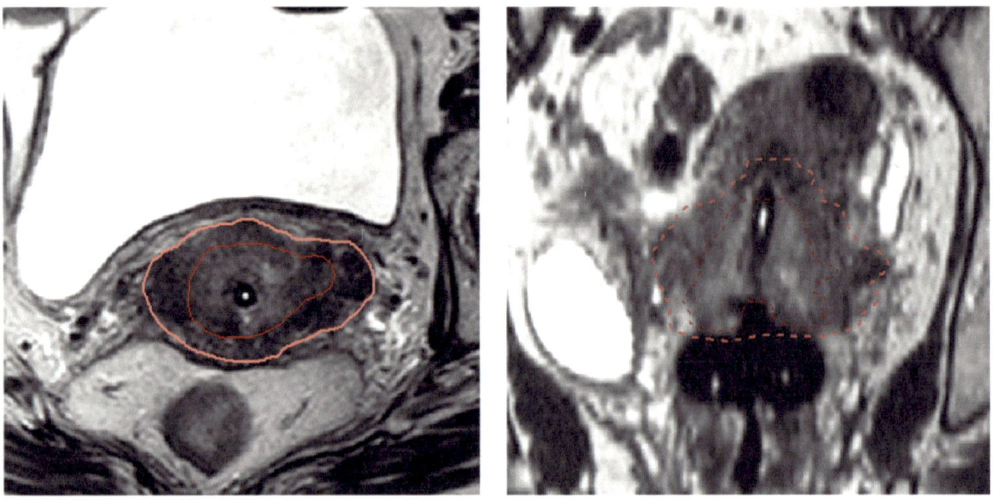

Figure 2. HR-CTV (pink and outer line) and GTV (red and inner line) of extensive disease delineated on axial image (original) and coronal image (reconstructed).

4. IGABT procedure (Kobe University Hospital)

4.1. Anesthesia

To perform more appropriate IGABT, appropriate anesthesia is very important. There are four types of anesthesia and combinations as follows: general anesthesia, lumbar subarachnoid spinal nerve block, sacral epidural block, and intravenous sedation. Intravenous sedation is inadequate to perform appropriate IGABT and therefore should only be performed in patients who cannot safely receive other anesthesia modalities. Lumber subarachnoid spinal nerve block seems to be better than sacral epidural block. However, sacral epidural block may be better for patients receiving anticoagulation therapy. In addition, anesthesia should be performed by an anesthetist for patient safety. Lumber subarachnoid spinal nerve block or sacral epidural block is performed most frequently. In our institution, the first choice for IGABT is a lumbar subarachnoid spinal nerve block. A sacral epidural block is the second choice for patients receiving anticoagulation therapy or those with severe medical complications.

4.2. Flow of IGABT

Applicator implantation should be performed using transrectal ultrasound. This is important for guidance during dilatation of the cervical canal and tandem implantation. X-ray is also useful. If available in the BT room, CT is very useful to verify the final position of the applicators, and also to perform needle implantation. Moreover, when CT-based planning is performed, the entire BT procedure (implant, imaging, planning, and irradiation) can be done in the same room. Therefore, if an institution is going to initiate IGABT, the most important thing is to place CT in the BT room.

When MRI-based IGABT is performed, patients must be transported to the MRI room. Transfer must be performed as quickly as possible for safety and the MRI protocol must be limited to that necessary for treatment. After acquisition of MR images, treatment planning, and irradiation is performed.

4.3. Imaging protocols

For the acquisition of MR images, a 1.5 or 3.0 T machine is recommended. T2-weighted images (WI) with transverse sections are necessary for treatment planning. Sagittal sections are also important. Diffusion-weighted images (DWI) are optional but are useful to define GTV. As an example, details of MRI performed at Kobe University Hospital are shown in **Table 1**.

Sequence	Slice thickness (mm)	No. of slices	Imaging time (seconds)
T2WI (transverse)	2	70	308
T2WI (sagittal)	2.5	40	85
DWI	5	25	263

Notes: T2WI: T2 weighted image, DWI: diffusion weighted image.

Table 1. MR imaging protocol at Kobe University.

5. Treatment

5.1. Treatment schedule and details of EBRT

The Japanese protocol for EBRT and BT for cervical cancer is shown in **Table 2a**. Most institutions, including Kobe University Hospital, still use this protocol. Most patients are treated with 3D conformal pelvic irradiation (PI), with a total dose of 50.4 Gy in 28 fractions. At first, whole pelvic irradiation (WPI) is performed, and then WPI with a CS technique is performed. Generally, BT is initiated at the end of the WPI period and before the start of PI with a CS technique. Most patients are treated with three or four sessions of BT given once or twice a week. Regarding combined WPI and CS technique, 30.6 Gy in 17 fractions of WPI and 19.8 Gy in 11 fractions with CS technique are used for International Federation of Gynecologists and Obstetricians (FIGO) stage IB to IIB disease. For more advanced disease, 41.4 Gy in 23 fractions of WPI and 9.0 Gy in 5 fractions with CS technique are used. Paraaortic regional irradiation is added for patients with gross metastases. For lymph node metastases, an additional 10 Gy in 5 fractions is usually applied to each metastatic region.

In contrast with the Japanese protocol, many foreign institutions such as Medical University of Vienna deliver EBRT consisting of 45 Gy in 25 fractions without using a CS technique; at the end of EBRT, 4 fractions of BT are administered. IMRT is usually performed. The treatment schedules at representative institutions are also shown in **Table 2b** for direct comparison with the Japanese protocol. CS technique is not used by all institutions [8–12].

5.2. Treatment planning for BT

5.2.1. Applicator reconstruction

Fusion of CT and MR images is necessary for BT treatment planning, even for MRI-based IGABT, if the positions of the sources cannot be identified correctly due to the lack of simulated sources compatible with MRI (**Figure 3a**). To achieve true MRI-based treatment planning, home-made catheters using flexible tubes filled with normal saline solution for interstitial BT that were compatible with MRI were used as simulated sources (**Figure 3b**). Using these catheters, positions of the sources could be described very clearly. By using the system included in the Oncentra Brachy applicator placement technique and these catheters, it is possible to achieve true MRI-based treatment planning for patients treated with IC-BT (**Figure 4**).

5.2.2. Delineation of target and OAR

The GTV and HR-CTV are delineated based on the recommendations from GYN GEO-ESTRO [1]. The intermediate risk clinical target volume (IR-CTV) is automatically delineated with a 5–15 mm margin from the HR-CTV, excluding the OAR.

FIGO stage, tumor size	WPI (Gy)	CS technique (Gy)	HDR-BT (to point A)
Ib1, II (small)	20	30	6 Gy × 4 fractions
Ib2, II (large), III	30	20	6 Gy × 4 fractions
	40	10	6 Gy × 3 fractions
IVA	40	10	6 Gy × 3 fractions
	50	0	6 Gy × 2 fractions

Notes: WPI: whole pelvic irradiation, CS: central shielding, HDR-BT: high dose rate brachytherapy.

Table 2a. Details of Japanese treatment protocol for cervical cancer.

http://dx.doi.org/10.5772/67382

Institutions	WPI (Gy)	CS technique (Gy)	HDR-BT (to HRCTV)
Medical University of Vienna [8]	45	0	7 Gy × 4 fractions
University Medical Center Utrecht [9]	45	0	7 Gy × 4 fractions
University of Pittsburgh Medical Center [10]	45	0	25–30 Gy in 5 fractions
Leiden University Medical Center [11]	46 or 45–50.4	0	7 Gy × 3 or, 8.5 Gy × 2 fractions
University of California San Diego [12]	45	0	25–30 Gy in 3–5 fractions

Notes: WPI: whole pelvic irradiation, CS: central shielding, HDR-BT: high dose rate brachytherapy, HRCTV: high risk clinical target volume.

Table 2b. Details of treatment protocols for cervical cancer at the representative institutions.

The rectum, bladder, sigmoid colon, and small bowel are delineated using MR images. The bladder is usually filled with 100 mL of normal saline solution to avoid high doses to the small bowels before the acquisition of images. If necessary, the urethra is also delineated.

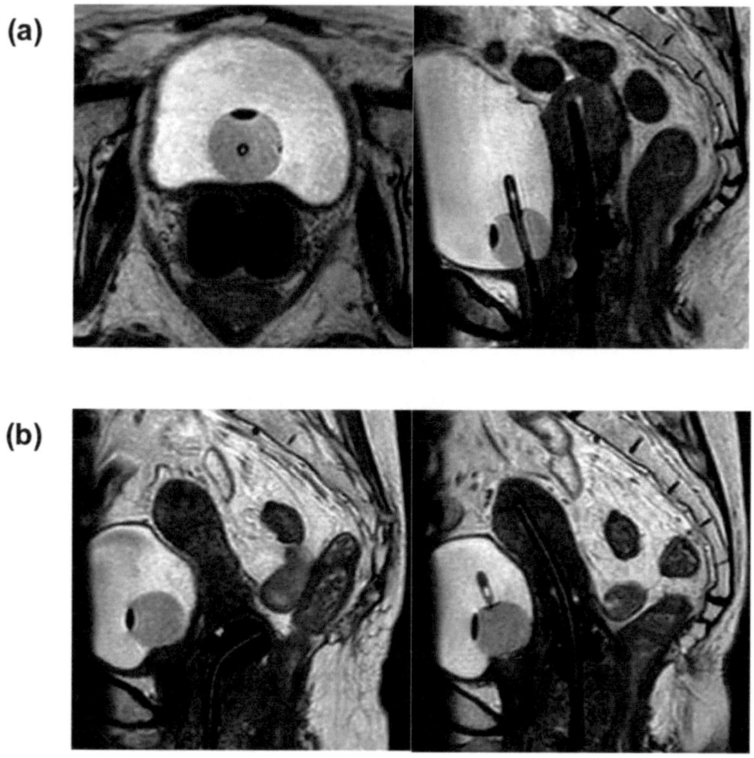

Figure 3. (a) MR images for treatment planning without simulated sources. (b) MR images for treatment planning with simulated sources consisting of flexible tube for interstitial BT.

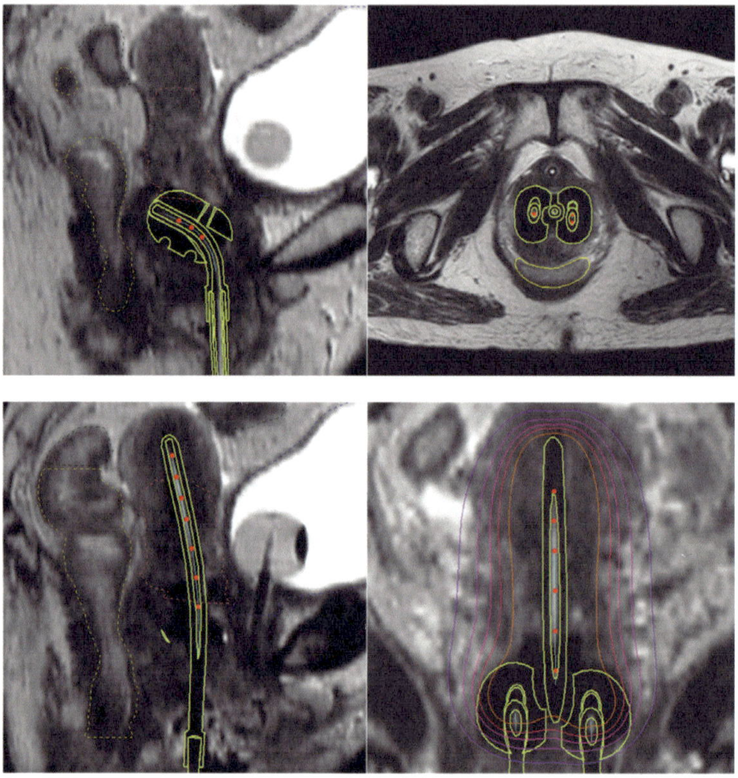

Figure 4. MRI-based treatment planning of intracavitary BT using simulated sources and applicator placement technique.

5.2.3. Treatment aim for dosimetric parameters

5.2.3.1. HR-CTV

The most important dosimetric parameter of the target is the HR-CTV D90. Our primary treatment aim is that the HR-CTV D90 should be more than 7.0 Gy per implant with a total of 70–80 Gy equivalent dose in 2 Gy fractions (EQD2) calculated by using the following formula:

$$\text{EQD2} = n * d * ((d + \alpha/\beta)/(2 + \alpha/\beta)) \quad (1)$$

where n is the number of fractions, d is the single fraction dose, tumor $\alpha/\beta = 10$, normal tissue $\alpha/\beta = 3$.

Total HR-CTV D90s calculated from the single fraction dose and the number of fractions of IGABT and WPI are shown in **Table 3a**. Doses for pelvic irradiation with the CS technique are not included. At other representative institutions, the total HR-CTV D90 is usually aimed at more than 85 Gy in EQD2. In previous reports, Nomden et al. reported that the mean HR-CTV D90 in EQD2 was 84 Gy [9]. Simpson et al. reported that the mean HR-CTV D90 was 86.3 Gy [12]. Although our HR-CTV D90 per implant was equivalent to that in other institutions [8, 9],

HR-CTV D90 in IGABT single dose × fractions (Gy)	WPI: single dose × fractions (total) (Gy)			
	1.8 × 17 (30.6)	1.8 × 23 (41.4)	1.8 × 25 (45)	1.8 × 28 (50.4)
	Total HR-CTV D90 in 3/4 fractions (Gy, EQD2)			
6.5 × 3/4	56.9/65.8	67.5/76.5	71.1/80.0	76.4/85.3
7 × 3/4	59.8/69.8	70.5/80.4	74/83.9	79.3/89.2
7.5 × 3/4	62.9/73.8	73.5/84.5	77.1/88.0	82.4/93.3
8 × 3/4	66.1/78.1	76.7/88.7	80.3/92.3	85.6/97.6
8.5 × 3/4	69.4/82.5	80.0/93.1	83.4/96.7	88.9/102.0
9 × 3/4	72.8/87.1	83.5/97.7	87.0/101.3	92.3/106.6

Notes: HR-CTV: high risk clinical target volume, EQD2: equivalent dose in 2 Gy fractions, IGABT: image-guided adaptive brachytherapy, WPI: whole pelvic irradiation.

Table 3a. Total HR-CTV D90 (EQD2) calculated from the single dose and number of fractions of IGABT and WPI.

the goal of total D90 was set lower because the use of the CS technique might hinder delivery of higher D90.

5.2.3.2. OAR

For the OAR, D2cc is recognized as the most important dosimetric parameter. In clinical IGABT, bladder, rectum, sigmoid colon, and small bowel D2cc must be calculated and recorded for every implant. The proposed upper limit of the total bladder dose is 85 Gy with a maximum of 90 Gy in EQD2. Those of the total rectum, sigmoid colon, and small bowel are 70 Gy with a maximum of 75 Gy in the EQD2. The upper limit of single OAR doses (non-EQD2) in IGABT calculated from the total OAR D2cc and WPI dose are shown in **Table 3b**. Doses from PI with the CS technique are not included. As for these OARs, many previous studies used similar criteria [8–10, 12].

Total D2cc in EQD2 (Gy)	WPI: single dose × fractions (total) (Gy)			
	1.8 × 17 (30.6)	1.8 × 23 (41.4)	1.8 × 25 (45)	1.8 × 28 (50.4)
	Upper limit of single OAR dose in 3/4 fractions (Gy, non-EQD2)			
Bladder				
85	8.2/6.9	7.3/6.1	6.9/5.8	6.4/5.4
90	8.6/7.3	7.7/6.5	7.4/6.2	6.9/5.8
Rectum and other bowels				
70	6.8/5.7	5.7/4.8	5.3/4.4	4.6/3.9
75	7.3/6.1	6.3/5.3	5.9/4.9	5.3/4.4

Notes: EQD2: equivalent dose in 2 Gy fractions, OAR: organ at risk, WPI: whole pelvic irradiation.

Table 3b. Upper limit of single OAR doses (non-EQD2) in IGABT calculated from the total OAR D2cc and WPI dose.

5.2.4. Dose prescription and optimization

5.2.4.1. Intracavitary BT

The basic treatment plan prescribed to point A according to Japanese guidelines is first created for every implant. The point A dose is 6.0 Gy. Then, graphical optimization is performed to achieve the treatment aim for both the HR-CTV and the OAR.

5.2.4.2. Combined intracavitary/interstitial BT

Similar to intracavitary BT, a basic plan prescribed to point A (6.0 Gy) is first created. Next, optimization of the intracavitary applicator is performed to reduce the doses to the OAR. Then, the interstitial needles are activated to increase the target coverage. Additional optimization is usually performed to achieve the treatment aim.

5.3. Limitations of CT-based planning

In performing CT-based planning, the most important limitation is inaccurate delineation of the HR-CTV. CT-based delineation is often very different from MRI-based delineation (**Figure 5**). The HR-CTV D90 may be significantly affected by the difference in imaging modality at BT (MRI or CT). Hegazy et al. reported that CT-based HR-CTV contouring based on FIGO stage led to a large overestimation of the width and volume. They concluded that if only CT was available, a minimum two-third of the uterine height might be a good surrogate for the height of the HR-CTV [13]. Clinical gynecologic examination and acquisition of MR images just before the start of BT can help to improve the accuracy of delineation.

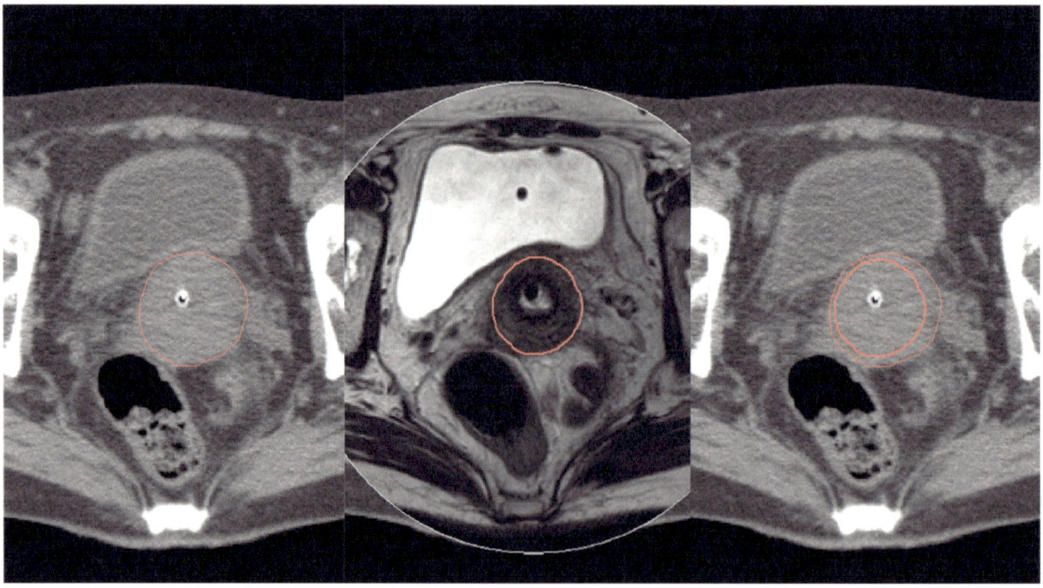

Figure 5. Comparison of CT-based and MRI-based delineation of HRCTV. CT-based delineation is quite large compared to MRI-based delineation.

6. Reported treatment results

There are an increasing number of published reports regarding treatment results of IGABT for cervical cancer as shown in **Table 4** [8–12, 14–17]. In 2011, Pötter et al. retrospectively analyzed 156 patients with FIGO stage IB to IVA cervical cancer treated by IGABT at Medical University of Vienna [8]. A combined IC/IS approach was used in 44% of the patients with residual disease at the time of BT. They reported the three-year overall survival (OS) rates for stage IB, IIB, and IIIB disease were 74, 79, and 45%, respectively. They also reported that three-year local control (LC) rates for stage IB, IIB, and IIIB disease were 100, 96, and 86%, respectively. These results indicate that IGABT can achieve excellent LC rates even in cases of unfavorable advanced disease, such as stage IIIB disease, by using interstitial needles.

In a recent large multicenter study called RetroEMBRACE, Sturdza et al. analyzed 731 patients [17]. They reported that three-year overall survival rates for stage IB, IIB, and IIIB patients

Author (year)	No. of patients	median follow up (months)	Imaging	mean HRCTV D90 (SD) in EQD2 (Gy)	LC rate (%)	CSS rate (%)	OS rate (%)
Pötter et al. (2011) [8]	156	42	MRI	93 (13)	95 (3-year)	74 (3-year)	68 (3-year)
Lindegaard et al. (2013) [14]	140	36	MRI	91	91 (3-year)	87 (3-year)	79 (3-year)
Nomden et al. (2013) [9]	46	41	MRI	84 (9)	93 (3-year)	74 (3-year)	65 (3-year)
Gill et al. (2014) [10]	128	24.4	MRI	83.2 (2.7)	91.6 (3-year)	85.4 (3-year)	76.6 (3-year)
Rijkmans et al. (2014) [11]	83	42.3	MRI	80.8	NA	NA	86 (3-year)
Castelnau-Marchand et al. (2015) [15]	225	38.8	MRI	80.4 (10.3)	86.4 (3-year)	NA	76.1 (3-year)
Simpson et al. (2015) [12]	76	17	CT	86.3 (8.1)	NA	NA	75 (2-year)
Ribeiro et al. (2016) [16]	170	37	MRI	85 (8.4)	96 (3-year)	NA	73 (3-year)
Sturdza et al. (2016) [17]	731	43	MRI/CT	87 (15)	91 (3-year)	79 (3-year)	74 (3-year)

Notes: IGABT: image-guided adaptive brachytherapy, HR-CTV: high risk clinical target volume, LC: local control, CSS: cancer specific survival, OS: overall survival.

Table 4. Reported treatment results of IGABT for cervical cancer.

were 88, 78, and 56%, respectively. They also reported that three-year LC rates were 98, 93, and 79%, respectively. These results indicate that IGABT is an indispensable treatment tool to achieve excellent LC rates. Lindegaard et al. compared the treatment results of MRI-guided IGABT to X-ray-based BT [14]. Both OS and cancer-specific survival (CSS) rates were significantly better in the patient group treated with MRI-guided IGABT.

The mean total HR-CTVs in these reports ranged from 80.3 to 93 Gy in EQD2. All of the total HR-CTV D90s were more than 80 Gy. In our experience with IGABT for 50 cervical cancer patients, the mean total HR-CTV D90 was 77.0 Gy, lower than that at the representative centers. This difference was caused by the CS technique. According to other reports from Japan, although treatment outcomes were excellent, HR-CTV D90s were less than 70 Gy [18, 19]. These results are also lower than our findings. The studies used CT-based planning, which also accounted for the large difference when combined with CS technique. It is likely that a larger HR-CTV delineated using CT and a lower WPI dose combined with CS technique resulted in a significantly lower D90. MRI-based planning without CS technique might achieve HR-CTV D90 comparable to that in foreign institutions. More institutions in Japan should perform MRI-based planning because it may become the global standard. Use of CS technique should also be discussed.

In summary, the use of IGABT can help achieve excellent LC even in advanced stage cervical cancer with the help of interstitial needles. Survival results with IGABT showed superiority to those achieved with traditional X-ray-based BT. HR-CTV D90 can be easily affected by imaging modality and variability of EBRT dosing. However, 45 Gy of WPI and MRI-based treatment planning aiming for a total HR-CTV D90 from 80 to 85 Gy should be considered the most appropriate treatment regimen.

7. Treatment-related adverse events

Late bladder, gastrointestinal, and vaginal toxicities have been reported by previous studies. In the Retro-EMBRACE study [17], five-year Grade 3–5 toxicity in the bladder, gastrointestinal tract, and vagina among 610 patients affected 5, 7, and 5%, respectively. Ribeiro et al. also reported Grade 3–4 late rectal, urinary, sigmoid, and vaginal morbidity rates were 5, 6, 2, and 5%, respectively, in their long-term treatment outcome study [16]. They also identified a correlation between rectal $D2cm^3 > 65$ Gy and Grade > 3 late morbidity. Among patients treated at Kobe University Hospital, Grade 3 rectal toxicity occurred in two (4%) patients. No Grade 3 or greater late bladder and vaginal toxicities have occurred to date.

Acute toxicities are rarely reported in published studies. According to our experience, hematological toxicity is the most frequent, especially in patients treated with concurrent chemoradiotherapy (CCRT). Among the 50 patients treated at Kobe University Hospital, Grade 3 or greater acute hematologic toxicity occurred in 36 (72%) patients. Procedure-related complications should also be reported. In the early period, mild pressure ulcers around the buttocks occurred in five patients. Respiratory suppression occurred in one patient who received intravenous sedation. In addition, interstitial needles may cause severe complications. The most common is bleeding. It is sometimes difficult to manage extravaginal bleeding caused by laceration of the vaginal wall. It is also important to be aware of possible intraabdominal bleeding.

This may be caused by injury to the uterine arteries. Performing CT immediately after removal of the applicators may be useful for the early detection of intraabdominal bleeding.

In summary, according to the results from previous studies and our experience, Grade ≥3 late treatment-related toxicity occurs in approximately 5% of patients. Acute severe hematologic toxicity frequently occurs in patients treated with CCRT. The role of the CS technique performed for the protection of OAR from higher doses should be discussed from the aspect of toxicity. Monitoring is essential for procedure-related complications. Interstitial needles can cause severe complications. It is necessary to improve procedures, including needle implantation, to prevent complications.

8. Conclusions

In this chapter, an overview of our experience of MRI based-IGABT for cervical cancer was described. IGABT using MRI has been widely accepted, especially in European countries, and the combination of 45 Gy in 25 fractions of EBRT without using a CS technique and more than 7 Gy × 4 fractions for HR-CTV is the most standard protocol. Pelvic IMRT has been increasingly performed. The total EQD2 delivered in this protocol is usually more than 85 Gy. Interstitial needles are often implanted for large tumors using a Vienna ring applicator, which is very suitable for combined IC/IS BT because the ring part has the source pathway and can be used as the template of the needles. Tandem and ovoid applicator which had function for the template of the interstitial needles were also reported [7]. Increasing numbers of treatment results have been reported, and the impressive role of IGABT, especially in LC, has been demonstrated when delivering more than 80 Gy as a mean total HR-CTV D90s. Therefore, many representative institutions aimed at least more than 80 Gy [9–13]. Although MRI-based IGABT has been performed since September 2014 at Kobe University, CT-based IGABT still has been performed at most Japanese institutions because of various circumstances, and interstitial needles are less frequently used. CT-based IGABT is well established; however, considerable differences in the delineation of HR-CTV can occur as compared to MRI-based BT. In addition, we continue to use a CS technique with EBRT and pelvic IMRT has not been accepted in the definitive RT for cervical cancer. Therefore, although successful outcomes were reported [18, 19], RT for cervical cancer in Japan is still different from that in European countries in both BT and EBRT. In the immediate future, a new treatment protocol (MRI-or CT-based? with or without the CS technique? 3D-CRT or IMRT?), which is closer to the global standard, should be established for the further development of RT treatment of cervical cancer in Japan.

Author details

Kenji Yoshida[1]*, Ryo Nishikawa[1], Daisuke Miyawaki[1], Yasuhiko Ebina[2] and Ryohei Sasaki[1]

*Address all correspondence to: kyoshi@med.kobe-u.ac.jp

1 Division of Radiation Oncology, Kobe University Graduate School of Medicine, Kobe, Japan

2 Department of Gynecology, Kobe University Graduate School of Medicine, Kobe, Japan

References

[1] Haie-Meder C, Pötter R, Van Limbergen E, Briot E, De Brabandere M, Dimopoulos J, Dumas I, Hellebust TP, Kirisits C, Lang S, Muschitz S, Nevinson J, Nulens A, Petrow P, Wachter-Gerstner N. Gynaecological (GYN) GEC-ESTRO Working Group. Recommendations from Gynaecological (GYN) GEC-ESTRO Working Group (I): concepts and terms in 3D image based 3D treatment planning in cervix cancer brachytherapy with emphasis on MRI assessment of GTV and CTV. Radiother Oncol. 2005 Mar;74(3):235–245. Review.

[2] Pötter R, Dimopoulos J, Bachtiary B, Sissolak G, Klos B, Rheinthaller A, Kirisits C, Knocke-Abulesz TH. 3D conformal HDR-brachy- and external beam therapy plus simultaneous cisplatin for high-risk cervical cancer: clinical experience with 3-year follow-up. Radiother Oncol. 2006 Apr;79(1):80–86. Epub 2006 Mar 3.

[3] International Commission on Radiation Units and Measurements. Dose and volume specification for intracavity therapy in gynecology. 1985, ICRU report 38. ICRU, Washington

[4] Pötter R, Haie-Meder C, Van Limbergen E, Barillot I, De Brabandere M, Dimopoulos J, Dumas I, Erickson B, Lang S, Nulens A, Petrow P, Rownd J, Kirisits C; GEC ESTRO Working Group. Recommendations from Gynaecological (GYN) GEC ESTRO working group (II): concepts and terms in 3D image-based treatment planning in cervix cancer brachytherapy-3D dose volume parameters and aspects of 3D image-based anatomy, radiation physics, radiobiology. Radiother Oncol. 2006 Jan;78(1):67–77. Epub 2006 Jan 5.

[5] Dimopoulos JC, Petrow P, Tanderup K, Petric P, Berger D, Kirisits C, Pedersen EM, van Limbergen E, Haie-Meder C, Pötter R. Recommendations from Gynaecological (GYN) GEC-ESTRO Working Group (IV): basic principles and parameters for MR imaging within the frame of image based adaptive cervix cancer brachytherapy. Radiother Oncol. 2012 Apr;103(1):113–22. doi: 10.1016/j.radonc.2011.12.024. Epub 2012 Jan 30.

[6] Kirisits C, Lang S, Dimopoulos J, Berger D, Georg D, Pötter R. The Vienna applicator for combined intracavitary and interstitial brachytherapy of cervical cancer: design, application, treatment planning, and dosimetric results. Int J Radiat Oncol Biol Phys. 2006 Jun 1;65(2):624–30.

[7] Jürgenliemk-Schulz IM, Tersteeg RJ, Roesink JM, Bijmolt S, Nomden CN, Moerland MA, de Leeuw AA. MRI-guided treatment-planning optimisation in intracavitary or combined intracavitary/interstitial PDR brachytherapy using tandem ovoid applicators in locally advanced cervical cancer. Radiother Oncol. 2009 Nov;93(2):322–30. doi: 10.1016/j.radonc.2009.08.014.

[8] Pötter R, Georg P, Dimopoulos JC, Grimm M, Berger D, Nesvacil N, Georg D, Schmid MP, Reinthaller A, Sturdza A, Kirisits C. Clinical outcome of protocol based image (MRI) guided adaptive brachytherapy combined with 3D conformal radiotherapy with or without chemotherapy in patients with locally advanced cervical cancer. Radiother Oncol. 2011 Jul;100(1):116–23. doi: 10.1016/j.radonc.2011.07.012. Epub 2011 Aug 5.

[9] Nomden CN, de Leeuw AA, Roesink JM, Tersteeg RJ, Moerland MA, Witteveen PO, Schreuder HW, van Dorst EB, Jürgenliemk-Schulz IM. Clinical outcome and dosimetric parameters of chemo-radiation including MRI guided adaptive brachytherapy with tandem-ovoid applicators for cervical cancer patients: a single institution experience. Radiother Oncol. 2013 Apr;107(1):69–74. doi: 10.1016/j.radonc.2013.04.006. Epub 2013 Apr 29.

[10] Gill BS, Kim H1, Houser CJ, Kelley JL, Sukumvanich P, Edwards RP, Comerci JT, Olawaiye AB, Huang M, Courtney-Brooks M, Beriwal S. MRI-guided high-dose-rate intracavitary brachytherapy for treatment of cervical cancer: the University of Pittsburgh experience. Int J Radiat Oncol Biol Phys. 2015 Mar 1;91(3):540–7. doi: 10.1016/j.ijrobp.2014.10.053. Epub 2015 Jan 30.

[11] Rijkmans EC, Nout RA, Rutten IH, Ketelaars M, Neelis KJ, Laman MS, Coen VL, Gaarenstroom KN, Kroep JR, Creutzberg CL. Improved survival of patients with cervical cancer treated with image-guided brachytherapy compared with conventional brachytherapy. Gynecol Oncol. 2014 Nov;135(2):231–8. doi: 10.1016/j.ygyno.2014.08.027. Epub 2014 Aug 27.

[12] Simpson DR, Scanderbeg DJ, Carmona R, McMurtrie RM, Einck J, Mell LK, McHale MT, Saenz CC, Plaxe SC, Harrison T, Mundt AJ, Yashar CM. Clinical outcomes of computed tomography-based volumetric brachytherapy planning for cervical cancer. Int J Radiat Oncol Biol Phys. 2015 Sep 1;93(1):150–7. doi: 10.1016/j.ijrobp.2015.04.043. Epub 2015 May 4.

[13] Hegazy N, Pötter R, Kirisits C, Berger D, Federico M, Sturdza A, Nesvacil N. High-risk clinical target volume delineation in CT-guided cervical cancer brachytherapy: impact of information from FIGO stage with or without systematic inclusion of 3D documentation of clinical gynecological examination. Acta Oncol. 2013 Oct;52(7):1345–52. doi: 10.3109/0284186X.2013.813068. Epub 2013 Aug 2.

[14] Lindegaard JC, Fokdal LU, Nielsen SK, Juul-Christensen J, Tanderup K. MRI-guided adaptive radiotherapy in locally advanced cervical cancer from a Nordic perspective. Acta Oncol. 2013 Oct;52(7):1510–9. doi: 10.3109/0284186X.2013.818253. Epub 2013 Aug 21.

[15] Castelnau-Marchand P, Chargari C, Maroun P, Dumas I, Del Campo ER, Cao K, Petit C, Martinetti F, Tafo-Guemnie A, Lefkopoulos D, Morice P, Haie-Meder C, Mazeron R. Clinical outcomes of definitive chemoradiation followed by intracavitary pulsed-dose rate image-guided adaptive brachytherapy in locally advanced cervical cancer. Gynecol Oncol. 2015 Nov;139(2):288–94. doi: 10.1016/j.ygyno.2015.09.008. Epub 2015 Sep 11.

[16] Ribeiro I, Janssen H, De Brabandere M, Nulens A, De Bal D, Vergote I, Van Limbergen E. Long term experience with 3D image guided brachytherapy and clinical outcome in cervical cancer patients. Radiother Oncol. 2016 May 2. pii: S0167-8140(16):31050-57. doi: 10.1016/j.radonc.2016.04.016. [Epub ahead of print]

[17] Sturdza A, Pötter R, Fokdal LU, Haie-Meder C, Tan LT, Mazeron R, Petric P, Šegedin B, Jurgenliemk-Schulz IM, Nomden C, Gillham C, McArdle O, Van Limbergen E, Janssen H, Hoskin P, Lowe G, Tharavichitkul E, Villafranca E, Mahantshetty U, Georg P, Kirchheiner K, Kirisits C, Tanderup K, Lindegaard JC. Image guided brachytherapy in locally advanced cervical cancer: Improved pelvic control and survival in RetroEMBRACE, a multicenter cohort study. Radiother Oncol. 2016 Apr 29. pii: S0167-8140(16):31018-0. doi: 10.1016/j.radonc.2016.03.011. [Epub ahead of print]

[18] Murakami N, Kasamatsu T, Wakita A, Nakamura S, Okamoto H, Inaba K, Morota M, Ito Y, Sumi M, Itami J. CT based three dimensional dose-volume evaluations for high-dose rate intracavitary brachytherapy for cervical cancer. BMC Cancer. 2014 Jun 17;14:447. doi: 10.1186/1471-2407-14-447.

[19] Ohno T, Noda SE, Okonogi N2, Murata K, Shibuya K, Kiyohara H, Tamaki T, Ando K, Oike T, Ohkubo Y, Wakatsuki M, Saitoh JI, Nakano T. In-room computed tomography-based brachytherapy for uterine cervical cancer: results of a 5-year retrospective study. J Radiat Res. 2016 Dec 15. [Epub ahead of print]

Chapter 6

Re-irradiation for Recurrent Head and Neck Cancer

Viktoras Rudzianskas and
Rita Kupcinskaite-Noreikiene

Additional information is available at the end of the chapter

http://dx.doi.org/10.5772/67060

Abstract

After radical treatment of head and neck cancer about 20–50% of patients are diagnosed with the locoregional recurrence during first two years. The main treatment for recurrent disease is salvage surgery, but in most cases, surgery is not feasible due to the high risk of complications and morbidity, and only 20% of patients are suitable for surgical salvage. Reirradiation is an effective treatment method with acceptable toxicity, but this treatment method is limited to normal tissue tolerance to a total dose. When chemotherapy is administered for recurrence, the response rate is up to 40%, so with the advancement of technical measures, after introduction of intensity-modulated radiotherapy, fractionated stereotactic body radiation therapy, high-dose-rate brachytherapy, proton beam reirradiation, a reirradiation is increasingly more often used for head and neck cancer relapse treatment. In this chapter, we will discuss about reirradiation with curative intent using new different radiation techniques (intensity-modulated radiotherapy (IMRT), stereotactic body radiation therapy (SBRT), high-dose-rate brachytherapy (HDR-BRT) and proton beam reirradiation (PBRT) for previously irradiated head and neck cancer and present recommendations for retreatment of head and neck cancer relapse using reirradiation alone or with systemic chemotherapy/biologic therapy.

Keywords: reirradiation, head and neck cancer, brachytherapy, proton beam therapy, stereotactic body radiation

1. Introduction

Despite the sophisticated methods of cancer diagnosis, more than 50% of cases are still diagnosed when the disease has reached III/IV stage. After radical treatment of head and neck cancer, about 20–50% of patients are diagnosed with the locoregional recurrence during first two years [1–3]. The main treatment for recurrent disease is salvage surgery, but in most cases, surgery is not feasible due to the high risk of complications and morbidity, and only 15–30%

of patients are suitable for surgical salvage [4–8], and 5-year overall survival is 16–36% [9–14]. When chemotherapy is administered for recurrence, the response rate is up to 35–40%, and median overall survival is about 10% [15–17]. The results of retrospective studies presented in literature, using reirradiation by three-dimensional radiotherapy (3D-RT) for head and neck cancer recurrence, according to a 2-year overall survival and toxicity, are poor: overall survival reached 15.2–40%, the rate of severe late toxicities (grade 3 and 4) reached 1.4–47%, the rate of degree 5 (lethal) complications reached 7.6% [18–21]. However, with the advancement of technical measures, after introduction of intensity-modulated radiotherapy (IMRT), fractionated stereotactic body radiation therapy (F-SBRT), high-dose-rate brachytherapy (HDR-BRT), proton beam reirradiation (PBRT), a reirradiation is increasingly more often used for head and neck cancer relapse treatment [6, 18, 22–24].

In this chapter, we will discuss about reirradiation with curative intent using new different radiation techniques (IMRT, SBRT, HDR-BRT and PBRT) for previously irradiated head and neck cancer and present recommendations for retreatment of head and neck cancer relapse using reirradiation alone or with systemic chemotherapy/biologic therapy.

2. Reirradiation techniques and outcomes

2.1. Intensity-modulated radiotherapy and stereotactic body radiotherapy reirradiation

When comparing IMRT and F-SBRT against 3D-RT technique, it is possible to apply a larger radiation total dose during IMRT and F-SBRT, better protect adjacent tissues, while also achieving a better dose homogeneity. Lee et al. published results of 105 patients treated for head and neck cancer relapse using external beam radiation therapy [25]. Study included 74 (70%) patients treated with IMRT, 16 (15%) patients received conformal 3D radiation therapy and 15 (15%) patients received 2D radiation therapy. Prior to reirradiation, surgical treatment was performed on 36 (34%) patients, chemotherapy (mostly platinum-based) was administered to 75 (71%) patients, including 45 (43%) cases combined with radiation therapy. The median reirradiation dose was 59.4 Gy (range 30–70 Gy), median cumulative dose was 121.4 Gy (range 88–137 Gy). The 1-year and 2-year overall survival was 56% and 37%, respectively; locoregional control was 48% and 42%, respectively. The frequencies of early and late grade 3 and 4 toxicities were 23% and 15% (early and late, respectively). Sulman et al. conducted a retrospective analysis of 74 patients who were treated for head and neck cancer relapse and secondary cancer by applying IMRT to the previously irradiated area [24]. Before the reirradiation, 20 (27%) patients underwent surgery, 36 (48.6%) patients received chemotherapy: 23 patients received concurrent chemotherapy, four (11.1%) patients received induction chemotherapy, one (2.8%) patient received adjuvant chemotherapy, seven (19.4%) patients received induction and concurrent chemotherapy and one patient received concurrent and adjuvant chemotherapy. Platinum-based chemotherapy was administered to nine (25%) patients, 23 (64%) patients received a combined platinum- and taxane-based chemotherapy, three (8.3%) patients received platinum- and 5-fluorouracil-based treatment and one patient was administered a medication based on platinum with taxanes and lonafarnib (farnesyltransferase inhibitor). Median survival was 27.6 months; 2-year overall survival and locoregional control were 58% and 64%, respectively. Severe late toxicity (grade 3 and 4) was observed in 15 (20%) patients; one patient died (grade 5 toxic reaction). Duprez et al. published medical results based on 84 patients treated for recurrent or secondary head and neck cancer using IMRT [26]. Concurrent platinum-based chemotherapy was administered to 17 (20%) patients, 19 patients underwent surgical treatment and IMRT. Median dose delivered by IMRT was 69 Gy, median cumulative dose was 130 Gy (range 71–138 Gy). Median survival was 13.4 months; 1-year, 2-year and 5-year overall survival was 54%, 35%, and 20%, respectively; progression-free survival was 58%, 42%, and 29%, respectively. Severe early toxicity occurred in 26 (31%) patients, late toxicity occurred in 52 (62%) patients (grade 3 and 4 in 11 (13.1%) patients). Late grade 5 reactions occurred in two (2.4%) patients. It was determined during this study that T4 ($p = 0.013$), >2 years time interval between primary radiation therapy and reirradiation ($p = 0.011$), and hypopharyngeal cancer ($p = 0.013$) are statistically significant unfavorable factors impacting the overall survival, while the concurrent chemotherapy ($p = 0.0009$) is related to higher frequency of severe complications (grade 3 and 4). Chen et al. completed a retrospective study which included 21 patients [27]. All patients were diagnosed with recurrent head and neck cancer or secondary tumor, and IMRT was used in combination with image-guided radiation therapy (IGRT). The 1-year and 2-year overall survival was 65% and 40%, respectively. The authors identified severe acute toxicity frequencies: skin desquamation in 12 (57%) patients, dysphagia in 9 (42%) patients and mucositis in 5 (23%) patients. Late reactions: 2 patients were diagnosed with trismus, 1 patient was diagnosed with brachial plexopathy and gastrostomy was performed on 12 (57%) patients to manage swallowing disorder following the radiation therapy. Similar results were published for application of fractional stereotactic body radiation therapy (F-SBRT). Roh et al. treated 36 patients (44 areas) diagnosed with head and neck cancer relapse [28]. Median total dose was 30 Gy (range 18–40 Gy), delivered in 3–5 fractions over 3–5 days prescribed to the 65–85% isodose line. The 1-year and 2-year progression-free survival was 61% and 52.2%, respectively, while 1-year overall survival was 52.1%, 2-year survival was 30.9%. Early grade 3 reactions were diagnosed in 13 patients; late complications (grade 3 and 4) were diagnosed in 3 (8.6%) patients. Cengiz et al. used F-SBRT to treat 46 patients diagnosed with unresectable recurrent head and neck cancer [22]. Median total dose was 30 Gy (range 18–35 Gy), delivered mostly in five fractions (range 1–5 fractions). Overall 1-year survival and progression-free survival was 47% and 41%, respectively. Frequency of early toxicity was 4.4%: one patient was diagnosed with grade 3 dermatitis and grade 1–3 mucositis according to RTOG criteria; grade 5 complication frequency was 4.4%. Late reactions were diagnosed in six (13.3%) patients: two patients were diagnosed with soft tissue necrosis, two patients had osteonecrosis of the mandible and two patients were also diagnosed with grade 2 dysphagia. Five (11%) patients died due to bleeding from the carotid artery. Siddiqui et al. used stereotactic radiation therapy to treat 44 patients (55 areas), including 21 patients (29 cases) diagnosed with head and neck cancer relapse in primary tumor location or adjacent location [23]. Patients who were diagnosed with the relapse in regional neck lymph nodes where not included in this group. Delivered total dose was 36 Gy in 6 fractions or 48 Gy in 8 fractions, 2–3 fractions/week or 16–18 Gy single fraction. In this group of patients, 1-year and 2-year overall survival was 38.1% and 14.3%, respectively, local control was 60.6% and 40.4%, respectively. Early grade 3 toxicity was diagnosed in one patient; grade 4 complications were diagnosed in three patients.

In conclusion, it can be stated that the results of external beam reirradiation therapy used to treat head and neck cancer relapse, according to the treatment techniques, are: using IMRT, 2-year overall survival was 35–58%, locoregional control was 42–64%, 2-year progression-free survival reaches 42%, while the frequency of grade 3 and 4 toxicity was 13.1–20%, frequency of grade 5 radiotherapy reactions up to 2.8% [16, 25, 26, 28]. Results from F-SBRT studies: 2-year overall survival was 14.3–40%, local control 40.4%, progression-free survival was 52.2%, frequency of late severe complications was 8.6–14%, frequency of grade 5 complications was 2.8–14% [16, 22, 23, 28] (**Table 1**). During most of these studies, prognostic factors have been determined which influence the overall survival, locoregional control and progression-free survival; these factors were: longer time interval between initial radiation therapy and reirradiation; chemotherapy or biological therapy, administered in combination

Author	N	Treatment	Late toxicity grade 3–4	Results
Lee et al. [25]	105	(a) IMRT/(n = 74) (b) 3D-RT/(n = 16) (c) 2D-RT/(n = 15) 75 pts. received platinum-based CHT Median dose 59.4 Gy (30–70 Gy)	15%	1 y OS—56% 2 y OS—37% 1 y LRC—48% 2 y LRC—42%
Sulman et al. [24]	74	(a) Surgery + IMRT/(n = 20) (b) IMRT + CHT/(n = 36) (c) IMRT/(n = 48) Median dose 63 Gy (48.8–70 Gy)	20% Grade 5—2.8%	2 y OS—58% 2 y LRC—64%
Duprez et al. [26]	84	(a) OP + IMRT/(n = 19) (b) IMRT + CHT/(n = 17) (c) IMRT/(n = 48) Median dose 69 Gy	13.1% grade 5—2.4%	1 y OS—54% 2 y OS—35% 5 y OS—20% 1 y DFS—58% 2 y DFS—42% 5 y DFS—29%
Chen et al. [27]	21	IMRT, median dose 66 Gy (60–70 Gy)	Dysphagia—57%, trismus—9.5%, brachial plexopathy—4.8%	1 y OS—65% 2 y OS—40%
Roh et al. [28]	36	F-SBRT, median dose 30 Gy (18–40 Gy)	8.6% grade 5—2.8%	1 y OS—52.1% 2 y OS—30.9% 1 y LRC—61% 2 y LRC—52.2%
Cengiz et al. [22]	46	F-SBRT, median dose 30 Gy (18–35 Gy)	13.3% grade 5—11%	1 y OS—47% 1 y DFS—41%
Siddiqui et al. [23]	21*	F-SBRT/(n = 10): (a) 36 Gy/6 fx (b) 48 Gy/8 fx S-SBRT/(n = 11): Single-fraction 13–18 Gy	Grade 4—14%	1 y OS—38.1% 2 y OS—14.3% 1 y LC—60.6% 2 y LC—40.4%

Notes: 3D-RT, three-dimensional conformal radiotherapy; 2D-RT, two-dimensional radiotherapy; IMRT, intensity-modulated radiotherapy; CHT, chemotherapy; F-SBRT, fractionated stereotactic body radiation therapy; S-SBRT, radiosurgery; OS, overall survival; LRC, locoregional control; DFS, disease free survival; LC, local control.

* 44 patients participated in study, but results are presented only for 21 patient treated for disease relapse.

Table 1. Summary of published data on IMRT and SBRT for recurrence from head and neck cancer.

with reirradiation therapy; total dose of reirradiation therapy ≥50 Gy and surgical treatment prior to reirradiation therapy. Frequency of severe toxicity (grade 3 and higher) statistically significantly depended on the following factors: chemotherapy, administered in combination with reirradiation therapy; total dose of reirradiation therapy >60 Gy.

Results of the discussed studies prove that it is possible to achieve good locoregional control with acceptable toxic reactions through application of external beam reirradiation therapy. Using IMRT method, the number of late radiation reactions was lower compared with 3D-RT or F-SBRT.

Recommendations for IMRT (**Figure 1**):

1. To use repeated IMRT to treat patients with good functional status (Karnofsky Performance Score ≥ 60) in combination with chemotherapy or biological therapy after surgery, when there are positive resection margins, extracapsular nodal spread, perineural or lymphovascular infiltration.
2. Minimal time interval between initial radiation therapy and reirradiation 6–12 months.
3. Reirradiation volume: PTV = GTV + 5 mm, total dose ≥50–60 Gy, using conventional fractionation (1.8–2 Gy/fx).

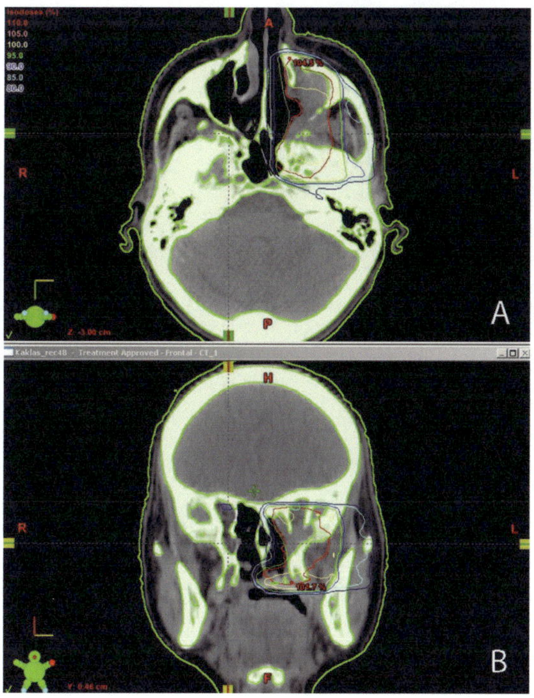

Figure 1. Representative isodose plan for patient undergoing reirradiation: (A) axial and (B) coronal CT slice. The patient had recurrent grade 3 adenoid cystic carcinomas of hard palate previously treated to 60 Gy with concurrent cisplatin. A local recurrence developed after 15 months, and the patient underwent reirradiation with IMRT to 48 Gy. The clinical and planning target volumes are showed in red, the total cumulative dose to brainstem was 51.54 Gy, spinal cord—42.1 Gy, chiasma—50.4 Gy, n. opticus left—51.2 Gy. No late toxicity was observed after 1 year.

Recommendations for F-SBRT (**Figure 2**):

1. To use repeated F-SBRT to treat patients with good functional status (Karnofsky Performance Score ≥ 60) in combination with chemotherapy or biological therapy after surgery, when there are positive resection margins, extracapsular nodal spread, perineural or lymphovascular infiltration.

2. F-SBRT is not recommended to treat laryngeal and hypopharyngeal site of recurrence due to higher frequency of late reactions.

3. Recommended total dose 35–42 Gy in 7 fractions prescribed to the 80–85% isodose line, over 2.5 weeks (total dose must not exceed 44 Gy).

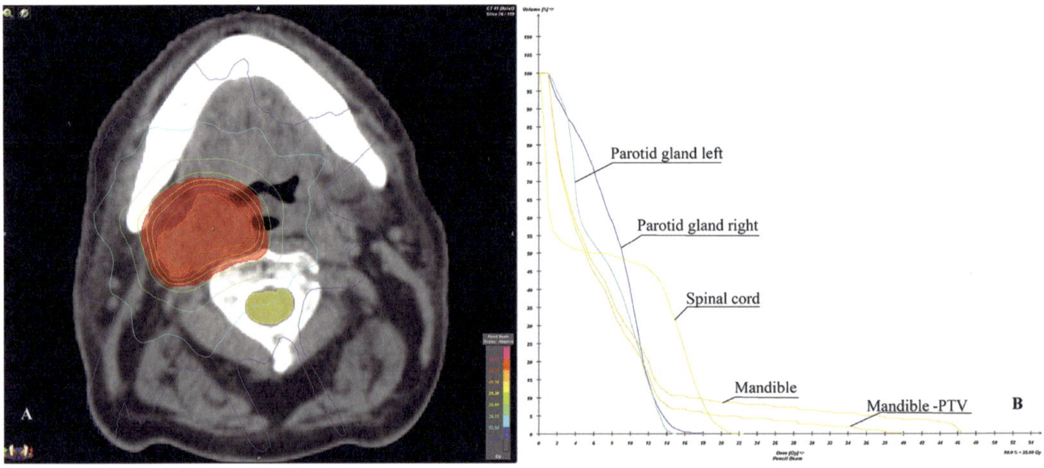

Figure 2. Dosimetric plan (A) used for reirradiation of a patient with recurrent oropharyngeal squamous cell carcinoma; dose-volume histogram is showed in apex (B). The patient underwent radical chemoradiotherapy as primary treatment (total dose 68 Gy/34 fx), after local recurrence developed approximately 21 months later, and the patient underwent reirradiation with F-SBRT—35 Gy/7 fx prescribed to the 80% isodose. The total cumulative dose to spinal cord was 57.8 Gy, mandible—93 Gy, larynx—72.4 Gy, parotid gland left—36 Gy, parotid gland right—72.4 Gy. No late toxicity was observed after 1.6 year.

2.2. High-dose-rate brachytherapy reirradiation

When using brachytherapy, it is possible to directly irradiate the tumor and deliver sufficient dose while also reducing the frequency of severe complications, such as trismus or severe xerostomia [29, 30]. In published studies, which involved patients with the diagnosis of head and neck cancer relapse and who were treated using HDR-BRT, different treatment regimens have been selected.

Hepel et al. published results of study involving 30 patients diagnosed with head and neck cancer relapse and treated using 192I-HDR-BRT [31]. All patients were treated using external beam radiation therapy, delivering mean dose of 59 Gy (range 23–75 Gy), with minimal 1-year follow-up. Adjuvant chemotherapy was administered to 43% patients, 36% were treated using hyperthermia therapy. Using HDR-BRT, two daily fractions have been prescribed with minimum 6-hour separation interval. In patients with implant volume adjoined to mucosa 3 Gy/fraction was delivered, and 4 Gy/fraction in other patients. Average administered total dose was 34 Gy (range 18–48 Gy), average implant volume 85 cm^3 (range 34–265 cm^3). Dose distribution was evaluated according to dose-volumes histogram (DVH), also ensuring that implant volume irradiated by 200% of the prescribed dose (V200) would not exceed 10% PTV. The 1-year and 2-year overall survival was 56% and 37%, respectively, local control was 69% and 67%, respectively, progression-free survival was 54% and 45%, respectively. Medium grade mucositis was diagnosed in most patients; late reactions (grade 3 and 4) were diagnosed in five (16%) patients: two were diagnosed with soft tissue necrosis, one had esophago-cutaneous fistula, one had lower jaw bone necrosis and one patient was diagnosed with tongue atrophy and fibrosis along with speech disorder. No grade 5 complications occurred. Tselis et al. used the accelerated hypofractionated 192Ir-HDR-BRT to treat 74 diagnosed with isolated head and neck cancer relapse in neck [7]. Patients had previously received radiation therapy or chemoradiation therapy; administered median total dose was 60 Gy (range 22–72 Gy). Due to primary tumor, surgery was performed on 43 (58%) patients; lymphadenectomy was performed at the same time on 33 of these patients (45%). Median time interval after primary treatment until isolated relapse was 12 months (range 3–207 months). Median target volume was 64.7 cm^3 (range 6.4–622 cm^3). Prior to HDR-BRT, 9 (12%) patients have been treated using external beam radiation therapy, administered median dose 40 Gy (range 20–70 Gy); 48 (65%) patients received chemotherapy; five (8%) received surgical treatment. Median time interval between external beam reirradiation therapy, last palliative chemotherapy course, or surgery and the beginning of HDR-BRT was 221 days (range 68–476 days), 53 days (range 22–819 days) and 149 days (range 94–251 days), respectively. A total of 12 (16%) patients were not additionally treated following primary treatment until procedures of HDR-BRT. During HDR-BRT, median Karnofsky Performance Score was 80 (range 60–100). When performing HDR-BRT, 71 (96%) patients were prescribed two daily fractions with minimum 6-hour separation interval, and median delivered single fraction dose was 3 Gy (range 2–5 Gy). For remaining three (4%) patients, the median delivered single fraction dose was 6 Gy (range 6–10 Gy) delivered in one daily fraction. All patients were administered a median total dose of 30 Gy (range 10–36 Gy). A total of 69 (93%) patients were treated using stand-alone HDR-BRT; five (7%) patients received this treatment in combination with external beam radiation therapy; median prescribed dose was 30.6 Gy (range 20–45 Gy). Dose distribution was evaluated according to DVH with consideration of D90, and dose heterogeneity was assessed according to V100, V150 and V200. In 60 (81%) patients who were prescribed with single fraction dose of 3 Gy, evaluated dosimetric parameters were as follows: D90 = 2.9 Gy (range 2.1–3.7 Gy) = 96.7% of the administered dose. Resulting dosimetric parameters for all the patients: median D90—97.7% (range 70–123.3%); V100 = 88.8% (range 68.8–96.9%); V150 = 58% (range 42–76%) and V200 = 38% (range 21–58%). Radiotherapy toxicity was evaluated according to RTOG/EORTC criteria. Median overall survival was 42 weeks; 1-year, 2-year and 3-year overall survival reached 42%, 19% and 6%, respectively. The 1-year local control was 67%, 2-year—67% and 3-year—67%; 1-year, 2-year and 3-year progression-free survival was 42%, 37% and 19%, respectively. After determining that the median target volume was ~65 cm^3, patients were divided into two groups, and it was found that in patients with target volume <65 cm^3 survival reached 13 months compared to 6 months in patients with target volume ≥65 cm^3

($p = 0.0001$). In patients who were prescribed with a treatment dose of <32.5 Gy based on calculated EQD2, median survival was 9 months, while in patient group with accordingly calculated EQD2 ≥ 32.5 Gy median survival was 13 months ($p = 0.098$). In the scope of this study, no statistically significant difference has been found between patient survival and factors such as primary tumor location, histological type of tumor, T and N stages of the primary tumor. Also, no statistical significant difference has been determined between local control and primary tumor location, histological type of tumor, T and N stages of the primary tumor, tumor relapse volume, KPS or prescribed dose. Acute toxicity (grade 3 and 4) was diagnosed in 5% of patients; frequency of late complications (grade 3 and 4) reached 8%, including three diagnosed with fistula. No grade 5 complications were diagnosed. Narayana et al. used HDR-BRT to treat 30 patients diagnosed with recurrent head and neck cancer [32]. About 77% of all patients had been diagnosed with local or regional relapse in previously irradiated location. Prior to HDR-BRT, 18 patients received surgical treatment, and they were prescribed with a total dose of 34 Gy administered in two 3.4 Gy daily fractions. A total of nine patients were treated using stand-alone HDR-BRT; a total dose prescribed was 40 Gy in two 4 Gy daily fractions. Remaining three patients received external beam radiation therapy 40–50 Gy and HDR-BRT 20 Gy, delivering two 4 Gy daily fractions. Toxicity was evaluated according to RTOG and NCI-CTC Version 3 toxicity criteria. The 2-year overall survival and local control were 63% and 71%, respectively. In group of patients who received surgical treatment and HDR-BRT, 2-year local control was better compared to remaining patients (88% vs. 40%, $p = 0.05$), although no statistically significant difference has been found when comparing the overall survival in these groups (70% vs. 43%, $p = 0.66$). Early complications (grade 3 and 4) were diagnosed in four patients; late grade 2 toxicity was diagnosed in six (20%) patients, late grade 3 toxicity was diagnosed in four (13%) patients: soft tissue fibrosis in two cases, one patient was diagnosed with trismus and one patient was diagnosed with a strong constant pain requiring nerve blockade to suppress it. No toxic reactions grade 4 and 5 occurred. Pellizzon et al. published results from a retrospective study which involved 21 patients diagnosed with head and neck cancer relapse in neck lymph nodes [33]. A total of 15 patients (71.4%) previously had been treated using external beam radiation therapy, with median total administered dose of 52 Gy (range 30–66 Gy). Median time between initial and repeated treatments was 32 months (range 14–86 months). All patients received surgical treatment; median time between surgery and HDR-BRT was 5 days (range 4–12 days). 192Ir-HDR-BRT treatment planning and optimization has been carried out in accordance with the Paris System principles, ensuring that the "hot spots" in the quarter of PTV would not exceed 135% of prescribed dose, and the skin-affecting dose would not exceed 60% of prescribed dose. Median prescribed total dose was 35 Gy (range 12–48 Gy), number of fractions 3–16 (median—8 fractions). After HDR-BRT, patients underwent external beam radiation therapy; median time between these treatment stages was seven days (range 1–37 days). Median prescribed total dose was 45 Gy (range 30–66 Gy), and in patients who already had been treated using external beam radiation therapy median dose was 30 Gy (range 25–50 Gy). The 5-year and 8-year overall survival was 50% and 42.9%, respectively, disease free survival was 42.5% and 28.6%, respectively. During this study, only a single factor has been determined which influences overall survival and progression-free survival in statistically meaningful way ($p = 0.0002$ and p = 0.0007, respectively), and this prognostic factor is the condition of resection margin (positive vs. negative resection margin). About four (19.4%) patients were diagnosed with early radiation reactions, and four patients had severe late complications: three were diagnosed with local non-healing wounds, one patient had wide-neck tissue fibrosis. There were no cases of soft-tissue necrosis. Schiefke et al. treated 18 patients diagnosed with locally advanced head and neck cancer; treatment was carried out by performing tumor resection and delivering 192Ir-HDR-BRT [34]. A total of 5 patients were treated for primary head and neck cancer; 13 patients were treated for relapse. Out of 13, 10 patients who were diagnosed with cancer recurrence had radical tumor resection during initial treatment, eight of them had lymphadenectomy performed simultaneously; following surgery, external beam radiation therapy was administered with a total prescribed dose 59.4–69.9 Gy; one patient received adjuvant chemotherapy. All the patients included in this study received surgery by performing partial tumor resection and implantation of brachytherapy catheters, ensuring that the post-operative bed including 5 mm margin is covered by 100% isodose. Median time between surgery and HDR-BRT was 6 days (range 4–41 days), median total dose was 30 Gy (range 15–44.8 Gy), with median prescribed single fraction dose of 3 Gy (1.5–3.5 Gy); two daily fractions were prescribed with minimal interval of 8 hours. Median PTV volume was 103.1 cm^3 (range 25.4–220 cm^3). A total of eight patients additionally received external beam radiation therapy, total dose 6–49.6 Gy (median 45 Gy); 7 patients received chemotherapy. In patients treated for relapse, median survival was 22.8 months (range 2.4–43.8 months) and 2-year overall survival and progression-free survival was 59.8 and 64.8%, respectively. Median progression-free survival was 12.8 months (range 4–27 months). Severe late toxicity was diagnosed in four (22.2%) patients: one patient experienced bleeding from the carotid artery, one patient experienced abnormal healing of operating wounds and was diagnosed with fistula, two patients were diagnosed with osteonecrosis.

In published studies involving application of HDR-BRT to treat head and neck cancer relapse, 3 Gy fractions to total dose of 30 Gy, or 4 Gy fractions to total dose of 40 Gy have been delivered. Using these treatment regimens, 2-year overall survival was 19–63%, local control was 67–71%, progression-free survival was 37–64.8%, and the frequency of late grade 3 and 4 toxicity was 8–22.2%. No grade 5 reactions were diagnosed (**Table 2**).

Application of HDR-BRT is limited by technical possibilities to implant brachytherapy catheters, and therefore this method of therapy is suitable to treat lip, oral cavity, oropharyngeal cancers, and also is suitable for inoperable recurrent cervical lymphadenopathy.

Recommendations for HDR-BRT (**Figure 3**):

1. High-dose-rate brachytherapy is effective and safe method of treatment, which can be applied to treat local head and neck cancer relapse diagnosed in previously irradiated area, delivering total dose of 30–40 Gy in 3–4 Gy/fraction, in two daily fractions separated by minimum 6-hour interval.

2. High-dose-rate brachytherapy is recommended to treat head and neck cancer relapse if the relapse volume does not exceed 30–40 cm^3.

3. In order to avoid severe late radiotherapy complications and to ensure local control, it is recommended that: PTV volume is ≥5 mm away from bone structures; PTV volume irradiated by 200% of prescribed dose (V200) does not exceed 10% of total PTV; skin-affecting dose does not exceed 60% of prescribed dose; homogeneity index (HI) is no less than 0.6–0.7; dose non-uniformity ratio (DNR) is not higher than 0.25–0.35.

Author	N	Treatment	Late toxicity grade 3-4	Results
Hepel et al. [31]	22	192Ir-HDR-BRT median dose 34 Gy (18–48 Gy)/3–4 Gy/fx	16%	1 y OS—56% 2 y OS—37% 1 y DFS—54% 2 y DFS—45%
Narayana et al. [32]	39	(a) Surgery + 192Ir-HDR-BRT 34 Gy/(n = 18) (b) 192Ir-HDR-BRT 40 Gy/(n = 9) (c) RT 40–50 Gy + 192Ir-HDR-BRT 20 Gy/(n = 3)	13% No grade 4 toxicity	2 y OS—63% 2 y LC—71%
Tselis et al. [7]	100	(a) 192Ir-HDR-BRT, median dose 30 Gy (30–36 Gy)/(n = 69) (b) 192Ir-HDR-BRT+RT, median dose 30.6 Gy (20–45 Gy)/(n = 5)	8%	1 y OS—42% 2 y OS—19% 3 y OS—65% 1 y LC—67% 2 y LC—67% 3 y LC—67% 1 y DFS—42% 2 y DFS—37% 3 y DFS—19%
Pellizzon et al. [33]	84	(a) Surgery + 192Ir-HDR-BRT, median dose 35 Gy (12–48 Gy)/3–4 Gy/fx + RT, median dose 45 Gy (30–60 Gy)/(n = 6) (b) Surgery + 192Ir-HDR-BRT median dose 35 Gy (12–48 Gy)/3–4 Gy/fx + RT, median dose 30 Gy (25–50 Gy)/(n = 15)	19.4%	5 y OS—50% 8 y OS—42.9% 5 y DFS—42.5% 8 y DFS—28.6%
Schiefke et al. [34]	23	(a) Surgery+192Ir-HDR-BRT, median dose 30 Gy (15–44.8 Gy)/(n = 10) (b) Surgery+192Ir-HDR-BRT, median dose 30 Gy (15–44.8 Gy)+RT, median dose 45 Gy (6–49.6 Gy)/(n = 8)	22.2%	2 y OS—59.8% 2 y DFS—64.8%

Notes: 192Ir, iridium 192; HDR-BRT, high dose rate brachytherapy; RT, external beam radiotherapy; OS, overall survival; DFS, disease free survival; LC, local control.

Table 2. Summary of published data on interstitial high-dose-rate brachytherapy for head and neck cancer relapses.

2.3. Reirradiation with proton beam therapy

External beam radiation therapy extends survival in patients diagnosed with head and neck cancer; however, occurring xerostomia, dysphagia, impaired ability to sense taste, post-radiation caries worsens the quality of life [35]. It is likely that delivering repeated external beam radiation therapy in patients diagnosed with head and neck cancer relapse would lead to higher frequency of late reactions. Because of advantages associated with dosimetric parameters of proton therapy compared with IMRT and F-SBRT, this therapy is used for reirradiation treatment with aim to reduce treatment-related toxicity and to protect previously irradiated healthy tissues. So far only several studies have been published involving

http://dx.doi.org/10.5772/67060

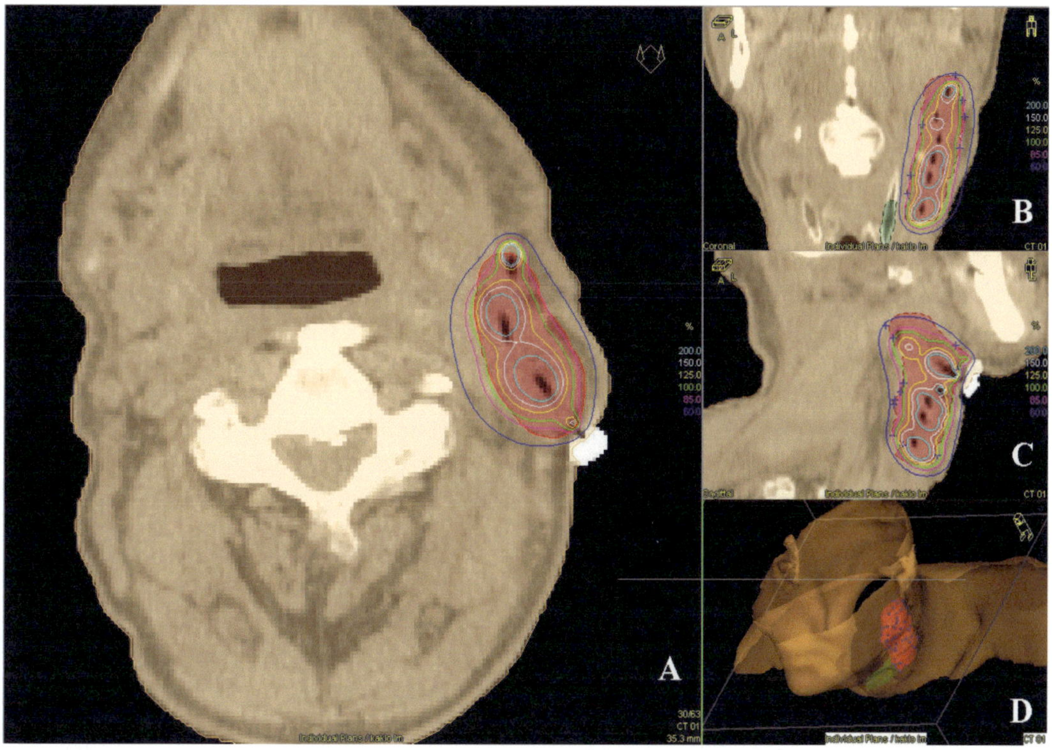

Figure 3. HDR-BRT dosimetric plan shown on axial (A), coronal (B) and sagittal (C) CT slice, 3D view of PTV (red) (D) for a patient with isolated neck recurrence of tonsil squamous cell carcinoma. PTV volume was 37.85 cm^3, V100 = 85.89%, V150 = 32.28%, V200 = 12.1%, HI = 0.62, DNR = 0.37.

application of proton beam therapy to treat head and neck cancer relapse. Romesser et al. published results of a multi-institutional study during which 92 patients were treated using proton beam therapy [36]. Median follow-up was 13.3 months (range 8.2–19.2 months) for surviving patients, and 10.4 months for all patients (range 5.3–17.5 months). In total, 65 (70.7%) men and 27 (29.3%) women were included in this study with a median age of 63 years (range 51.5–70 years); 70.7% of patients had Karnofsky Performance Score 80 and higher. Median time between initial radiotherapy and proton beam therapy was 34.4 months (range 8.2–19.2 months). Study subject group was very heterogeneous according to tumor localization: oropharynx—17 (18.5%), nasal cavity and paranasal sinuses—12 (13%), larynx or hypopharynx—10 (10.9%), salivary glands—11 (12%) and nasopharynx—9 (9.8%); also, there were included five patients with skin, eight patients with skull base tumors and eight patients diagnosed with tumors in other locations. Most of subjects—52 (56.5%)—had histologically confirmed diagnosis of squamous cell carcinoma. Prior to proton beam therapy, 36 (39.1%) patients received surgical treatment; median prescribed dose was 60.6 Gy (range 50–66.1 Gy). About 44 (47.8%) patients received concurrent biological therapy based on cetuximab. The 12-month regional control was 25.1%; skull base was the most frequent location of local recurrence. The 12-month overall survival reached 65.2%, freedom-from-distant metastasis was 84%. Late grade 3 and higher toxic skin reactions and dysphagia were diagnosed in six (8.7%)

and four (7.1%) patients, respectively, two (2.9%) patients were diagnosed with treatment-related bleeding (grade 5 toxicity). Phan et al. used proton beam therapy to treat 60 patients, including 55 diagnosed with head and neck cancer relapse and five diagnosed with secondary tumor [37]. Largest segment (16 patients) consisted of recurrent oropharyngeal tumors, five nasopharyngeal tumors, 11 sinonasal tumors, eight parotid gland tumors. A total of 40 (66.7%) patients had histologically confirmed squamous cell carcinoma; median time between initial radiation therapy and proton beam therapy was 47.1 months (range 7.3–438.2 months), median follow-up was 13.6 months (range 0–50 months). A total of 35 (58%) patients received surgical treatment, 44 (73%) received proton beam therapy in combination with chemotherapy. Median prescribed dose of adjuvant proton beam therapy was 61.5 Gy (range 50–70 Gy); in patients who received a definitive PBRT median dose was 66 Gy (range 50–70 Gy). The 1-year and 2-year locoregional control was 68.4% and 55.9%, overall survival—81.3% and 69%, progression-free survival—60.1% and 48.2%, distant metastasis-free survival—75% and 63.7%, respectively. Frequency of late grade 3 toxicity was 20% (12 patients); no grade 4 toxicity was diagnosed, yet death of two (3%) patients was potentially treatment related.

PBRT is an effective treatment method for patients diagnosed with head and neck cancer relapse; however, results of this treatment method are difficult to compare with other radiotherapy regiments (**Table 3**). Study groups were highly heterogeneous according to the primary tumor location, different cancer types have been included (squamous cell carcinoma, sarcoma, adenocarcinoma, etc.), part of patients received surgical treatment before proton beam therapy, others received combined chemotherapy or biological therapy. It is therefore necessary to conduct further studies with aim to assess advantages of proton beam therapy compared with IMRT or F-SBRT.

Recommendations for PBRT:

1. Proton beam therapy is recommended for patients with good functional status, deciding individually and comparing treatment planning dosimetric parameters of PBRT and IMRT or F-SBRT to each other.

2. Proton beam therapy is recommended for patients if relapse volume does not exceed 50 cm^3.

Author	N	Treatment	Late toxicity grade 3–4	Results
Romesser et al. [36]	92	(a) Surgery+PBRT (n = 36) (b) Biological therapy+PBRT (n = 44) Median dose 60.6 Gy (50–66.1 Gy)	Dysphagia—7.1%, skin reactions—8.7% grade 5—2.9%	1 y OS—65.2% 1 y DFS—84%
Phan et al. [37]	60	(a) Surgery+PBRT/(n = 35) (b) PBRT+CHT/(n = 44) Median dose 61.5 Gy (50–70 Gy)	20% Grade 5—2.8%	1 y OS—81.3% 2 y OS—69% 1 y LC—68.4% 2 y LC—55.9% 1 y DFS—75% 2 y DFS—63.7%

Notes: PBRT, proton beam therapy; CHT, chemotherapy; OS, overall survival; DFS, disease free survival; LC, local control.

Table 3. Summary of published data on PBRT for recurrent head and neck cancer.

http://dx.doi.org/10.5772/67060

2.4. Organs at risk

2.4.1. Spinal cord and brain stem

In some studies, the cumulative dose limit was ≤60 Gy, delivered in 2 Gy/fraction, 5 days/week (biologically equivalent dose [BED] 120 Gy_2). There were no cases of myelopathy in these studies, and a minimal time interval between primary therapy and reirradiation was 6 months [27, 38, 39]. When applying fractionation regimen of 2 Gy/day, and after irradiating the full cord cross-section to a total dose of 50, 60 and ~69 Gy, the frequency of myelopathy was 0.2%, 6% and 50%, respectively [39]. However, most authors recommend not to exceed the cumulative dose of 50 Gy [19, 24, 26]. When using the hypofractionated stereotactic body radiation therapy, it is recommended not to exceed the cumulative dose of 25 Gy (2 Gy—equivalent dose, $\alpha/\beta = 2$), when the total dose of primary radiotherapy does not exceed 50 Gy and the minimal time between two radiotherapy courses is 5 months [40].

2.4.2. Mandible

Up to this date there are no clear volume and dose limitations when using the reirradiation therapy, although osteoradionecrosis is one of the possible late toxic reactions. Studies published by De Crevoisier et al. and Duprez et al. indicate osteoradionecrosis frequencies of 8% and 3.6%, when administering total cumulative dose of 130 Gy, using conventional radiotherapy [10, 26]. In a research conducted by Salama et al., the total cumulative dose was 135 Gy, and frequency of osteoradionecrosis was 11% [41]. When using repeated stereotactic body radiation therapy in patients who received a total dose of 66–70.2 Gy during the primary radiotherapy, it is recommended not to exceed 25–40 Gy/5 fractions (BED 40–90 Gy_2) [40].

2.4.3. Larynx/hypopharynx

In study conducted by Tanvetyanon et al., frequency of laryngeal toxicities of grade 3 and higher was 7.8%, when administering a total cumulative dose of 124 Gy [21]. Takiar et al. completed a 15-year analysis and published its results, which include: chondroradionecrosis after delivering 140 Gy total cumulative dose; non-healing ulcer and stenosis requiring surgery after ≥120 Gy [42]. It is therefore recommended that the total cumulative dose for larynx and hypopharynx does not exceed 120 Gy.

It is recommended to reduce (according to possibilities) the total dose which involves such organs as base of tongue, carotid arteries, jugular veins, oral cavity, sternocleidomastoid muscle, parotid and submandibular glands; however, there is no dose limit established for these body structures.

3. Conclusions

Reirradiation therapy is suitable and safe method of treatment for patients diagnosed with head and neck cancer relapse. It is important to take into consideration the functional status of the patient, recurrence location and volume, and time interval between initial radiotherapy and reirradiation. Surgical treatment, chemotherapy or biological therapies are more efficient methods of treatment when combined with reirradiation. Currently there is a lack of randomized clinical trials comparing effectiveness and toxicity of different radiotherapy methods, so for each case the potential of reirradiation therapy must be evaluated individually, considering recommendations presented here.

Author details

Viktoras Rudzianskas* and Rita Kupcinskaite-Noreikiene

*Address all correspondence to: wictoras@hotmail.com

Institute of Oncology, Medical Academy, Lithuanian University of Health Sciences, Kaunas, Lithuania

References

[1] Brockstein B, Haraf DJ, Rademaker AW, Kies MS, Stenson KM, Rosen F, et al. Patterns of failure, prognostic factors and survival in locoregionally advanced head and neck cancer treated with concomitant chemoradiotherapy: a 9-year, 337-patient, multi-institutional experience. Ann Oncol. 2004;**15**:1179–86. DOI: 10.1093/annonc/mdh308

[2] Wong SJ, Machtay M, Li Y. Locally recurrent, previously irradiated head and neck cancer: concurent re-irradiation and chemotherapy, or chemotherapy alone? J Clin Oncol. 2006;**24**:2653–8. DOI: 10.1200/JCO.2005.05.3850

[3] Platteaux N, Dirix P, Vanstraelen B, Nuyts S. Outcome after re-irradiation of head and neck cancer patients. Strahlenther Oncol. 2011;**187**:23–31. DOI: 10.1007/s00066-010-2139-9

[4] Grégoire V, Lefebvre JL, Licitra L, Felip E, EHNS-ESMO-ESTRO Guidelines Working Group. Squamous cell carcinoma of the head and neck: EHNS-ESMO-ESTRO clinical practice guidelines for diagnosis, treatment and follow-up. Ann Oncol. 2010;**21**:v184–6. DOI: 10.1093/annonc/mdq185

[5] Vermorken JB, Specenier P. Optimal treatment for recurrent/metastatic head and neck cancer. Ann Oncol. 2010;**21**:vii252–61. DOI: 10.1093/annonc/mdq453

[6] Chopra S, Gupta T, Agarwal JP, Budrukkar A, Ghosh-Laskar S, Dinshaw K. Re-irradiation in the management of isolated neck recurrences: current status and recommendations. Radiother Oncol. 2006;**81**:1–8. DOI: 10.1016/j.radonc.2006.08.017

[7] Tselis N, Ratka M, Vogt HG, Kolotas C, Baghi M, Baltas D, et al. Hypofractionated accelerated CT-guided interstitial ^{192}Ir-HDR-Brachytherapy as re-irradiation in inoperable recurrent cervical lymphadenopathy from head and neck cancer. Radiother Oncol. 2011;**98**:57–62. DOI: 10.1016/j.radonc.2010.10.025

[8] McDonald MW, Lawson J, Garg MK, Quon H, Ridge JA, Saba N, et al. ACR appropriateness criteria retreatment of recurrent head and neck cancer after prior definitive radiation expert panel on radiation oncology-head and neck cancer. Int J Radiat Oncol Biol Phys. 2011;**80**:1292–8. DOI: 10.1016/j.ijrobp

[9] Biagioli MC, Harvey M, Roman E, Raez LE, Wolfson AH, Mutyala S, et al. Intensity-modulated radiotherapy with concurrent chemotherapy for previously irradiated, recurrent head and neck cancer. Int J Radiat Oncol Biol Phys. 2007;**69**:1067–73. DOI: 10.1016/j.ijrobp.2007.04.057

[10] De Crevoisier R, Domenge C, Wibault P, Koscielny S, Lusinchi A, Janot F, et al. Full dose reirradiation combined with chemotherapy after salvage surgery in head and neck carcinoma. Cancer. 2001;**91**:2071–6. DOI: 10.1002/1097-0142(20010601)91:11<2071::AID-CNCR1234>3.0.CO;2-Z

[11] Kao J, Garofalo MC, Milano MT, Chmura SJ, Citron JR, Haraf DJ. Reirradiation of recurrent and second primary head and neck malignancies: a comprehensive review. Cancer Treat Rev. 2003;**29**:21–30. DOI: 10.1016/S0305-7372(02)00096-8

[12] Parsons JT, Mendenhall WM, Stringer SP, Cassisi NJ, Million RR. Salvage surgery following radiation failure in squamous cell carcinoma of the supraglottic larynx. Int J Radiat Oncol Biol Phys. 1995;**32**:605–9. DOI: 10.1016/0360-3016(95)00527-6

[13] Ganly I, Patel SG, Matsuo J, Singh B, Kraus DH, Boyle JO, et al. Results of surgical salvage after failure of definitive radiation therapy for early-stage squamous cell carcinoma of the glottic larynx. Arch Otolaryngol Head Neck Surg. 2006;**132**:59–66. DOI: 10.1001/archotol.132.1.59

[14] Teman S, Pape E, Janot F, Wibault P, Julieron M, Lusinchi A, et al. Salvage surgery after failure of very accelerated radiotherapy in advanced head-and-neck squamous cell carcinoma. Int J Radiat Oncol Biol Phys. 2005;**62**:1078–83. DOI: 10.1016/j.ijrobp.2004.12.062

[15] Gibson MK, Li Y, Murphy B, Hussain MH, DeConti RC, Ensley J, Forastiere AA, Eastern Cooperative Oncology Group. Randomized phase III evaluation of cisplatin plus fluorouracil versus cisplatin plus paclitaxel in advanced head and neck cancer (E1395): an intergroup trial of the Eastern Cooperative Oncology Group. J Clin Oncol. 2005;**23**:3562–7. DOI: 10.1200/JCO.2005.01.057

[16] Vermorker JB, Mesia R, Rivera F, Remenar E, Kawecki A, Rottey S, et al. Platinum-based chemotherapy plus cetuximab in head and neck cancer. N Engl J Med. 2008;**359**:1116–27. DOI: 10.1056/NEJMoa0802656

[17] Vermorker JB, Remenar E, van Herpen C, Gorlia T, Mesia R, Degardin M, et al. Cisplatin, fluorouracil, and docetaxel in unresectable head and neck cancer. N Engl J Med. 2007;**357**:1695–704. DOI: 10.1056/NEJMoa071028

[18] Hoebers F, Heemsbergen W, Moor S, Lopez M, Klop M, Tesselaar M, et al. Reirradiation for head-and-neck cancer: delicate balance between effectiveness and toxicity. Int J Radiat Oncol Biol Phys. 2011;**81**:e111–8. DOI: 10.1016/j.ijrobp.2011.01.004

[19] Spencer SA, Harris J, Wheeler RH, Machtay M, Schultz C, Spanos W, et al. Final report of RTOG 9610, a multi-institutional trial of reirradiation and chemotherapy for unresectable recurrent squamous cell carcinoma of the head and neck. Head Neck. 2008;**30**:281–8. DOI: 10.1002/hed.20697

[20] Langer CJ, Harris J, Horwitz EM, Nicolaou N, Kies M, Curran W, et al. Phase II study of low-dose paclitaxel and cisplatin in combination with split-course concomitant twice-daily reirradiation in recurrent squamous cell carcinoma of the head and neck: results of Radiation Therapy Oncology Group Protocol 9911. J Clin Oncol. 2007;**25**:4800–5. DOI: 10.1200/JCO.2006.07.9194

[21] Tanvetyanon T, Padhya T, McCaffrey J, Zhu W, Boulware D, Deconti R, et al. Prognostic factors for survival after salvage reirradiation of head and neck cancer. J Clin Oncol. 2009;**27**:1983–91. DOI: 10.1200/JCO.2008.20.0691

[22] Cengiz M, Özyiğit G, Yazici G, Doğan A, Yildiz F, Zorlu F, et al. Salvage reirradiaton with stereotactic body radiotherapy for locally recurrent head-and-neck tumors. Int J Radiat Oncol Biol Phys. 2011;**81**:104–9. DOI: 10.1016/j.ijrobp.2010.04.027

[23] Siddiqui F, Patel M, Khan M, McLean S, Dragovic J, Jin JY, et al. Stereotactic body radiation therapy for primary, recurrent, and metastatic tumors in the head-and-neck region. Int J Radiat Oncol Biol Phys. 2009;**74**:1047–53. DOI: 10.1016/j.ijrobp.2008.09.022

[24] Sulman EP, SchwartzDL, Le TT, Ang KK, Morrison WH, Rosenthal DI, et al. IMRT reirradiation of head and neck cancer-disease control and morbidity outcomes. Int J Radiat Oncol Biol Phys. 2009;**73**:399–409. DOI: 10.1016/j.ijrobp.2008.04.021

[25] Lee N, Chan K, Bekelman JE, Zhung J, Mechalakos J, Narayana A, et al. Salvage re-irradiation for recurrent head and neck cancer. Int J Radiat Oncol Biol Phys. 2007;**68**:731–40. DOI: 10.1016/j.ijrobp.2006.12.055

[26] Duprez F, Madani I, Bonte K, Boterberg T, Vakaet L, Derie C, et al. Intensity-modulated radiotherapy for recurrent and second primary head and neck cancer in previously irradiated territory. Radiother Oncol. 2009;**93**:563–9. DOI: 10.1016/j.radonc.2009.10.012

[27] Chen AM, Farwell DG, Luu Q, Cheng S, Donald PJ, Purdy JA. Prospective trial of high-dose reirradiation using daily image guidance with intensity-modulated radiotherapy for recurrent and second primary head-and-neck cancer. Int J Radiat Oncol Biol Phys. 2011;**80**:669–76. DOI: 10.1016/j.ijrobp.2010.02.023

[28] Roh KW, Jang JS, Kim MS, Sun DI, Kim BS, Jung SL, et al. Fractionated stereotactic radiotherapy as reirradiation for locally recurrent head and neck cancer. Int J Radiat Oncol Biol Phys. 2009;**74**:1348–55. DOI: 10.1016/j.ijrobp.2008.10.013

[29] Mazeron JJ, Ardiet JM, Haie-Méder C, Kovács G, Levendag P, Peiffert D, et al. GEC-ESTRO recommendations for brachytherapy for head and neck squamous cell carcinomas. Radiother Oncol. 2009;**91**:150–6. DOI: 10.1016/j.radonc.2009.01.005

[30] Kovács G. Modern head and neck brachytherapy: from radium towards intensity modulated interventional brachytherapy. J Contemp Brachytherapy. 2015;**6**:404–16. DOI: 10.5114/jcb.2014.47813

[31] Hepel JT, Syed AMN, Puthawala A, Sharma A, Frankel P. Salvage high-dose-rate (HDR) brachytherapy for recurrent head-and-neck cancer. Int J Radiat Oncol Biol Phys. 2005;**62**:1444–50. DOI: 10.1016/j.ijrobp.2004.12.078

[32] Narayana A, Cohen GN, Zaider M, Chan K, Lee N, Wong RJ, et al. High-dose-rate interstitial brachytherapy in recurrent and previously irradiated head and neck cancers—preliminary results. Brachytherapy. 2007;**6**:157–63. DOI: 10.1016/j.brachy.2006.12.001

[33] Pellizzon AC, Salvajoli JV, Kowalski LP, Carvalho AL. Radiat Oncol. Salvage for cervical recurrences of head and neck cancer with dissection and interstitial high dose rate brachytherapy. 2006;**1**:27. DOI: 000294864

[34] Schiefke F, Hilderbrandt G, Pohlmann S, Heinicke F, Hemprich A, Frerich B. Combination of surgical resection and HDR-brachytherapy in patients with recurrent or advanced head and neck carcinomas. J Craniomaxillofac Surg. 2008;**36**:285–92. DOI: 10.1016/j.jcms.2007.08.009

[35] Rudžianskas V, Inčiūra A, Vaitkus S, Padervinskis E, Rudžianskiene M, Kupčinskaite-Noreikiene R, et al. Reirradiation for patients with recurrence head and neck squamous cell carcinoma: a single-institution comparative study. Medicina. 2014;**50**:92–9. DOI: 10.1016/j.medici.2014.06.006

[36] Romesser PB, Cahlon O, Scher ED, Hug EB, Sine K, DeSelm C, et al. Proton beam reirradiation for recurrent head and neck cancer: multi-institutional report on feasibility and early outcomes. Int J Radiat Oncol Biol Phys. 2016;**95**:386–95. DOI: 10.1016/j.ijrobp.2016.02.036

[37] Phan J, Sio TT, Nguyen TP, Takiar V, Gunn GB, Garden AS, et al. Reirradiation of head and neck cancers with proton therapy: outcomes and analyses. Int J Radiat Oncol Biol Phys. 2016;**96**:30–41. DOI: 10.1016/j.ijrobp.2016.03.053

[38] Langendijk JA, Kasperts N, Leemans CR, Doornaert P, Slotman BJ. A phase II study of primary reirradiation in squamous cell carcinoma of head and neck. Radiother Oncol. 2006;**78**:306–12. DOI: 10.1016/j.radonc.2006.02.003

[39] Kirkpatrick JP, van der Kogel AJ, Schultheiss TE. Radiation dose-volume effects in the spinal cord. Int J Radiat Oncol Biol Phys. 2010;**76**:S42–9. DOI: 10.1016/j.ijrobp.2009.04.095

[40] Mantel F, Flentje M, Guckenberger M. Stereotactic body radiation therapy in the re-irradiation situation—a review. Radiat Oncol. 2013;**8**:7. DOI: 10.1186/1748-717X-8-7

[41] Salama JK, Vokes EE, Chmura SJ, Milano MT, Kao J, Stenson KM, et al. Long-term outcome of concurrent chemotherapy and reirradiation for recurrent and second primary head-and-neck squamous cell carcinoma. Int J Radiat Oncol Biol Phys. 2006;**64**:382–91. DOI: 10.1016/j.ijrobp.2005.07.005

[42] Takiar V, Garden AS, Ma D, Morrison WH, Edson M, Zafereo ME, et al. Reirradiation of head and neck cancers with intensity modulated radiation therapy: outcomes and analyses. Int J Radiat Oncol Biol Phys. 2016;**95**:1117–31. DOI: 10.1016/j.ijrobp.2016.03.015

Chapter 7

Radiation Therapy with a Simultaneous Integrated Boost

Despina Katsochi

Additional information is available at the end of the chapter

http://dx.doi.org/10.5772/67326

Abstract

Radiotherapy has an established role in the treatment of cancer and represents a definitive, less invasive approach for various cancer types. Its main aim is to deliver the maximum dose to the tumor with minimal toxicity on neighboring healthy tissues. Therefore, the precise determination of the target and its spatial relation to critical surrounding organs is of main importance. New imaging modalities such as the CT, MRI, and PET/CT offer more anatomical detail and facilitate the accurate delineation of the target volume and the organs at risk. The recent advances in 3D-CRT and IMRT radiation techniques offer high accuracy in tumor targeting and ensure safe dose escalation. Moreover, the introduction of IGRT offers the opportunity to safely apply a supplementary dose to the macroscopic tumor. In trials conducted, a simultaneous integrated boost (SIB) has proved to be feasible in various cancer localizations, to safely increase the total delivered dose, shorten the total treatment time and results in increased tumor control while keeping the side effects low at the same time. However, more trials need to be conducted to establish an acceptable protocol.

Keywords: radiation therapy, simultaneous integrated boost, fractionation, radiation dose escalation, image guided radiotherapy

1. Introduction

Radiation therapy is the core treatment strategy with curative intent and organ preservation for many inoperable cancer types. The main aim of radiation therapy is the local control of the tumor.

With open field conventional 2D RT, both healthy tissue and tumors are irradiated with a similar dose per fraction of 1.8–2 Gy. Now, the 3D-CRT is the new standardized procedure. The target volumes are defined on CT or PET-CT or other high-definition imaging such as the MRI. During the treatment planning, a 3-D projection of the area of interest provides the opportunity to match the high-dose radiation region to the target volume while minimizing the radiation dose to the surrounding healthy tissue. More refined radiation techniques, which lead to enhanced conformity, can be performed with the use of these generation machines. 3-D techniques have given way to IMRT or volumetric modulated arc therapy (V-MAT) [1–4].

High conformity is generally accepted as a way to reduce toxicity and allows dose escalation to produce better results and long-term tumor control. This is only possible through IGRT, which involves real-time imaging of the treatment target and normal organs during each treatment, in order to avoid uncertainty about patient positioning and tumor targeting and to also reduce the irradiated volumes without missing any of the targets [5].

Trials have investigated different fractionation schedules to also increase local control, which has become of high importance in clinical oncology patient management. Randomized clinical trials have established equivalent outcomes between radical surgery and organ-preservation treatment with an RT backbone for appropriately selected patients.

The radiation oncologist's main concern is local recurrence after definitive radiation therapy. The combined chemo-radiation protocols have led to the increased tumor control and survival rates, but the results have remained unchanged for a long time. All eyes are now on radiation therapy for a more targeted improvement of local tumor control and diminishment of the odds of local recurrence [6].

The newly developed approach of applying different radiation doses to different areas in one single session is called SIB or simultaneous integrated boost-intensity-modulated radiotherapy (SIB-IMRT). By increasing the dose per fraction focally to the tumor itself while maintaining lower dose to the elective areas of interest, a more accurate dose distribution can be achieved, in order to improve local tumor control without putting the neighboring organs at risk. The advances, improvements and clinical usage of this technique will be expanded in full detail [7].

2. Simultaneous integrated boost–radiation therapy strategy and procedure

The radiation therapy strategy is an evidence-based treatment, personalized to the particular needs of each individual patient. The 3D-CRT is the minimum standard for the delivery of a radiation dose that conforms to the target volume and controls the exposure to surrounding tissue (**Figure 1**). The evolution of the 3D-CRT is the IMRT technique. It optimizes the radiation intensity distribution within each beam in order to achieve a higher rate of conformity and target coverage especially for irregularly shaped tumors, using nonuniform radiation beam intensities to maximize the delivery of radiation to the planned target volume while minimizing irradiation of normal tissue outside the target. It requires a precise definition of anatomy, a treatment planning system that can calculate the dose in three dimensions, and a treatment device that can deliver the specified dose. Randomized studies demonstrate reduced side effects with IMRT (particularly that of xerostomia in patients with head and neck tumors) in comparison with older 3D-CRT techniques even in the setting of concurrent chemotherapy.

http://dx.doi.org/10.5772/67326

The delivery of each dose to the tumor has become much faster with the introduction of the VMAT where the gantry moves around the patient as the beam is being modulated (**Figure 2**). Typically, IMRT plans require 20–25 min for delivery of the daily treatment while a VMAT plan can now be delivered in approximately 3–5 min (approximately 1.5 min per gantry rotational arc), which is easier on patients (**Figure 3**) [8–10].

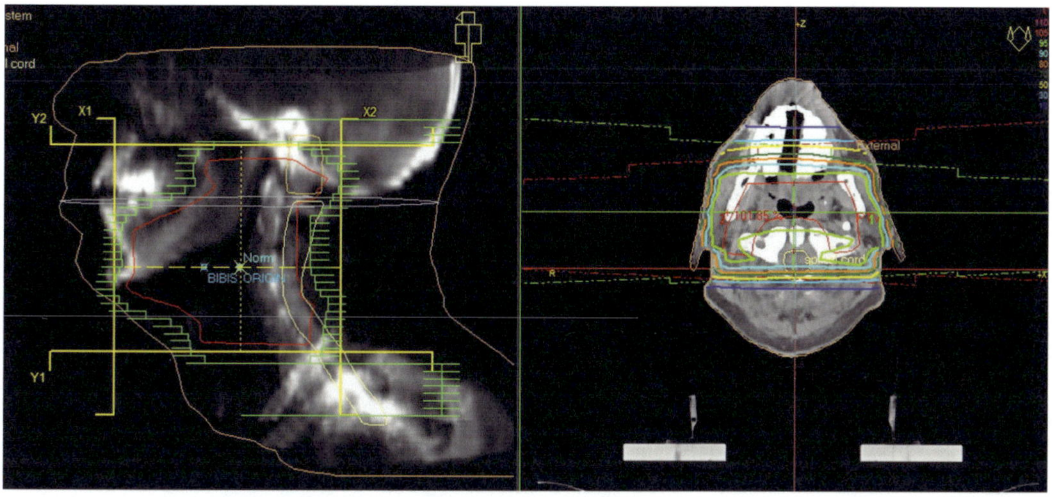

Figure 1. 3D-CRT RT with multileaf collimator shielding.

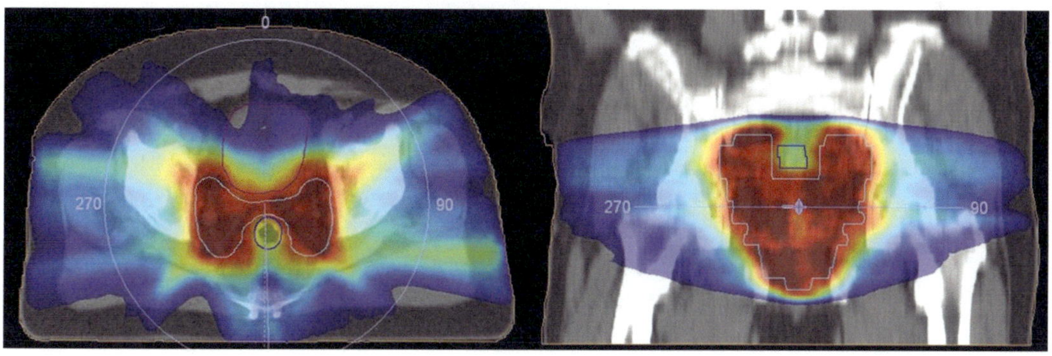

Figure 2. IMRT: Gradient dose distribution is achieved in the different parts of the target volume, and the surrounding healthy tissue is less exposed to the total radiation dose.

Treatment planning is the most important procedure. Target delineation is the main concern of the radiation oncologist. The definition of the extension of the infiltrated tissue is often an interdisciplinary procedure where the surgeon, pathologist, radiologist and radiation oncologist have to collaborate in order to decide on the most appropriate treatment plan. The precise determination of the target and its spatial relation to critical surrounding organs is of main importance. The reference imaging modality for RT treatment planning is the CT with which we can fuse additional medical images (MRI PET/CT scans) for accurate treatment planning, dosimetric calculations and ensure safe dose escalation. The PET/CT images can change gross tumor volume (GTV) delineation in 35–60% of patients treated and show a better treatment outcome (31 months vs. 16 months) and can increase the 1-year survival rate from 8 to 17% (**Figure 4**) [11–15].

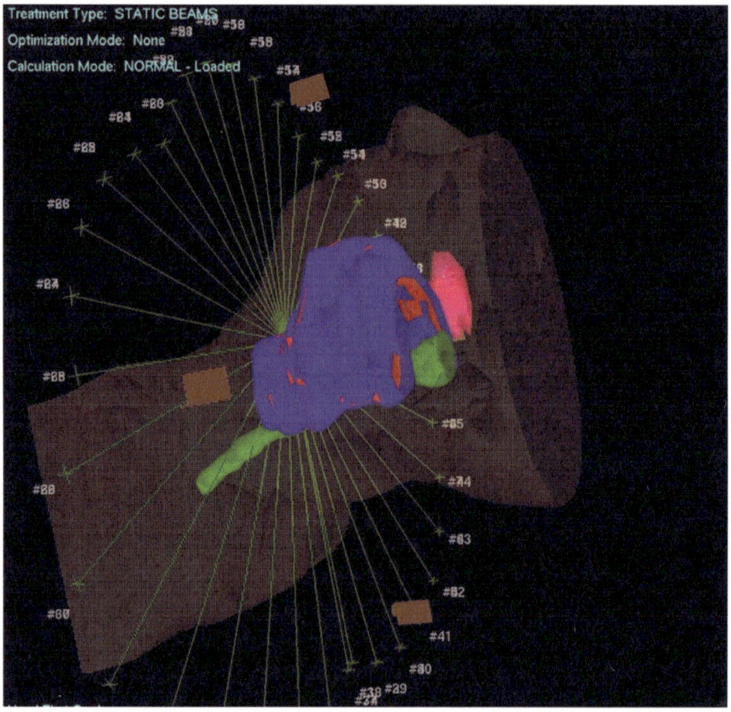

Figure 3. VMAT where the gantry moves around the patient as the beam is being modulated.

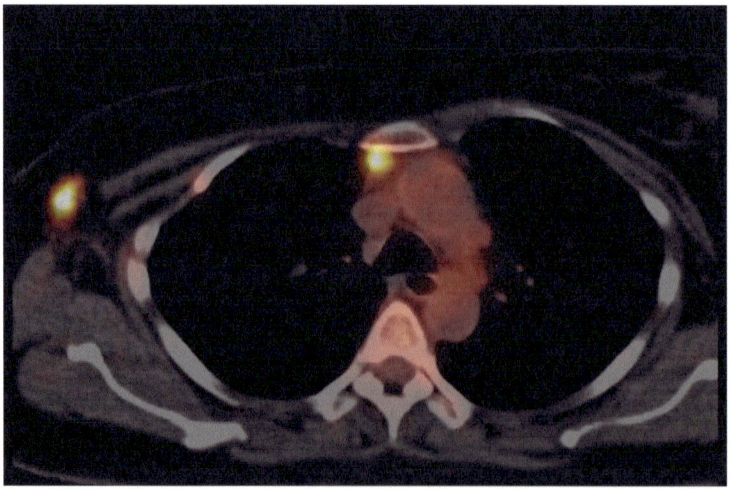

Figure 4. PET/CT gives information about the metabolic tumor activity.

For accurate 3D-CRT and IMRT delivery, every day patient set up and verification systems are required, i.e., CBCT scanners, which produce 3-D images of the treatment area (**Figure 5**) [10, 11].

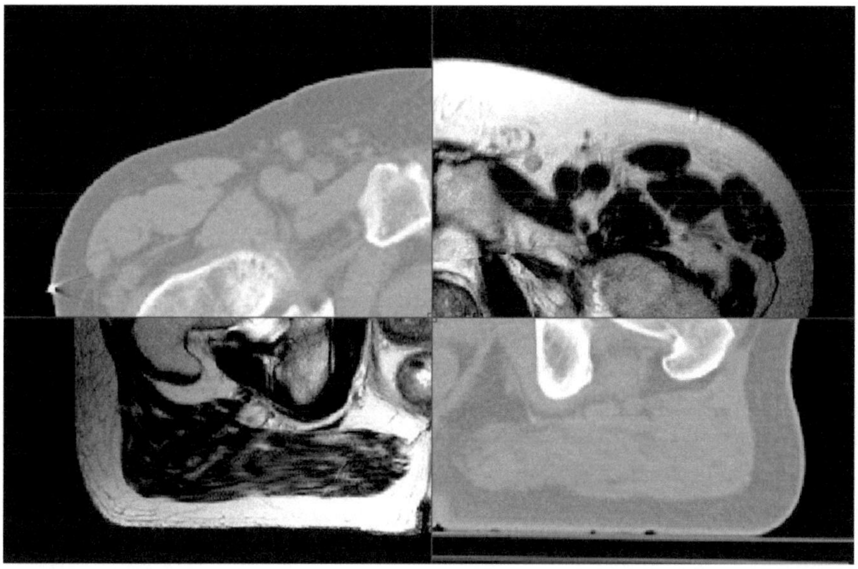

Figure 5. IGRT real-time imaging of the treatment area fused with the computer tomography image used for the planning.

According to ICRU-83, the GTV represents the palpable or visible (on imaging) tumor, whereas the so-called clinical target volume (CTV) is an additional volume with a certain probability of microscopic (subclinical) malignant disease. The irradiated planning target volume (PTV) is a geometrical concept. The PTV is defined according to the ICRU 62 report and includes GTV, CTV and takes into account the internal organ motion and set up errors [16, 17].

In the past, radiation therapy was applied using a shrinking field approach or sequential boost, starting with large fields and shrinking gradually depending on the pre-planned total dose to each region. Inevitably, the high-risk target volume or GTV, the intermediate risk target volume or CTV and the low risk volume or PTV were exposed to different total doses, which have been delivered sequentially (SeqB-IMRT intensity-modulated radiotherapy sequential boost). This risk adaptive strategy now is modified to deliver a single efficient treatment plan with dose levels and intensities appropriate for each elected region. The SIB-IMRT is more conformal and potentially enables a slightly higher dose escalation to high-risk volumes compared to the SeqB-IMRT. Higher conformity in combination with smaller PTV allows 25% RT dose escalation and increases the effectiveness of therapy. A dose escalation of 10 Gy to lung cancer patients treated with 3D-CRT is correlated with 36% decrease in local failure rates [18–20].

The concomitant boost technique is a variant of accelerated fractionation, whereby the boost is delivered as a second daily fraction during the basic treatment course to reduce the total duration of treatment. The incorporation of boost at the same session of RT is the SIB, which involves the CTV with a prophylactic dose and the GTV with a curative dose.

Simultaneous accelerated radiation therapy (SMART) boost technique initially was described by Butler in 1999 [21]. The GTV was treated with large fractions of 2.4 Gy, while conventional fractions of 2 Gy were delivered to the PTV, which represent the regions at risk for microscopic disease up to a total dose of 60 and 50 Gy, respectively. The total treatment time was moderately shortened than previously. The term "simultaneous integrated boost" was introduced later to define such treatment, delivering different doses per fraction in different target regions, by Mohan, 2000 [22]. The initial proposed dose delivery was either the conventional 2 Gy per fraction to the lower or intermediate dose volumes, thereby enabling a higher dose per fraction to be delivered to the GTV, with as much as 2.4 Gy for gross disease. The SIB technique offers the biological advantage of shortened treatment duration, i.e., 70 Gy over 6 weeks, which has been shown to significantly increase the loco-regional control compared to the same dose delivered in 7 weeks. According to the literature provided, an increase in the biological dose of 7.5% could be translated into an increase in loco-regional control in the order of 15%. In this context, the gain resulting from an increase in the equivalent dose can be achieved without any further increase in late normal tissue complications compared to standard treatment. Only the normal tissues embedded in the tumor volume and thus included in the PTV will be irradiated with a dose per fraction similar to that of the tumor itself. Provided that the dose per fraction to the organs at risk is limited to a maximum of 2 Gy per fraction, this increase in dose intensity will be achievable without undue damage to normal tissue (**Figure 6**) [23, 24].

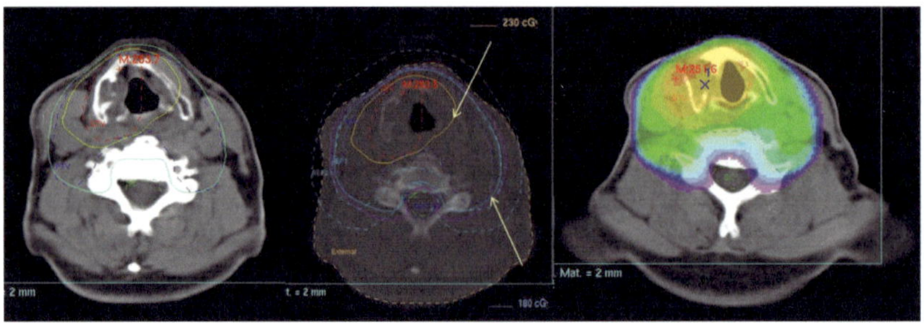

Figure 6. SIB-IMRT gradient dose distribution in the different parts of the target volume and the surrounding healthy issue in one single session.

In the following paragraphs, there are detailed examples of different cases where the SIB technique has been applied.

It is a fact that the treatment of **head and neck cancers** is influenced by fraction size, total dose and overall treatment time regarding the tumor control and toxicity. The total radiation dose has demonstrated a direct impact to the tumor response as well as to the acute or late adverse events.

The SIB-IMRT approach may be used to deliver a fraction size of 2.2 Gy to the boost volume and a fraction size of 1.8 Gy to the elective volume in the same treatment session. As a result, the high-risk volume is treated with fewer fractions compared to conventional protocols and leads to reduction in the overall treatment time (6 weeks compared to 7 weeks) (**Figure 7**).

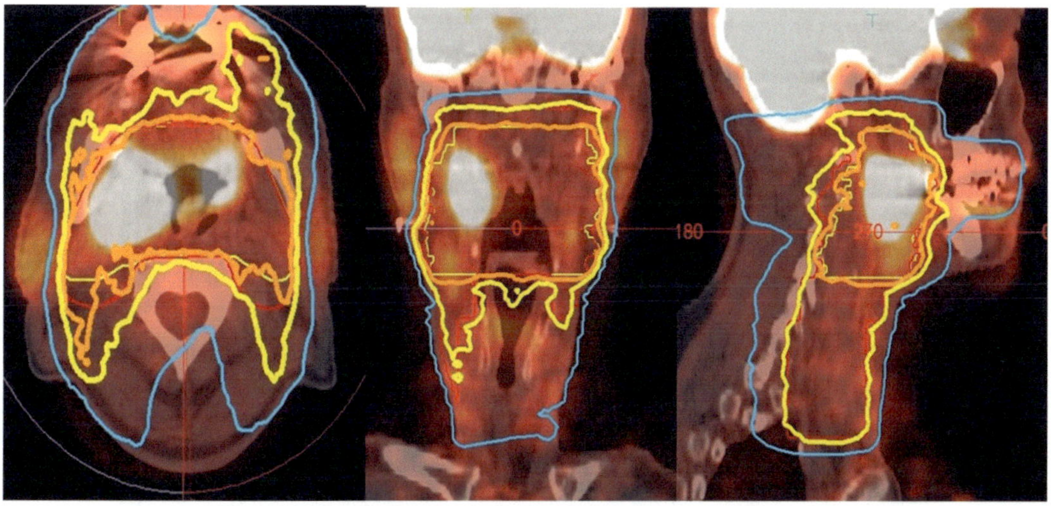

Figure 7. Head and neck tumor, metabolic image activity for better targeting of GTV gross tumor volume.

According to the RTOG H-0022 trial for oropharyngeal carcinomas SIB-IMRT in head and neck cancer, the use of 2.0, 2.11 or 2.2 Gy per session is highly effective and safe with respect to tumor response and tolerance. However, SIB with 2.2 Gy is not recommended for large tumors involving laryngeal structures [25–32].

Before the arrival of IMRT, the SeqB method was mostly used, within the 3D conformal irradiation technique to treat **high-grade gliomas**. With the SIB method, the dose per fraction to the PTV is lower when compared with the SEB, delivers an enhanced dose to the gross tumor volume and has a greater potential of sparing of organs at risk (**Figure 8**) [33–37].

Whole brain radiotherapy is the most common palliative treatment and has always been considered the standard treatment for patients with **brain metastases**. As opposed to surgery which was used in the past decades, today neurosurgical techniques such as radiosurgery have been combined with whole brain radiotherapy and have allowed for using more aggressive local treatment with the goal to increase local control probability and potentially overall survival. The literature reports a statistical advantage on overall survival probability in patients with a single brain metastasis treated with a combination of whole brain radiotherapy and radiosurgery compared with whole brain radiotherapy alone.

According to RTOG, the use of 20 Gy in five fractions to the WBRT can be considered an acceptable fractionation and is equivalent to 30 Gy in 2 weeks. Median survival (15–18 weeks) and overall response rates probability (75–80% for symptom palliation) are similar. The SIB together with this hypofractionated schedule in WBRT (20 Gy in five fractions) (40 Gy in five fractions) has proven to be feasible. This schedule offers the advantage of shorter treatment time, which could be very useful in oligometastatic patients that need systemic therapy (**Figure 9**) [38–43].

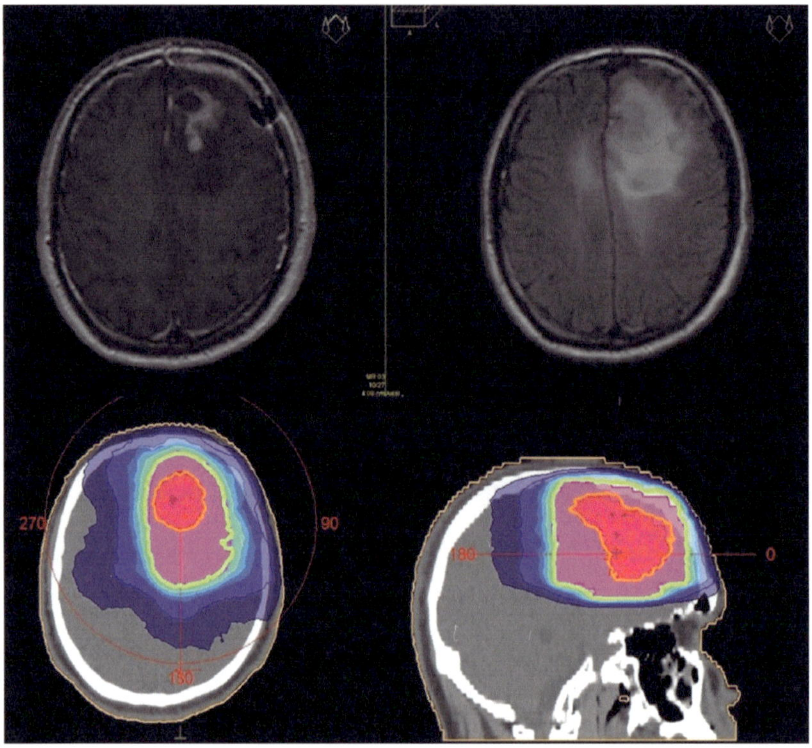

Figure 8. CT after excision of a brain tumor, SIB-IMRT.

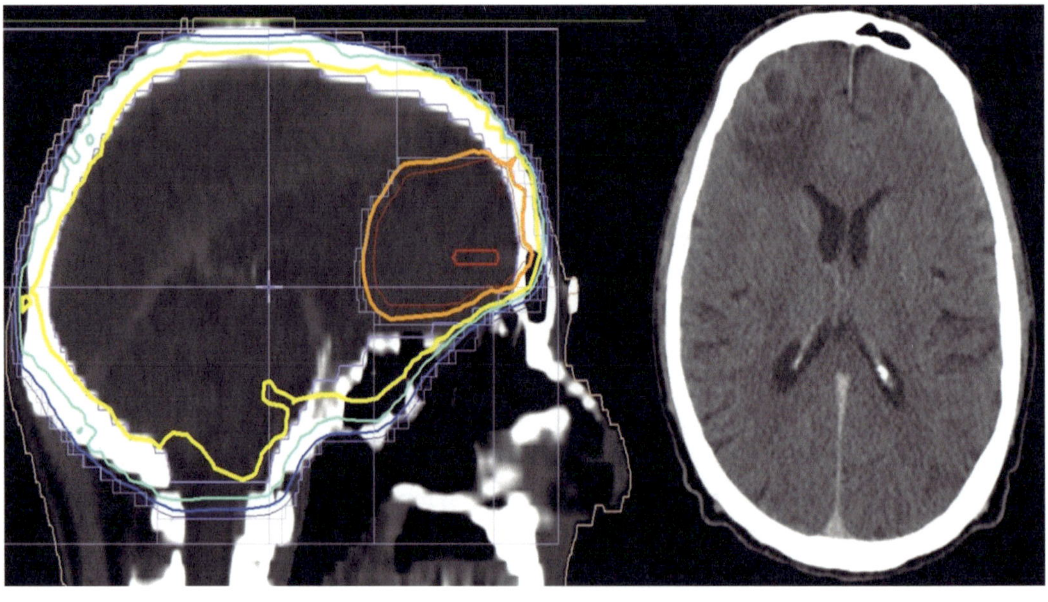

Figure 9. Single brain metastasis treated whole brain VMAT and SAB.

The true value of radiotherapy confined to the thorax is indisputable in the treatment of locally advanced **nonsmall cell lung cancer**. However, even with standard chemo-radiation, it is difficult to achieve durable local control, and this contributes to the high morbidity and mortality of patients with NSCLC. Results of RTOG 0617 clinical (Phase III) trial showed that the overall survival of stage III NSCLC patients given a high-dose (74 Gy) conformal radiation therapy with concurrent chemotherapy was no better than that of patients given the standard dose (60 Gy) [44–46]. The new idea is, instead of escalating the dose to the whole PTV, to selectively increase the treatment dose using SIB-IMRT to deliver a higher dose to the GTV and a relatively lower dose to the subclinical disease PTV [47–51].

Clinical outcomes of patients with NSCLC treated with SIB-IMRT have been retrospectively analyzed to evaluate the feasibility of this technology and to provide evidence in support of future clinical studies. The results so far should, at the very least, be considered encouraging (**Figure 10**).

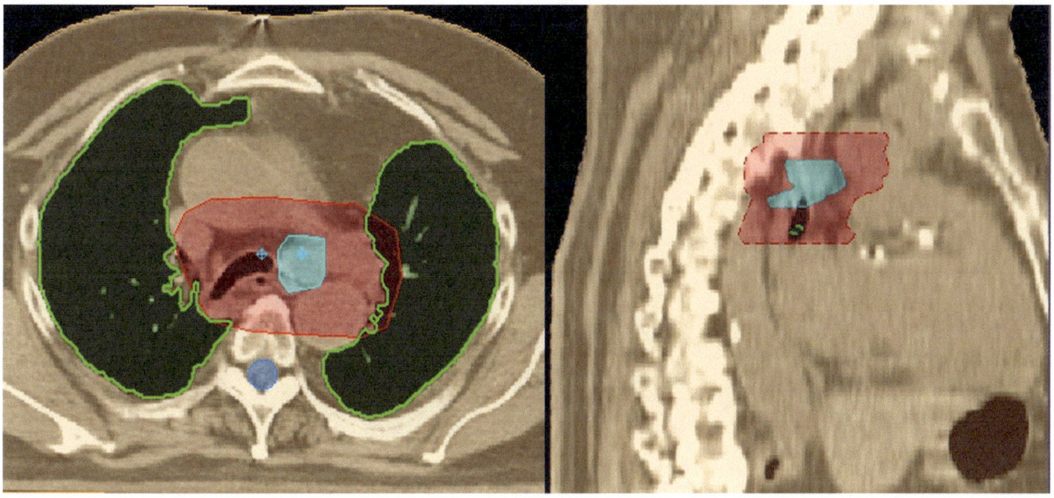

Figure 10. SIB treatment plan in lung cancer nodal recurrence.

Breast-conserving surgery followed by whole breast radiotherapy has become the standard approach for early stage **breast cancer** since the survival rates have proved to be similar to those with radical surgery. Local control can be improved by an additional boost of 16 Gy to the lumpectomy cavity after administration of 50 Gy to the whole breast. Breast irradiation with a boost to the tumor bed provides significantly higher local recurrence rates than whole breast irradiation alone, namely, 93.8% vs. 89.8% at 10 years. In the EORTC study 22881–10882, the absolute benefit of a boost in terms of local control was most pronounced in young patients [52–55].

A new technical perspective is to apply SIB to the whole breast 3D-CRT plan, in one integrated treatment schedule throughout the entire course of treatment. In this case, the whole breast represents the PTV and is exposed to a daily fraction of 1.8 Gy for 28 days, a total dose of 50,

40 Gy. Additionally, the tumor bed CTV is delineated, guided by the presence of the surgical clips, hematoma, seroma and/or other surgery-induced changes and is irradiated with a daily dose of 2.3 Gy (76.2%) or 2.4 Gy (23.8%) adding up to a total dose of 64.4 Gy or 67.2 Gy. These fractionation schemes are biologically equivalent to the sequential boost technique [56, 57].

The SIB technique is proposed for standard use in breast-conserving radiation therapy, because it can be easily implemented to reduce excess volumes of normal tissue irradiated, shorten the treatment course, decrease the dose per fraction for the breast, and increase the dose per fraction for the boost, with a relatively low incidence of acute skin toxicity (**Figure 11**).

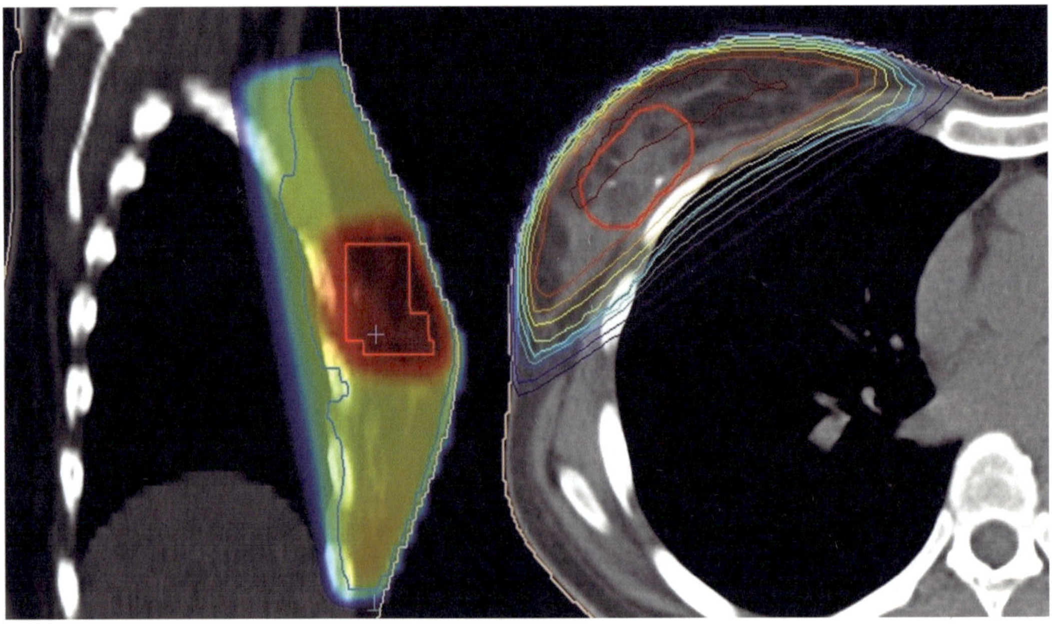

Figure 11. SIB breast cancer-tumor bed guided by the presence of the surgical clips.

The prospective RTOG 0529 phase II trial investigated the utility of IMRT in **anal cancer**. The two-year loco-regional control rate was 80%. In comparison with the results of RTOG 98–11, the use of IMRT reduced early G3 or higher gastrointestinal toxicity from 36 to 22%, and G3 or higher skin toxicity from 47 to 20%. However, until long-term control rates become available, concerns remain regarding potential compromise of tumor control rates using more conformal radiotherapy.

Several different SIB-IMRT schedules are described in various literatures. In the RTOG trial, the total dose varied according to T stage, in which 45 Gy/50.4 Gy was given to T1/T2 and 55–59 Gy/54 Gy to T3/4 tumors (RTOG 98–11, RTOG 0529). In contrast to tactics used in many US centers, where 59 Gy were administered regardless of T stage, with very few exceptions for very small primary tumors [58–62].

A new SIB-IMRT schedule is presented to treat patients with anal cancer in two series using moderate single doses from 1.5 to 2.0 Gy with a total dose of 59 Gy in combination with

http://dx.doi.org/10.5772/67326

mitomycin and 5FU 5FU/MMC. The results, in terms of loco-regional control and toxicity, are comparable to the results of other studies. Remarkably, the incidence of treatment interruptions was very low. Therefore, this regimen appears to be safe and favorable for clinical use.

The optimal technique of IMRT with or without SIB is still under debate, and up to date no standard SIB-IMRT schedule has been established.

The overall radiation therapy treatment time plays an important role, since every single one day prolongation of treatment beyond 30 days leads to 1% loss of tumor control in patients with **cervix carcinoma**. The presence of lymph node metastases in cervical cancer patients is a significant risk factor for disease recurrence. Currently available data showed that ^{18}FDG-PET\ CT detects more favorable results as far as regional disease when compared with the CT or MRI. PET/CT contributes to better disease control as far as better diagnosis of local and regional disease spread with consequent better delineation based on molecular data [63–66].

IMRT with simultaneous integrated boost (SIB) improves the therapeutic ratio and delivers different doses to different parts of the irradiated volume through dose painting. Further trials are needed in order to optimize the treatment procedure (**Figure 12**).

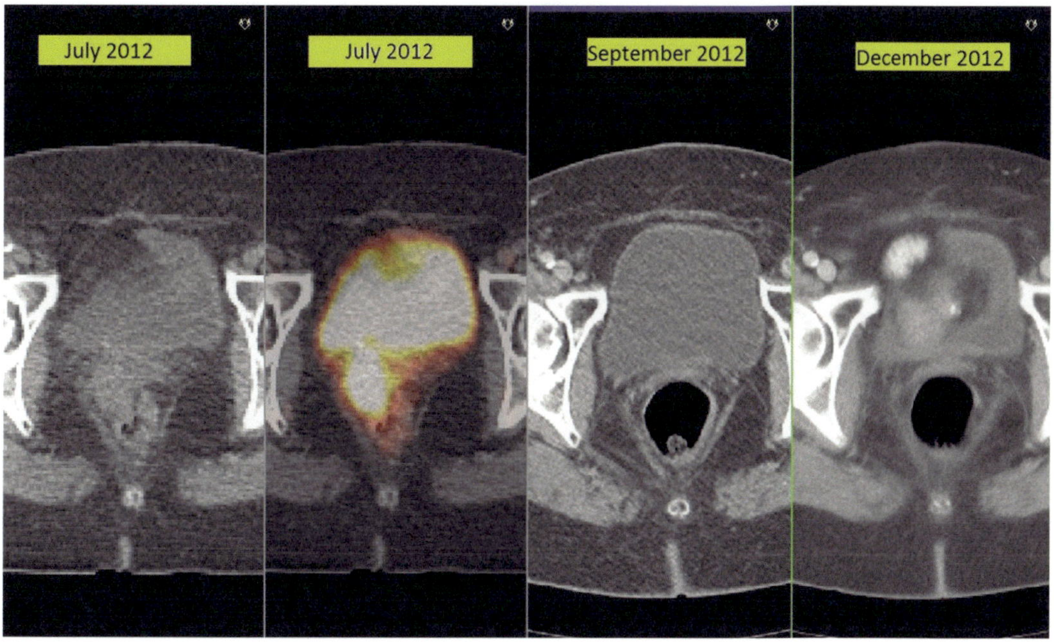

Figure 12. Follow-up of a patient treated with SIB-IMRT.

Local recurrences after external beam radiotherapy for **prostate cancer** are dose-dependent and mainly occur in the dominant intraprostatic lesion, i.e., the initial tumor site. Trials published demonstrated the feasibility and safety of delivering a SIB to the dominant intraprostatic lesion. No increase in acute and late GU or rectal toxicity was observed when performing a SIB up to an eight-year follow-up. The impact on outcome of focal boosting to the dominant intraprostatic lesion is currently evaluated in an ongoing phase 3 trial randomizing intermediate and high-risk prostate cancer patients to receive either 77 Gy (35 fractions) or 77 Gy to the prostate with an additional boost to the macroscopic tumor up to 95 Gy [67–71].

3. Conclusion

The SIB-IMRT or SMART is feasible and time sparing with encouraging loco-regional results and controlled side effects. From a radiobiological point of view, it appears to be an effective RT strategy for the primary treatment of H&N cancers, and also for various other cancer types. Many different SIB schedules have been employed so far, but a standard regimen has not yet been defined. Based on the available published studies on the SIB-IMRT, the short-term clinical outcome is very promising. However, very few data on late effects are available as of yet, due to the short follow-up time in the majority of the reported studies. However, further data are awaited shortly from ongoing clinical trials in order to determine the most efficient protocol.

For the past 5 years, our department has been using the SIB method where it is applicable. All images shown in this chapter are actual images of patients we personally have treated.

Acknowledgements

To our medical physicist, radiologist and nurses without whose assistance none of this would have been possible. We are privileged to have our devoted, attentive, not to mention excellently trained personnel as well as the state-of-the-art technological equipment our facilities have to offer, at our disposal.

Conflicts of interest statement

Nothing to declare.

Author details

Despina Katsochi

Address all correspondence to: dkatsochi@aktinotherapeia.com
Hygeia Hospital, Athens, Greece

References

[1] Brahme A. Design principles and clinical possibilities with a new generation of radiation therapy equipment. A review. Acta Oncol. 1987;26:403.

[2] Bortfeld T, Bürkelbach J, Boesecke R, Schlegel W. Methods of image reconstruction from projections applied to conformation radiotherapy. Phys Med Biol. 1990;35:1423.

[3] Guerrero Urbano MT, Nutting CM. Clinical use of intensity-modulated radiotherapy: Part I. Br J Radiol. 2004;77:88. DOI:10.1259/bjr/54028034

[4] Scorsetti M, Fogliata A, Castiglioni S. Early clinical experience with volumetric modulated arc therapy in head and neck cancer patients. Radiat Oncol. 2010;5:93. DOI:10.1186/1748-717X-5-93

[5] Stützel J, Oelfke U, Nill S. Linac integrated kV-cone beam CT: Technical features and first applications. Med Dosim. 2006;31:62–70. DOI:10.1016/j.meddos.2005.12.008

[6] Dandekar V, Morgan T, Turian J. Patterns-of-failure after helical tomotherapy-based chemoradiotherapy for head and neck cancer: Implications for CTV margin, elective nodal dose and bilateral parotid sparing. Oral Oncol. 2014;50:520–526. DOI:10.1016/j.oraloncology.2014.02.009

[7] Lauve A, Morris M, Schmidt-Ullrich R. Simultaneous integrated boost intensity-modulated radiotherapy for locally advanced head-and-neck squamous cell carcinomas: II-clinical results. Int J Radiat Oncol Biol Phys. 2004;60:374–387.

[8] Bourhis J, Overgaard J, Audry H. Hyperfractionated or accelerated radiotherapy in head and neck cancer: A meta-analysis. Lancet. 2006;368:843. DOI:10.1016/S0140-6736(06)69121-6

[9] Marks LB, Yorke ED, Jackson A. Use of normal tissue complication probability models in the clinic. Int J Radiat Oncol Biol Phys. 2010;376:S10–S976. DOI:10.1016/j.ijrobp.2009.07.1754

[10] Schäfer M, Münter M, Sterzing F, Häring P, Rhein B, Debus J. Measurements of characteristics of time pattern in dose delivery in step-and-shoot IMRT. Strahlenther Onkol. 2005;181:587. DOI:10.1007/s00066-005-1289-7

[11] Grégoire V, Haustermans K, Geets X, Roels S, Lonneux M. PET-based treatment planning in radiotherapy: A new standard? J Nucl Med. 2007;48:68S–77S.

[12] Garden AS, Morrison WH, Wong PF, Tung SS, Rosenthal DI, Dong L, Mason B, Perkins GH, Ang KK. Disease-control rates following intensity-modulated radiation therapy for small primary oropharyngeal carcinoma. Int J Radiat Oncol Biol Phys. 2007;67:438. DOI:10.1016/j.ijrobp.2006.08.078

[13] Morin O, Gillis A, Chen J, Aubin M, Bucci K, Roach M, Pouliot J. Megavoltage cone-beam CT: System description and clinical applications. Med Dosim. 2006;31:51–61. DOI:10.1016/j.meddos.2005.12.009

[14] Mac Manus M, Hicks RJ, Everitt S. Role of PET-CT in the optimization of thoracic radiotherapy. J Thorac Oncol. 2006;1(1):81–84. DOI:org/10.1016/S1556-0864(15)31519-7

[15] Hicks RJ, Kalff V, MacManus MP, Ware RE, Hogg A, McKenzie AF, Matthews JP, Ball DL. PET provides high-impact and powerful prognostic stratification in staging newly diagnosed non-small cell lung cancer. J Nucl Med. 2001 Nov;42(11):1596-604

[16] Menzel HG. The International Commission on Radiation Units and Measurements (ICRU), since its inception in 1925, has had as its principal. J ICRU. 2010;10:83. DOI:10. 1016/j.ijrobp. 2009.07.1754

[17] Marks LB, Yorke ED, Jackson A. Use of normal tissue complication probability models in the clinic. Int J Radiat Oncol Biol Phys. 2010;76:S10–S19. DOI:10.1016/j.ijrobp.2004.04.013

[18] Rengan R, Rosenzweig KE, Venkatraman E, Koutcher LA, Fox JL, Nayak R, Amols H, Yorke E, Jackson A, Ling CC, Leibel SA. Improved local control with higher doses of radiation in large-volume stage III non-small-cell lung cancer. Int J Radiat Oncol Biol Phys. 2004;60(3):741–747.

[19] Dogan N, King S, Emami B, Mohideen N, Mirkovic N, Leybovich LB, Sethi A. Assessment of different IMRT boost delivery methods on target coverage and normal-tissue sparing. Int J Radiat Oncol Biol Phys. 2003;57:1480–1491.

[20] Fu KK, Pajak TF, Trotti A. A Radiation Therapy Oncology Group (RTOG) phase III randomized study to compare hyperfractionation and two variants of accelerated fractionation to standard fractionation radiotherapy for head and neck squamous cell carcinomas: First report of RTOG 9003. Int J Radiat Oncol Biol Phys. 2000;48:7. DOI:10.1016/j. ijrobp.2004.03.010

[21] Butler EB, Teh BS, Grant WH, Woo S. Smart (simultaneous modulated accelerated radiation therapy) boost: a new accelerated fractionation schedule for the treatment of head and neck cancer with intensity modulated radiotherapy – What is the price for speeding? Int J Rad Oncol Biol Phy. 1999;45(1):21–32. DOI: 10.1016/S1470-2045(11)70346-1

[22] Mohan R, Wu Q, Manning M, Schmidt-Ullrich R. Radiobiological considerations in the design of fractionation strategies for intensity-modulated radiation therapy of head and neck cancers. Int J Radiat Oncol Biol Phys. 2000;46:619.

[23] Bourhis J, Sire C, Graff P. Concomitant chemoradiotherapy versus acceleration of radiotherapy with or without concomitant chemotherapy in locally advanced head and neck carcinoma (GORTEC 99–02): An open-label phase 3 randomised trial. Lancet Oncol. 2012;13:145.

[24] Denis F, Garaud P, Bardet E. Final results of the 94–01 French Head and Neck Oncology and Radiotherapy Group randomized trial comparing radiotherapy alone with concomitant radiochemotherapy in advanced-stage oropharynx carcinoma. J Clin Oncol. 2004;22:69.

[25] Marcial VA, Pajak TF, Chang C. Hyperfractionated photon radiation therapy in the treatment of advanced squamous cell carcinoma of the oral cavity, pharynx, larynx, and sinuses, using radiation therapy as the only planned modality: (preliminary report) by the Radiation Therapy Oncology Group (RTOG). Int J Radiat Oncol Biol Phys. 1987;13:41.

[26] Beck-Bornholdt HP, Dubben HH, Liertz-Petersen C, Willers H. Hyperfractionation: Where do we stand? Radiother Oncol. 1997;43:1.

[27] Eisbruch A, Harris J, Garden AS. Multi-institutional trial of accelerated hypofractionated intensity-modulated radiation therapy for early-stage oropharyngeal cancer (RTOG 00–22). Int J Radiat Oncol Biol Phys. 2010;76:1333–1338. DOI:10.1016/j.ijrobp.2009.04.011

[28] Songthong AP, Kannarunimit D, Chakkabat C. A randomized phase II/III study of adverse events between sequential (SEQ) versus simultaneous integrated boost (SIB) intensity modulated radiation therapy (IMRT) in nasopharyngeal carcinoma; preliminary result on acute adverse events. Radiat Oncol. 2015;10:166. DOI:10.1186/s13014-015-0472-y

[29] Koom WS, Kim TH, Shin KH, Pyo HR, Kim JY, Kim DY, Yoon M, Park SY, Lee DH, Ryu JS, Jung YS, Lee SH, Cho KH. Smart (Simultaneous Modulated Accelerated Radiotherapy) for locally advanced nasopharyngeal carcinomas. Head Neck. 2008;10:159–169. DOI:10.1002/hed.20667

[30] Nguyen-Tan PF, Zhang Q, Ang KK. Randomized phase III trial to test accelerated versus standard fractionation in combination with concurrent cisplatin for head and neck carcinomas in the Radiation Therapy Oncology Group 0129 trial: Long-term report of efficacy and toxicity. J Clin Oncol. 2014;32:3858. DOI:10.1200/JCO.2014.55.3925

[31] Beitler JJ, Zhang Q, Fu KK, Trotti A, Spencer SA, Jones CU, Garden AS, Shenouda G, Harris J, Ang KK. Final results of local-regional control and late toxicity of rtog 9003: A randomized trial of altered fractionation radiation for locally advanced head and neck cancer. Int J Radiat Oncol Biol Phys. 2014;89:13–20. DOI:10.1016/j.ijrobp.2013.12.027

[32] Xiao C, Hanlon A, Zhang Q. Risk factors for clinician-reported symptom clusters in patients with advanced head and neck cancer in a phase 3 randomized clinical trial: RTOG 0129. Cancer. 2014;120:848. DOI:10.1002/cncr.28500

[33] Stupp R, Mason WP, van den Bent MJ, Weller M, Fisher B, Taphoorn MJ. Radiotherapy plus concomitant and adjuvant temozolomide for glioblastoma. N Engl J Med. 2005;352: 987–996. DOI:10.1056/NEJMoa043330

[34] Farzin M, Molls M, Astner S, Rondak IC, Oechsner M. Simultaneous integrated vs. sequential boost in VMAT radiotherapy of high-grade gliomas. Strahlenther Onkol. 2015;191:945–952. DOI: 10.1056/NEJMoa043330

[35] Sultanem K, Patrocinio H, Lambert C, Corns R, Leblanc R, Parker W. The use of hypofractionated intensity-modulated irradiation in the treatment of glioblastoma multiforme: Preliminary results of a prospective trial. Int J Radiat Oncol Biol Phys. 2004;58:247–252.

[36] Monjazeb AM, Ayala D, Jensen C, Case LD, Bourland JD, Ellis TL. A phase I dose escalation study of hypofractionated IMRT field-in-field boost for newly diagnosed glioblastoma multiforme. Int J Radiat Oncol Biol Phys. 2012;82:743–748. DOI:10.1016/j.ijrobp.2010.10.018

[37] Truc G, Bernier V, Mirjolet C, Dalban C, Mazoyer F, Bonnetain F, Blanchard N, Lagneau É, Maingon P, Noël G. A phase I dose escalation study using simultaneous integrated-boost IMRT with temozolomide in patients with unifocal glioblastoma. Cancer/Radiothérapie. 2016:20;193–198. DOI:10.1016/j.canrad.2015.12.005

[38] Giaj N, Gianluisa L, Alba S, Sergio F, Ricchetti F, Mazzola R, Naccarato S, Ruggieri R, Filippo A. Whole brain radiotherapy with hippocampal avoidance and simultaneous integrated boost for brain metastases: A dosimetric volumetric-modulated arc therapy study. Radiol Med. 2016;121:60–69. DOI:10.1007/s11547-015-0563-8.

[39] Mehta MP, Tsao MN, Whelan TJ, Morris DE, Hayman JA, Flickinger JC, Mills M, Rogers CL, Souhami L. The American society for therapeutic radiology and oncology (ASTRO) evidence based review of the role of radiosurgery for brain metastasis. Int J Radiat Oncol Biol Phys. 2005;63:37–46. DOI:10.1016/j.ijrobp.2005.05.023.

[40] Kondziolka D, Patel A, Lunsford LD, Kassam A, Flickinger JC. Stereotactic radiosurgery plus whole brain radiotherapy versus radiotherapy alone for patients with multiple brain metastases. Int J Radiat Oncol Biol Phys. 1999;45:427–434.

[41] Andrews DW, Scott CB, Sperduto PW. Whole-brain radiation therapy with or without stereotactic radiosurgery boost for patients with one to three brain metastases: Phase III results of the RTOG-9508 randomized trial. Lancet. 2004;363:1665–1672. DOI:10.1016/S0140-6736(04)16250-8

[42] Prokic V, Wiedenmann N, Fels F, Schmucker M, Nieder C, Grosu AL. Whole brain irradiation with hippocampal sparing and dose escalation on multiple brain metastases: A planning study on treatment concepts. Int J Radiat Oncol Biol Phys. 2013;85:264–270. DOI:10.1016/j.ijrobp.2012.02.036

[43] Lagerwaard FJ, van der Hoorn EA, Verbakel WF, Haasbeek CJ, Slotman BJ, Senan S. Whole-brain radiotherapy with simultaneous integrated boost to multiple brain metastases using volumetric modulated arc therapy. Int J Radiat Oncol Biol Phys. 2009;75:253–259. DOI:10.1016/j.ijrobp.2009.03.029

[44] Barraclough LH, Swindell R, Livsey JE, Hunter RD, Davidson SE. External beam boost for cancer of the cervix uteri when intracavitary therapy cannot be performed. Int J Radiat Oncol Biol Phys. 2008;71:772–778. DOI:10.1016/j.ijrobp.2007.10.066

[45] Van de Bunt L, Jurgenliemk-Schulz IM, de Kort GA, Roesink JM, Tersteeg RJ, van der Heide UA. Motion and deformation of the target volumes during IMRT for cervical cancer: What margins do we need? Radiother Oncol. 2008;88:233–240. DOI:10.1016/j.radonc.2007.12.017

[46] Kaatee RS, Olofsen MJ, Verstraate MB, Quint S, Heijmen BJ: Detection of organ movement in cervix cancer patients using a fluoroscopic electronic portal imaging device and radiopaque markers. Int J Radiat Oncol Biol Phys. 2002;54:576–583.

[47] Van Baardwijk A, Wanders S, Boersma L. Mature results of an individualized radiation dose prescription study based on normal tissue constraints in stages I to III non-small-cell lung cancer. J Clin Oncol. 2010;28:1380–1386. DOI:10.1200/JCO.2009.24.7221

[48] Bradley JD, Paulus R, Komaki R. Standard-dose versus high-dose conformal radiotherapy with concurrent and consolidation carboplatin plus paclitaxel with or without cetuximab for patients with stage IIIA or IIIB non-small-cell lung cancer (RTOG 0617): A randomised, two-by-two factorial phase 3 study. Lancet Oncol. 2015;16:187–199.

[49] Vera P, Bohn P, Edet-Sanson A. Simultaneous positron emission tomography (PET) assessment of metabolism with (18)F-fluoro-2-deoxy-d-glucose (FDG), proliferation with (18)F-fluoro-thymidine (FLT), and hypoxia with (18)fluoro-misonidazole (F-miso) before and during radiotherapy in patients with non-small-cell lung cancer (NSCLC): A pilot study. Radiother Oncol. 2011;98:109–116. DOI:10.1016/j.radonc.2010.10.011

[50] Even AJG, van der Stoep J, Zegers CML, Reymen B, Troost EGC, Lambin P, van Elmpt W. PET-based dose painting in non-small cell lung cancer: Comparing uniform dose escalation with boosting hypoxic and metabolically active sub-volumes. Radiother Oncol. 2015;116(2):281–286. DOI:10.1016/j.radonc.2015.07.013.

[51] Han D, Qin Q, Hao S, Huang W, Wei Y, Zhang Z, Wang Z, Li B. Feasibility and efficacy of simultaneous integrated boost intensity-modulated radiation therapy in patients with limited-disease small cell lung cancer. Radiat Oncol. 2014;11(9):280. DOI:10.1186/s13014-014-0280-9.

[52] Bartelink H, Horiot JC, Poortmans PM, Struikmans H, Van den Bogaert W, Fourquet A. Impact of a higher radiation dose on local control and survival in breast-conserving therapy of early breast cancer: 10-year results of the randomized boost versus no boost EORTC 22881–10882 trial. J Clin Oncol. 2007;25:3259–3265. DOI:10.1200/JCO.2007.11.4991.

[53] Bentzen SM, Agrawal RK, Aird EG, Barrett JM, Barrett-Lee PJ, Bliss JM. The UK Standardisation of Breast Radiotherapy (START) Trial A of radiotherapy hypofractionation for treatment of early breast cancer: A randomised trial. Lancet Oncol. 2008;9:331–341. DOI:10.1016/S1470-2045(08)70077-9

[54] Dellas K, Vonthein R, Zimmer J, Dinges S, Boicev AD, Andreas P. Hypofractionation with simultaneous integrated boost for early breast cancer: Results of the German multicenter phase II trial (ARO-2010-01). Strahlenther Onkol. 2014;190:646–653. DOI:10.1007/s00066-014-0658-5

[55] Sedlmayer F, Sautter-Bihl ML, Budach W, Dunst J, Fastner G, Feyer P. DEGRO practical guidelines: Radiotherapy of breast cancer I: Radiotherapy following breast conserving therapy for invasive breast cancer. Strahlenther Onkol. 2013;189:825–833. DOI:10.1007/s00066-013-0437-8

[56] Alford SL, Prassas GN, Vogelesang CR, Leggett HJ, Hamilton CS. Adjuvant breast radiotherapy using a simultaneous integrated boost: Clinical and dosimetric perspectives. J Med Imaging Radiat Oncol. 2013;57:222–229. DOI:10.1111/j.1754-9485.2012.02473.x

[57] Bantema-Joppe EJ, Schilstra C, de Bock GH, Dolsma WV, Busz DM, Langendijk JA. Simultaneous integrated boost irradiation after breast-conserving surgery: Physician-rated toxicity and cosmetic outcome at 30 months' follow-up. Int J Radiat Oncol Biol Phys. 2012;83:e471–e477. DOI:10.1016/j.ijrobp.2012.01.050

[58] Hsu A, Hara W, Pawlicki J. IMRT in the treatment of anal cancer: A dosimetric comparison of conventional 3D, IMRT, and IMRT with integrated boost. Proc Am Soc Ther Radiol Oncol. 2006;66:674.

[59] Ajani JA, Winter KA, Gunderson LL. Intergroup RTOG 98–11: A phase III randomized study of 5-fluorouracil (5-FU), mitomycin, and radiotherapy versus 5-fluorouracil, cisplatin and radiotherapy in carcinoma of the anal canal. Proc Am Soc Clin Oncol. 2012;26:18. DOI:10.1200/JCO.2012.43.8085

[60] Chen YJ, Liu A, Tsai PT, Vora NL, Pezner RD, Schultheiss TE, Wong JY. Organ sparing by conformal avoidance intensity-modulated radiation therapy for anal cancer: Dosimetric evaluation of coverage of pelvis and inguinal/femoral nodes. Int J Radiat Oncol Biol Phys. 2005;63:274–281. DOI:10.1016/j.ijrobp.2005.05.052

[61] Kachnic LA1, Winter K, Myerson RJ, Goodyear MD, Willins J. Esthappan J, Haddock MG, Rotman M, Parikh PJ, Safran H, Willett CG. Radiation Therapy Oncology Group (RTOG). A Phase II Evaluation of Dose-Painted IMRT in Combination with 5-Fluorouracil and Mitomycin-C for Reduction of Acute Morbidity in Carcinoma of the Anal Canal, RTOG 05-29. RTOG, Philadelphia, PA. 2012. Int J Radiat Oncol Biol Phys. 2013 May 1;86(1):27–33. DOI:10.1016/j.ijrobp.2012.09.023

[62] Jani AB, Farrey KJ, Rash C, Heimann R, Chmura SJ, Milano MT. Intensity-modulated radiation therapy (IMRT) in the treatment of anal cancer: toxicity and clinical outcome. Int J Radiat Oncol Biol Phys. 2005;63:354–361. DOI:10.1016/j.ijrobp.2005.02.030

[63] Georg D, Kirisits C, Hillbrand M, Dimopoulos J, Potter R. Image-guided radiotherapy for cervix cancer: High-tech external beam therapy versus high-tech brachytherapy. Int J Radiat Oncol Biol Phys. 2008;71:1272–1278. DOI:10.1016/j.ijrobp.2008.03.032

[64] Lim K, Small W Jr, Portelance L, Creutzberg C, Jurgenliemk-Schulz IM, Mundt A, Mell LK, Mayr N, Viswanathan A, Jhingran A. Consensus guidelines for delineation of clinical target volume for intensity-modulated pelvic radiotherapy for the definitive treatment of cervix cancer. Int J Radiat Oncol Biol Phys. 2011;79:348–355. DOI:10.1016/j.ijrobp.2009.10.075

[65] Fyles A, Keane TJ, Barton M, Simm J. The effect of treatment duration in the local control of cervix cancer. Radiother Oncol. 1992;25:273–279.

[66] Molla M, Escude L, Mouet P, Popowski Y, Hidalgo A, Rouzaud M, Linero D, Miralbell R. Fractionated stereotactic radiotherapy boost for gynecologic tumors: An alternative to brachytherapy? Int J Radiat Oncol Biol Phys. 2005 May 1;62(1):118–24. DOI:10.1016/j.ijrobp. 2004.09.028

[67] Zelefsky MJ, Pei X, Chou JF, Schechter M, Kollmeier M, Cox B. Dose escalation for prostate cancer radiotherapy: Predictors of long-term biochemical tumor control and distant metastases-free survival outcomes. Eur Urol. 2011;60:1133–1139. DOI:10.1016/j.eururo.2011.08.029

[68] Fonteyne V, Villeirs G, Speleers B, De Neve W, De Wagter C, Lumen N. Intensity-modulated radiotherapy as primary therapy for prostate cancer: Report on acute toxicity after dose escalation with simultaneous integrated boost to intraprostatic lesion. Int J Radiat Oncol Biol Phys. 2008;72:799–807. DOI:10.1016/j.ijrobp.2008.01.040

[69] Ippolito E, Mantini G, Morganti AG, Mazzeo E, Padula GD, Digesu C. Intensity-modulated radiotherapy with simultaneous integrated boost to dominant intraprostatic lesion: Preliminary report on toxicity. Am J Clin Oncol. 2012;35:158–162. DOI:10.1097/COC.0b013e318209cd8f

[70] Lips IM, van der Heide UA, Haustermans K, van Lin EN, Pos F, Franken SP. Single blind randomized phase III trial to investigate the benefit of a focal lesion ablative micro-boost in prostate cancer (FLAME-trial): Study protocol for a randomized controlled trial. Trials. 2011;12:255. DOI:10.1186/1745-6215-12-255

[71] Cox JD, Stetz J, Pajak TF. Toxicity criteria of the Radiation Therapy Oncology Group (RTOG) and the European Organization for Research and Treatment of Cancer (EORTC). Int Radiat Oncol Biol Phys. 1995;31:1341–1346. DOI:10.1016/0360-3016(95)00060-C.

Chapter 8

Low-Dose Radiotherapy of Painful Heel Spur/Plantar Fasciitis as an Example of Treatment Effects in Benign Diseases

Robert Michael Hermann, Frank Bruns and
Mirko Nitsche

Additional information is available at the end of the chapter

http://dx.doi.org/10.5772/67058

Abstract

Degenerative changes in the plantar fascia may cause the so-called "painful heel" with typical projections of tenderness. This condition is often associated with a plantar heel spur. Radiotherapy with low doses (LD-EBRT) has been well known for its anti-inflammatory potential. In the recent years, several microbiological mechanisms were elucidated to explain immunomodulation by LD-EBRT. Furthermore, a randomized study proved the clinical efficacy of this therapy in plantar fasciitis. Two other trials defined a fractionation schedule of 6 × 0.5 Gy twice weekly as the new standard therapy. Taken together, LD-EBRT is an effective and safe therapeutic option for patients over 30 years of age and after exclusion of pregnancy. In case of an insufficient response, a second course can be offered to the patient. There are still open questions concerning target volume definition and fractionation of LD-EBRT. Furthermore, studies randomizing LD-EBRT with other conservative therapeutic approaches are missing.

Keywords: low dose radiotherapy, heel spur, plantar fasciitis, *reizbestrahlung*, target volume definition

1. Incidence and etiology of plantar fasciitis

About 7% of the population >65 years suffer from a painful heel, even though younger people are often affected, too [1]. The most common cause of this symptom is the so-called "plantar fasciitis" [2]. This term is widely used, although "plantar fasciopathy" or "plantar fasciosis" would be a better description to point out the degenerative nature of the disease. However, as more than 1100 citations in Pubmed quote "plantar fasciitis" (in comparison with only 50), we will use the traditional term in the following.

Plantar fasciitis has been associated with obesity, with acute or chronic work overload, or with work on hard surfaces [2, 3]. It seems that physiological degeneration of the fascia at the calcaneal insertion exacerbates due to repetitive microtraumas caused by vertical compression [4]. This causes inflammatory tissue reactions. As a result, the fascia is thickened with an associated fluid collection to 4.0 mm and more in ultrasonography [5]. Furthermore, this inflammation may trigger bone formation, the so-called "plantar heel spur." This process has been studied intensively by Kumai and Benjamin [6]. They proposed three stages of spur growth: "(a) an initial formation of cartilage cell clusters and fissures at the plantar fascia enthesis; (b) thickening of the subchondral bone plate at the enthesis as small spurs form; and (c) development of vertically oriented trabeculae buttressing the proximal end of larger spurs" [6]. The first description of this spur formation and correlation with the clinical symptoms was carried out by Plettner in 1900 [7]. However, not every heel spur is associated with heel pain, as these spurs are found in 11–16% of the normal asymptomatic population [4]. On the other hand, some patients with painful plantar fasciitis do not have a radiographic confirmation of a spur formation.

A similar mechanism (although caused by longitudinal traction and not by vertical compression) of bone formation has been described at the insertion of the Achilles tendon [8].

According to the American clinical practice guidelines from 2010, diagnosis is established by the typical anamnesis and the characteristic localizations of tenderness. Still, weight-bearing radiographs are also recommended [9].

2. Treatment with LD-EBRT

2.1. Biological effects of LD-EBRT on lymphocytes and inflammatory processes

Single doses of external beam radiotherapy (EBRT) in the range of 0.3–1 Gy are called "low dose EBRT" (LD-EBRT). These single fractions are applied two or three times a week until a total dose of about 3–6 Gy is reached. Such radiotherapeutic concepts are used for diverse nonmalignant conditions, e.g., osteoarthrosis, tendinopathy, epicondylitis, or bursitis. A comprehensive review of the historical developments in LD-EBRT for benign diseases is given by Trott [10].

In contrast, EBRT in oncology is characterized by much higher single and total doses. "Normofractionation" describes single doses of 1.8–2 Gy, applied about five times a week. To treat breast cancer, the total doses of about 62 Gy are necessary, in prostate cancer even more than 72 Gy. From a radiobiological point of view, these high cumulative doses are used to induce DNA double strand breaks. Due to errors in a repair mechanism (nonhomologous end joining), dicentric chromosomes can occur. These can result in unfinished mitoses, the so-called "mitotic catastrophe," the main mechanism to reduce clonogenic survival in tumor cells [11]. High doses of EBRT induce local inflammation and tissue reactions.

The much lower doses of LD-EBRT act via different mechanisms. In the last two decades, several anti-inflammatory effects have been discovered, contrary to the effects of the above-mentioned high EBRT doses.

(a) *In vitro* LD-EBRT has been shown to induce apoptosis in peripheral blood mononuclear cells (PBMC) [12]. Interestingly, there was not a linear correlation between dose and the amount of apoptotic cells. Instead, the maximal induction of apoptosis was observed after a single dose between 0.3 and 0.7 Gy, higher doses (up to 3 Gy) not being more effective [12].

(b) Furthermore, doses between 0.1 and 0.5 Gy reduced the adhesion of PBMC significantly to endothelial cells (ECs) *in vitro*, probably by suppressing the expression of L-selectin on the surface of PBMC [13]. This is a very important finding, as the adhesion of leukocytes to the cells of the vessel wall is the first event of tissue invasion in inflammatory processes [13]. Another reason for the reduced adhesion between PBMC and EC was identified by Rödel et al. [14]: In irradiated EC mRNA expression and protein secretion of transforming growth factor β1 (TGF-β1) were highest after 0.5 Gy, higher doses resulted in a decline to basal levels [14]. Neutralization TGF-β1 with specific antibodies restored the adhesion between PBMC and EC. These *in vitro* results were confirmed *in vivo* in a mouse model for 0.3 Gy [15]. TGF-β expression is dependent on activation of the nuclear factor-kappa B (NF-κB) [16]. Also, NF-kB DNA-binding activity showed a biphasic response to LD-EBRT with a first maximum at 0.5 Gy, a relative minimum between 0.6 and 0.8 Gy, and a second increase at 1 and 3 Gy [16]. The above-mentioned findings show a biphasic time course with reduced adhesion of PBMC 4 and 24 h after LD-EBRT, with a relative maximum of adhesion after 12h [17].

(c) A third mechanism was the suppression of nitric oxide (NO) production in activated macrophages by LD-EBRT between 0.3 and 1.25 Gy [18]. As the expression of inducible nitric oxide synthases (iNOS) proteins was not altered, the LD-EBRT seemed to act at the translational or posttranslational level. Furthermore, a dose of 0.5 Gy significantly reduced oxidative burst and superoxide production of stimulated macrophages [19]. A diminished release of reactive oxygen species (ROS) can also contribute to the anti-inflammatory effects of LD-EBRT.

Taken together, all of these pathways and mechanisms showed a similar dose dependence with a maximum effect between 0.3 and 0.7 Gy regarding a discontinuous dose-effect relation [20].

There are several *in vivo* studies in different animal models about the effects of LD-EBRT, especially on osteoarthritis. A comprehensive overview is given in Ref. [20], however, as they are not directly related to calcaneodynia, we will not further comment on them.

2.2. Results of randomized trials on radiotherapy for painful heel spur

Since 1937 [21] for decades, large retrospective studies on the efficacy of LD-EBRT in calcaneodynia have been published (overview in 22). In 1970, one negative randomized trial was reported and heavily criticized but had not been repeated [23]. Starting in the 1980s, patients were systematically clinically examined and interrogated in a structured manner to try to control for diverse risk factors and to compare the efficacy of different fractionation schemes and total doses [24].

It took until the past decade to perform and report prospectively randomized trials to proof the efficacy of LD-EBRT and to identify the optimal dose fractionation schedule. In the following, we report the design and the results of these trials. **Table 1** gives a short overview of the studied dose concepts and the results. Due to methodological reasons, we will describe the studies not following their publications dates, but according to a systematic order.

Author	Year	N	Standard arm	Experimental arm	Results	Conclusions
Niewald et al. [26]	2012	66	6 × 1 Gy twice a week	6 × 0.1 Gy	3 months: VAS/CS/ SF12 sig. better with standard	1. Dose-response relationship
					1 year: less second treatment series with standard	2. Proof of therapeutic effect of LD-EBRT
Heyd et al. [30]	2007	130	6 × 1 Gy twice a week	6 × 0.5 Gy	6 months: CS no sig. differences	6 × 0.5 Gy as standard fractionation
Ott et al. [32]	2014	457	6 × 1 Gy twice a week	6 × 0.5 Gy	6 weeks, 2.5 years: VAS/CS no sig. differences	6 × 0.5 Gy as standard confirmed
Niewald et al. [25]	2015	127	6 × 1 Gy twice a week	12 × 0.5 Gy thrice a week	3 months: VAS/CS/SF12 no sig. differences	Efficacy not increased with 12 × 0.5 Gy standard still 6 × 0.5 Gy

Table 1. Summary of contemporary randomized trials on LD-EBRT of painful heel spurs: tested schedules, results, and conclusions.

2.2.1. Clinical proof of the efficacy of LD-EBRT

Since the publication of the first randomized trial on LD-EBRT in 1970, the efficacy of LD-EBRT was questioned [23]. Goldie et al. randomized 399 patients, however, only nine patients suffered from calcaneodynia. This is why these results cannot be extrapolated to LD-EBRT of a painful heel spur. Furthermore, endpoints were not clearly defined, and therapy was started in an acute stage of the disease [25].

The landmark study to prove the efficacy of LD-EBRT was performed by the German cooperative group on the radiotherapy for benign diseases (GCGBD) under the responsibility of Niewald et al. [26]. A very low dose EBRT (6 × 0.1 Gy applied twice a week up to a total dose of 0.6 Gy) was randomized to a standard dose LD-EBRT (6 × 1 Gy twice a week up to a total dose of 6 Gy). In the case of an unfavorable response after 3 months, the patient was offered a second treatment series ("reirradiation") applying a standard dose. The dosage of the experimental arm was chosen to examine if very low doses are effective at all. Second, it acted as a placebo irradiation, as a sham irradiation was regarded unethical. LD-EBRT was applied using a linear accelerator (4- to 6-MV photons) using lateral parallel opposing fields.

Inclusion criteria were tenderness of the calcaneus with a limitation of the painless walking distance and duration of the symptoms for more than 6 months. Furthermore, a radiological proof of a heel spur was required, and the patients had to be least 40 years of age. Patients with previous traumata to the foot, rheumatic or vascular diseases, lymphatic edema, pregnancy, or breastfeeding were excluded. Concomitant therapy with oral analgesics was not limited. However, local injections with steroids during the study period were not permitted.

Initially, 200 patients were planned [27] to detect a difference of 10% in the quality of life (QOL) sum score (SF-12) [28] and calcaneodynia sum score (CS) [29] (**Table 2**) with a power of 80% and an error probability of 5%. Furthermore, the visual analogue scale (VAS) to evaluate pain intensity was used. However, after randomization of 66 patients and interim analysis of 62 patients (4 had to be excluded due to a withdrawal of informed consent or violation of the inclusion criteria), the differences in efficacy between the two treatment arms were so pronounced, that the trial was closed early.

Criteria	Extent of symptoms/alteration	Points
1. Pain symptoms	S = Pain at **strain**	6 / 4 / 2 / 0
(total: 30%)	N = Pain during **night time**	6 / 4 / 2 / 0
	D = Pain during **day time** (continuously)	6 / 4 / 2 / 0
	R = Pain at **rest** (following any kind of strain)	6 / 4 / 2 / 0
	I = Pain at **initiation of movement**/morning stiffness	6 / 4 / 2 / 0
per single criterion	none = 6 ; slight = 4 ; moderate = 2 ; severe = 0 points	
	⇨	
2. Use of appliances	None	15
(total: 15%)	Orthopedic shoe, insoles, heel cushion	10
	One cane or crutch	5
	Two canes or crutches	0
	⇨	
3. Professional activities	No limitation, maximum professional strain possible	20
(total: 20%)	Slight limitation, normal professional work possible	10
	Moderate limitation, reduced professional activity	5
	Severe limitation, daily professional work impossible	0
	⇨	
4. Daily/leisure activities	No limitation of daily and leisure activities and sports	15
(total: 15%)	Slightly limitation/reduced leisure activities and sports	10
	Moderate limitation/no leisure activities and sports	5
	Complete limitation of any daily and leisure activities	0
	⇨	
5. Gait/limp	No limp, normal walking is possible without a limitation	20
(total: 20%)	Slightly altered, limp after walking **> 1 km (2 blocks)**	10
	Moderately altered, limp after walking **< 1 km (2 blocks)**	5
	Severely altered, normal walking is impossible	0
	⇨	
Total score	**Sum of the single scores 1 + 2 + 3 + 4 + 5** ⇨	

Table 2. Calcaneodynia score of the GCG-BD [29], based on [31].

The mean age of patients was 54 years in the standard dose group and 58 years in the 6 × 0.1 Gy group. Sixty-one patients had a plantar, one patient a dorsal heel spur. In mean, patients in the standard dose group suffered for 15.3 months before the start of LD-EBRT, in the 6 × 0.1 Gy group for 18.8 months. Twenty-one patients had symptoms on both sides. In 28 patients the pain irradiated into the calf, only in 18 patients it was localized to the sole of the foot. Two patients had received surgery for LD-EBRT.

Three months after therapy VAS values, CS- and QOL-scores were significantly better after the standard dose in comparison with the very low dose treatment arm. The higher pain relief resulted in a better QOL. Twelve months after therapy about 64% of the patients after 6 × 0.1 Gy had to receive a second treatment series due to insufficient treatment results, in comparison with only 17% of the patients in the standard dose treatment group. As the second series was applied with a standard dose (6 × 1 Gy), patients in the 6 × 0.1 Gy group who were reirradiated showed equally favorable results compared with those in the standard-dose group who did not receive a second course [26]. This is why the second treatment series in this clinical setting acted as a "salvage therapy." Another interesting finding was that patients with a good response already at 3 months remained stable or even improved at 12 months. Furthermore, this underlines the long-lasting efficacy of LD-EBRT.

Acute side effects or long-term toxicity did not occur.

In conclusion, this randomized trial established a dose-response-relationship of the analgesic effect of LD-EBRT, thus providing a clinical and methodological proof of the efficacy of 6 × 1 Gy LD-EBRT on the clinical course of painful heel spurs. The early termination of the study was justified due the interim analysis showing significant differences in the clinical outcome between both treatment arms. Still, the trial was not blinded, so both the patients and the staff were aware of the received dose. With modern linear accelerators, a complete blinding of the staff is nearly impossible. The only option would be a shame irradiation with closed collimator jaws, reducing the dose to the unavoidable "leakage" radiation. A much easier and straight forward way was used in the above-mentioned study by application of a minimal physical dose with 0.1 Gy. Another critical point might be that only half of the patients were examined 12 months after therapy ($n = 36$). This reduces the reliability of the study results at this time point. However, this does not affect the results concerning treatment efficacy 3 months after LD-EBRT.

Another potential confounder not only in this study but also in all other published prospective and retrospective case series might be that a lot of the patients had received diverse and other conservative therapies before being referred to LD-EBRT. An interaction between one of these other treatments and LD-EBRT cannot be ruled out due to methodological reasons. This reflects clinical reality. Still, an interaction between one of these therapies and LD-EBRT is rather unlikely and counter-intuitive, as patients were referred to LD-EBRT after the clinical failure of all the other conservative treatments.

2.2.2. Looking for the minimum effective dose: optimization of fractionation and total dose of LD-EBRT

2.2.2.1. Single dose 0.5 vs. 1 Gy

Two randomized studies investigated the efficacy of 0.5 Gy single dose in comparison to 1 Gy.

The first trial was conducted by Heyd et al. [30]. They randomized 130 patients between 6 × 0.5 Gy twice weekly (low dose) and 6 × 1 Gy (standard dose). A linear accelerator was used, applying a single field technique.

Inclusion criteria were clinical signs of a painful heel spur, radiological evidence of spur formation, patient age ≥30 years and a relapse after previous conservative treatments, in patients >45 years LD-EBRT could be used as the primary treatment. Endpoints of the study were changes in the "original" calcaneodynia score [31], that was documented before LD-EBRT, at the end of the course, and 6 weeks and 6 months afterward.

One hundred and thirty patients were randomized. Mean age was 58.4 years. A 102 patients suffered from a plantar, one patient from a dorsal, and 27 patients from combined spurs. In mean, patients had been suffering from symptoms for 9.8 months. The symptoms had been present in 58 patients for less than 6 months, in 72 patients for a longer time. In 7 heels LD-EBRT was the first therapeutic approach.

At the end of LD-EBRT, 66% in the low dose group vs. 59% in the standard dose experienced an improvement in symptoms, 6 weeks later 80 vs. 85%. At this time point, 1.5% in each group reported an increase in symptoms, 19 vs. 14% no change. No statistically significant differences were noted. In case of insufficient treatment results patients were offered a second EBRT series. Thus 26 vs. 37% were treated a second time. Six weeks after that, 71 vs. 79% of these patients reported a further improvement. Six months after LD-EBRT 88% of the patients in both groups had an amelioration of their symptoms, the remaining patients reported no change. During the EBRT series a slight increase in pain was reported by 26 vs. 29% of the patients. No other acute or late toxicity occurred.

In conclusion, 6 × 0.5 Gy twice weekly was as effective as 6 × 1 Gy.

These results were confirmed by a second randomized trial [32, 33]. Ott et al. randomized 457 patients between 6 × 0.5 Gy (low dose) and 6 × 1 Gy (standard dose). In contrast to the above-cited "Heyd-study" [30] an X-ray unit (orthovoltage) and not linear accelerators was used. Patients received a single field (6 × 8 cm on the plantar calcaneus) with 150 kV, 15 mA, 1 mm Cu-filter, with source-to-skin distance (SSD) of 40 cm. Six weeks after the LD-EBRT a second series was offered to patients with an insufficient response. The endpoint was pain reduction. CS score and VAS values were measured before and at the end of LD-EBRT (early response), 6 weeks (delayed), and 2.5 years (long-term) afterward.

With a median follow-up of 32 months the mean VAS values before treatment, for early, delayed, and long-term response for the 0.5 and 1.0 Gy groups were 65.5 ± 22.1 and 64.0 ± 20.5 (p = 0.19), 34.8 ± 24.7 and 39.0 ± 26.3 (p =0.12), 25.1 ± 26.8 and 28.9 ± 26.8 (p =0.16), and 16.3 ± 24.3 and 14.1 ± 19.7 (p =0.68) [31]. Similar results were obtained for the CS score without any significant differences between both dose groups.

Taken together, the above-mentioned studies proofed an equivalent clinical efficacy of 6 × 0.5 Gy in comparison to 6 × 1 Gy, thus defining a new clinical treatment standard with six times 0.5 Gy twice weekly as the minimum effective dose.

Before proofing 0.5 Gy as the new standard single dose, another randomized study tried to increase efficacy in reaching the "old" cumulative dose of 6 Gy with a single dose of 0.5 Gy. Niewald et al. randomized between 6 × 1 Gy twice a week (old "standard dose") and 12 × 0.5 Gy three times a week ("experimental dose") [25]. The aim was not just to get comparable results, but to further improve the analgesic effects. Linear accelerators (6 MV photons) applying a lateral opposing field technique were used.

Inclusion and exclusion criteria were quite similar to the ones used in the landmark study [26]: Clinical evidence of a painful heel spur, and duration of the symptoms for more than 6 months; radiological proof of a spur formation; age at least 40 years; Karnofsky-Index at least 70%. Patients with previous radiotherapy or previous trauma to the foot, rheumatic or vascular diseases, lymphatic edema, pregnancy, breastfeeding, or severe psychiatric disorders were excluded. Concomitant therapy with analgesics was allowed. However, patients receiving surgery or shock wave therapy after randomization were excluded.

Endpoints were the SF-12 sum score, the CS sum score (**Table 2**), and VAS. Follow-up was scheduled every 6 weeks for 1 year.

Two-hundred and forty patients were calculated to detect a difference of 15% in the VAS and CS score, with a power of 80%, and an error probability of 5%. After randomization of 127 patients and an interim analysis of 107 patients, the study was closed early, as the intended increase in analgesic efficacy by the experimental treatment was very unlikely to be achieved.

The mean age of the patients in the standard group was 56.1 Gy in comparison with 58.1 Gy in the experimental group. The mean duration of symptoms before initiation of LD-EBRT was 17 vs. 16 months. In 98% of the standard group and 93% of the experimental group a plantar spur was treated, in 2 and 7% a combined (plantar and dorsal) spur.

Results after 3 months have been issued so far [25], longer follow-up has yet to be published. After 3 months, there were no significant differences neither in the VAS (standard 42.3 vs. experimental 44.4) nor the CS sum score (28 vs. 28.4) nor in the QOL (SF-12) scores. Although longer follow-up has to be awaited, a further increase in the analgesic effect by applying 12 × 0.5 Gy three times a week is unlikely. This is why this fractionation schedule is currently not recommended, as it does not follow the "as low as reasonable achievable" principle of radiation protection.

2.2.2.2. *Single dose 0.3 vs. 1 Gy*

Further reduced single doses in LD-EBRT (with the exception of 0.1 Gy [26]) have never been tested in a prospectively randomized clinical trial. In radiotherapy of degenerative joint disorders, single doses of about 0.3–0.4 Gy were established by von Pannewitz in the late 1920s and published in 1933 and 1970 [34, 35]. However, two studies on calcaneodynia have raised serious concerns on single doses as low as 0.3 Gy.

Seegenschmiedt et al. analyzed treatment efficacy in 141 patients (170 irradiated heels), who were treated from 1984–1994 with X-ray units (250 kV/200 kV, 20 mA, 40 cm SSD), applying a single field of 6 × 8 cm [24]. Seventy-two heels received 12 Gy with 6 × 1 Gy (three times a week) –6 weeks break – 6 × 1 Gy (group A), 50 heels were treated with 10 × 0.3 Gy every day (group B1), and 38 heels 10 × 0.5 Gy every day (group B2). The endpoint was the value of a semiquantitative pain score 3 months and in mean 4 years after LD-EBRT.

The median age of patients was 55 years in group A and 59 years in group B1/B2. The mean duration of symptoms before LD-EBRT was 8 months, in one-third, the symptoms persisted for more than 6 months.

Complete pain remission was achieved in 68–71% of the patients without significant differences between the treatment groups. However, there were differences in the clinical course of patients with partial remission of the symptoms: The best results in these patients were achieved during longer follow-up in group B1 (10 × 0.5 Gy), followed by group A (6 × 1–6 × 1 Gy), followed by group B2 (10 × 0.3 Gy). The latter group showed a significantly worse amelioration of symptoms than the other groups.

A reduced efficacy was also reported in another retrospective case series, comprising 673 heels treated with a single dose of 0.3 Gy three times weekly up to 1.5 Gy (X-ray) [36]. In case of insufficient treatment results the patients were offered a second course. After the first treatment, only 13% reported CR, nearly all patients had undergone a second LD-EBRT.

Taken together, to the best of our current knowledge a single dose of 0.5 Gy is standard of care and should only be modified in controlled clinical trials.

2.3. Risk factors potentially associated with treatment failure

In **Table 3** selected contemporary randomized trials and patient series are shown broken down into several factors that might be correlated with treatment efficacy. For a better overview, we did not differentiate between univariate and multivariate analyses. We did not try to collect all ever published data.

2.3.1. History of symptoms

Duration of symptoms before start of LD-EBRT has been shown to be correlated with treatment efficacy in numerous studies.

Muecke et al. analyzed in a retrospective multicenter study 502 patients [22]. Duration of symptoms ≤6 months was associated with 76% treatment success vs. 44% after a history >6 months. Also Seegenschmiedt et al. found in their large collectives a correlation between the duration of heel pain and treatment outcome [24]. A significant influence of duration of symptoms before LD-EBRT was also reported in 73 heels by Schneider et al. [37]. With a history of 3–6 months, the VAS value was reduced by 85%, 28 months after LD-EBRT in comparison with a reduction of 58% with a history > 6 months. Similar results were obtained by Hermann et al. in 285 heels comparing <12 month history of pain vs. >12 months [38].

In contrary, another study could not confirm these results [30].

2.3.2. Gender

To the best of our knowledge, in no study, an influence of gender on treatment outcome has been confirmed [22, 24, 30, 38, 39]. In contrast to radiotherapy for oncological indications with high doses, efficacy and tolerability of LD-EBRT seems to be the same concerning gender.

Study (citation)	[30]	[26]	[24]	[37]	[39]	[22]	[38]	[40]	[83]
Type	Rand	Rand	Prospect	Prospect	Retrospect	Retrospect	Retrospect	Retrospect	Retrospect
Number of heels	130	66	170	73	623	502	285	161	7947
Energy	MV	MV	KV	MV	KV	MV, KV	MV	KV	MV, KV
Target volume	calcaneus	calcaneus	calcaneus	entire dorsal and middle foot	insertion of plantar fascia	calcaneus	calcaneus vs. insertion of calcaneus	calcaneus	entire dorsal foot vs. calcaneus vs. insertion of plantar fascia
Dose	6 × 1 vs. 6 × 0.5 Gy	6 × 1 Gy vs. 6 × 0.1 Gy	12, 3, 5 Gy	5 Gy (increasing single dose)	1.5 (1–3) up to 9–12 Gy (1–45)	5–10 × 0.5–1 Gy	6 × 1 Gy6 × 0.5 Gy	6 × 1 Gy	0.3–1.5 Gy; 2–3x weekly 2.5–18.76 Gy
Potential factors									
History of symptoms	0	n.i.	+	+	0	+	+	+	+
Gender	0	n.i.	0	n.i.	0	0	0	n.i.	n.i.
Patient's age	0	n.i.	0	+	0	+	+	+	n.i.
Initial worsening of pain during LD-EBRT	n.i.	n.i.	n.i.	n.i.	n.i.	n.i.	n.i.	n.i.	n.i.
MV vs. KV	n.i.	n.i.	n.i.	n.i.	n.i.	+	n.i.	n.i.	0
Number of therapy series	n.i.	n.i.	n.i.	+	n.i.	+	n.i.	n.i.	+
Heel stress during LD-EBRT	n.i.	0	n.i.	+	n.i.	n.i.	n.i.	n.i.	n.i.

Note: 0: no correlation with treatment outcome; +: correlation with treatment outcome; n.i.: not investigated; prospect: prospective case series; rand: randomized clinical trial; retrospect: retrospective case series; KV: kilovoltage; MV: megavoltage.

Table 3. Factors associated with treatment efficacy in contemporary studies.

2.3.3. *Patients' age*

Several studies described a correlation between older age and better treatment results, at least 6 weeks after LD-EBRT [37]. Age somewhat over 50 years seems to be important: >50 years [40], > 53 [38], or > 58 [22]. For a possible explanation see Section 2.3.7.

However, other studies found no influence of this patient characteristic on treatment outcome [24, 30, 39].

2.3.4. *Initial increase in pain during LD-EBRT*

A very precise registration of changes in pain intensity (VAS) was done by Schneider at al. [37]. Sixty-two patients (73 treated heels) were prospectively scored every week during LD-EBRT, at the end of therapy, 6 weeks, 28 months, and 40 months later. Additionally, subjective mechanical heel stress during LD-EBRT was estimated. A linear accelerator (10 MV) was used, applying one single field with a size of 12 × 17 cm. Patients were treated twice a week to a total dose of 5 Gy, with increasing single fraction doses (0.25 – 0.25 – 0.5 – 1 – 1 – 1 – 1 Gy). Mean patient age was 54 years, and all had a radiologically proven plantar spurn, mean symptom duration before LD-EBRT was 6.5 months. Nearly all patients had received other conservative therapies before LD-EBRT with insufficient results.

Interestingly, VAS scores decreased continuously during LD-EBRT: before treatment the mean value was 6.3 ± 1.5, after the first week of LD-EBRT 6.2 ± 1.8, after the second week 5.5 ± 2 ($p <$ 0.05), after the third 4.7 ± 2.4, and 3.8 ± 2.1 at the end of therapy ($p < 0.001$). Six weeks later the value further decreased to 3 ± 2.5 ($p < 0.004$), 28 months after LD-EBRT to 1.6 ± 2.2 ($p < 0.01$). One year later no further decrease was noticed (1.8 ± 2.3). Only two patients reported intensification of pain during the LD-EBRT series. However, these data are not to be extrapolated, as increasing single doses (see above) were used to avoid this phenomenon.

In standard schedules with fixed single doses a slight increase in pain during the treatment series was reported by 26% (during 6 × 0.5 Gy) vs. 29% (6 × 1 Gy) of the patients [30]. Unfortunately, a possible correlation of this phenomenon with definite treatment results was not investigated.

Without further quantification, another study (6 × 1 vs. 6 × 0.1 Gy) stated, that this initial increase in symptoms "had no influence on the final pain relief 3 and 12 months after treatment" [26]. Older studies postulated a temporary reduction of the pH value in the irradiated tissues at the beginning of the treatment series, without consequences for the long-term efficacy of LD-EBRT [41].

This is contrasted by observations of LD-EBRT in peritendinitis humeroscapularis [42]. In 73 patients (86 shoulders) initial increase of pain during the treatment course was significantly associated with a good response.

2.3.5. *Use of megavoltage techniques/linear accelerators*

Muecke et al. analyzed in a retrospective multicenter study the influence of different treatment techniques in 502 patients [22]. Treatment failure was defined as pain persistence after

LD-EBRT and recurrence of pain during follow-up. Treatment with MV (6–10 MV) was a significant prognostic factor for pain relief in multivariate analysis, as MV was associated with an eight-year event-free probability of 68 vs. 61% after X-ray beams (175 kV). There are two possible explanations for this finding: besides the possibility of a random result, the authors postulate a more homogenous dose distribution with MV treatment in comparison with KV [22].

2.3.6. Number of therapy courses required

Schneider et al. reported an efficacy of just one-third after a second LD-EBRT course (so-called "re-irradiation") in comparison with the effects of the first course [37]. Out of 73 heels treated with 5 Gy LD-EBRT 18 heels received reirradiation due to insufficient treatment response. However, pain reduction measured by means of changes in VAS shortly after the second course and during long-term follow-up was significantly diminished in comparison with the efficacy of the first course (about 30% reduction in pain at the last evaluation vs. 86%).

Similar results were obtained in the large retrospective series (502 patients) by Muecke et al. [22]. Treatment failure was significantly associated with the number of treatment series: eight-year event-free probability was about 70% after the first course in comparison with just about 30% after reirradiation.

A systematic study on the efficacy of a reirradiation has been published by Hautmann et al. [43]. Eighty-three patients (101 heels) with insufficient response to the first course or recurrent pain afterward due to plantar fasciitis (83 heels), or achillodynia (28 heels) received a second LD-EBRT course in median 10 weeks (range 4 weeks to 63 months) after the first LD-EBRT. About 75% of the patients were treated with 6 × 1 Gy, the others 6 × 0.5 Gy. The pain was assessed using the numeric rating scale (NRS) before and at the end of LD-EBRT, 6, and 12 weeks, and 6, 12, and 24 months thereafter.

Before reirradiation NRS values were 6 (interquartile range 5–8), at the end of LD-EBRT 5 (2–6), 6 weeks later 2 (1–4), at 12 weeks 1 (0–3), at 6 months 0 (0–2), at 12 and 24 months 0 (0–1). Interestingly, not only the patients with recurrent pain after the first course but also patients with insufficient responses to the first course experienced a profound and long-lasting amelioration of their symptoms after the second course.

This is why a second treatment course should be recommended in case of insufficient efficacy of the first course.

2.3.7. Heel stress during LD-EBRT

A significant correlation between avoidance of heel stress during LD-EBRT and efficacy of LD-EBRT 6 weeks after therapy was reported by Schneider et al. in 73 heels [37]. With a Pearson's correlation coefficient of -0.467 ($p < 0.01$) there was an impressing influence of this variable on pain reduction measured by VAS values. However, this correlation was not seen 28 and 40 months after LD-EBRT.

An intuitive explanation is given by the authors [37]: As patient age was associated with positive treatment results, too, they proposed that older patients are often retired, thus being able to take more care of their heels.

2.3.8. *Spur size*

Interestingly, all randomized trials required the radiological proof of a heel spur before including patients into the studies. Furthermore, most of the prospective and retrospective series warranted such an objective sign. However, as a substantial part of the patients suffers from plantar heel pain without having developed a heel spur, LD-EBRT should be effective in these patients, too.

Hermann et al. analyzed treatment efficacy in 250 patients (285 heels), who received LD-EBRT predominantly with 6 × 1 Gy [38]. In this series, 33% of the treated heels were without radiological evidence of a spur. In 185 patients a spur was confirmed with a mean length of 6.5 mm (range 0.6–25 mm). Patients without evidence of a plantar heel spur had a significantly higher chance of CR after LD-EBRT (43 vs. 35%). Furthermore, the length of the spurs correlated directly with treatment outcome. Spurs >6.5 mm had just a 30% chance of experiencing CR in comparison with shorter ones. No statistical differences were found between treatment results of heels without spurs and those with spurs ≤6.5 mm.

Miszczyk et al. reported on 327 patients (623 LD-EBRT series) mostly treated with X-ray (180 kV, usually 1mm Cu filters) with single doses of 1.5 Gy (range 1–3 Gy) up to a total dose between 9 and 12 Gy (range 1–45 Gy) [39]. Mean spur size was 9 mm (range 1–30 mm). With a mean follow-up of 74 months, no correlation between spur size and duration of pain relief was found. Analysis concerning spur length and treatment outcome in itself were unfortunately not reported.

2.3.9. *The combination of different factors*

Multivariate logistic regression enables the identification of factors independently predicting treatment outcome. By combining these factors, models can be calculated, that predict treatment outcome with a high probability. An example from the study of Hermann et al. is given in **Table 4**: in 285 heels treated with 6 × 1 Gy/6 × 0.5 Gy the influences of the patient characteristics age, spur length, and duration of symptoms before LD-EBRT alone and in combination were calculated [38]. The best results were obtained for patients > 53 years, spur length <6 mm, and a duration of symptoms <12 months with a probability for CR of 55% (CI 36–73%) and PR of 38% (CI 22–58%). Without these characteristics, the chance for CR was just 18% (CI 9–33%), for PR 31% (17–48%).

2.4. Technique

In modern radiotherapeutic departments, X-ray sources are less and less available. This is why nowadays most patients are treated with linear accelerators, which were initially developed for the treatment of oncological diseases. However, these machines can be used in the treatment of benign diseases without any modifications or problems. Due to the high efforts in physical, technical, and organizational quality assurances for the operation of an accelerator or an X-ray source, the concentration on accelerators and their use for all indications is recommended.

Patient's age >53	No spur or spur ≤6.5 mm	Duration of symptoms <12 months	Probability of		
			No change	Partial remission	Complete remission
1	1	1	0.07 (0.03–0.14)	0.38 (0.22–0.58)	0.55 (0.36–0.73)
1	1	0	0.13 (0.07–0.28)	0.37 (0.21–0.57)	0.50 (0.30–0.70)
1	0	1	0.15 (0.06–0.24)	0.53 (0.33–0.72)	0.32 (0.17–0.53)
1	0	0	0.25 (0.13–0.45)	0.48 (0.27–0.69)	0.27 (0.13–0.48)
0	1	1	0.17 (0.10–0.31)	0.33 (0.19–0.50)	0.50 (0.33–0.66)
0	1	0	0.34 (0.20–0.53)	0.40 (0.24–0.59)	0.26 (0.13–0.45)
0	0	1	0.30 (0.20–0.46)	0.29 (0.18–0.43)	0.41 (0.27–0.56)
0	0	0	0.51 (0.35–0.69)	0.31 (0.17–0.48)	0.18 (0.09–0.33)

Table 4. Probabilities (95%-CI) for NC, PR and CR calculated by polytomous logistic regression in dependence of the risk factors age, spur length, and duration of symptoms before LD-EBRT according to Hermann et al. in a collective of 285 heels treated with 6 × 1/6 × 0.5 Gy (taken from [38]).

For irradiation of the heel, the patient has to be placed on the treatment couch with the feet toward the gantry of the accelerator (so-called "feet first"). Two different patient positions are widely used. He can be placed in supine position, with the irradiated leg is stretched out, while the other leg is angled. Another option is to place the patient in a lateral decubitus position on the side of the involved heel. Again, the symptomatic leg is stretched, while the contralateral leg is bent, with a cushion placed beneath the knee. Using X-rays, the ipsilateral knee is bent by 90% and the foot is positioned on the treatment table. One anterior-posterior (AP) beam is usually applied in this technique.

For the treatment itself, there are also two different options. Irradiation may be given as a single stationary field (SSD 100cm by convention). Alternatively, parallel opposing fields from 0° and 180° gantry position (in decubitus position) or lateral opposing fields (90° and 270° in supine position) are also applicable but take a little bit longer in daily clinical practice. The hypothetical advantage of using two opposing fields is a uniform dose distribution in the entire beam path in the calcaneus (**Figure 1**). However, there has never been a clinical proof, whether this theoretical assumption translates into any clinical advantage for the patient. When applying opposing fields, the dose is specified according to the ICRU 50 report, normally in the center of the calcaneus.

A third option is the so-called "plantar field" with the patient lying in prone position. A single field is positioned directly over the plantar insertion/calcaneus, potentially with rotations of the patient table and the gantry to compensate for inclinations of the patients surface in the irradiated field. However, this technique is regarded problematic when using linear accelerators due to the dose build-up effect in the critical tissue depth. This problem is illustrated in **Figure 2**: photons with 6 MV reach just the half of the prescribed dose at the skin level, 100% is reached at 1.5 cm tissue depth. This would result in an insufficient dose in the critical structures (plantar fascia and heel spur). To overcome this problem, a silicone flap of about 1 cm diameter must be positioned on the skin before radiation.

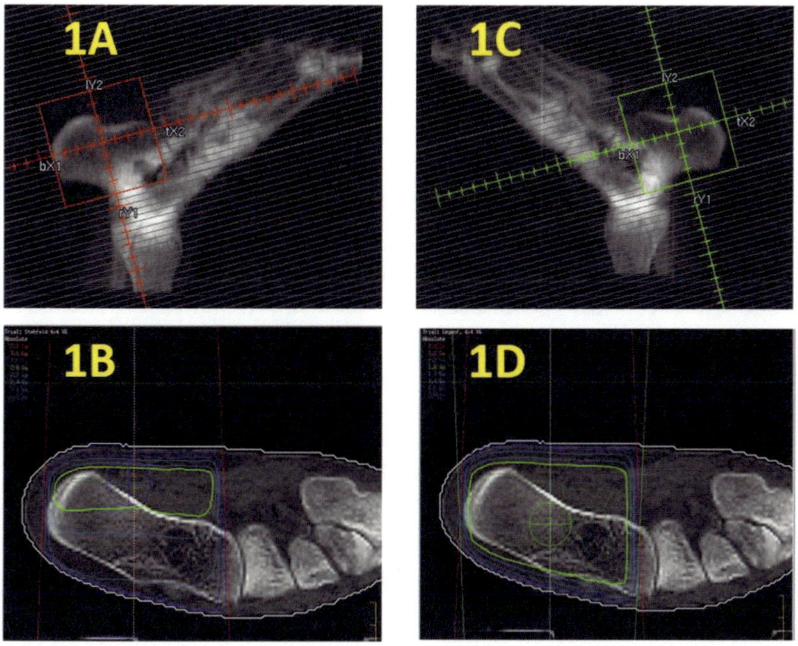

Figure 1. Dose distribution of two different treatment techniques generated in a treatment planning system (XIO®). In A and B just one single 6 MV photon field (8 × 8 cm) is applied, while C and D shows the dose distribution with two opposing fields from 0 and 180°. In the upper row, the so-called "beams eye views" are given, while in the lower row the respective dose distributions on an axial CT scan directly at the calcaneal insertion are shown. Note the more uniform dose distribution with opposing fields. The 95% isodose is given as a green line (2.85 Gy). This dose encompasses larger parts of the calcaneal bone in D (opposing fields) than in B (single field). More information is given in Section 2.4.

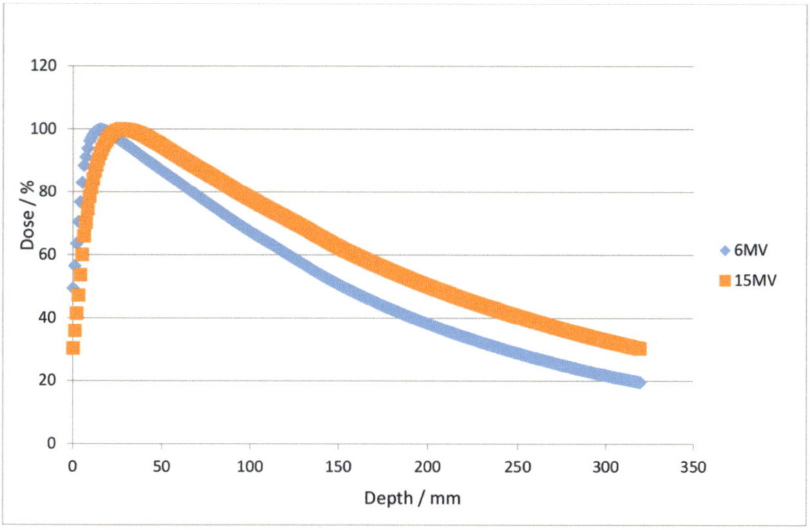

Figure 2. Depth curves of different megavoltage energies. Blue 6 MV photons, red 15 MV photons. At the surface of the body/skin (depth 0 mm), only half (or even less with 15 MV) of the prescribed dose is applied. By physical interactions between photons and the tissue/water, there is a steep increase in dose. A 100% is reached at 1.5 cm depth with 6 MV and at about 3 cm depth with 15 MV. KV-radiation reaches the maximum dose directly under the surface/skin (not shown). More information is given in Section 2.4.

3. Toxicity and potential risks of LD-EBRT

Patients are often sent to the radiotherapist after a long unsuccessful history of diverse conservative treatments. The reason for this is a widespread fear among general practitioners that LD-EBRT might be associated with severe side effects and risks. These fears are not substantiated, as reactions of the nerves or vessels require much higher doses than used for LD-EBRT. For example, a dose of 45 Gy in normofractionated oncological therapy is considered to be safe for the spinal cord and therefore daily clinical practice [44]. Peripheral nerves are even more radioresistant. Acute or chronic side-effects have never been reported in all contemporary studies on LD-EBRT.

3.1. Acute reactions of the skin

Acute side effects are negligible, as very low doses of ionizing radiation (in comparison with oncological treatments) are applied to a distal extremity. The total dose of LD-EBRT with 3 or 6 Gy is far too low to cause any acute or late reactions on the skin overlaying the calcaneus. During normofractionated EBRT (single doses of 1.8–2 Gy, treatment on 5 days a week) erythema and mild edema develop at about 30 Gy [45]. Hyperpigmentation occurs at about 45 Gy, moist epitheliolyses at about 50 Gy. A 50–60 Gy might cause telangiectasias years after the therapy. This is why there is no report on acute treatment side effects in LD-EBRT until now to the best of our knowledge.

3.2. Initial increase in pain during LD-EBRT

About one-third of the patients might experience a slight increase in pain during LD-EBRT. In the randomized trial by Heydt et al. this phenomenon was seen in 26% (during 6 × 0.5 Gy) vs. 29% (6 × 1 Gy) [30]. It does not seem to be correlated with treatment outcome; further detailed information is given in Section 2.3.4.

3.3. Impairment of gonad function

The dose scattered to the male gonads is somewhat higher than to the ovaries. Jansen et al. calculated for 6 × 0.5 Gy about 1.5 mSv received by the testes and 0.75 mSv to the ovaries [46]. Comparable results have repeatedly been measured in the past [47, 48].

Taken together, the dose received by the gonads is insignificant. As the distal extremity is irradiated, scattered dose to the gonads is comparable to normal diagnostic radiological imaging [49]. The hereditary effects of these doses are very small and very likely negligible [46].

Although spermatogonial cells are very radiosensitive, a single dose of at least 100 mSv is needed to induce a temporary failure of spermatogenesis [50]. A single dose of 1000 mSv (equivalent to 1 Gy photon irradiation) results in an azoospermia for 9–18 months [51]. Interestingly, fractionated doses harm these cells even more. A temporary oligospermia is reported after receiving several fractions up to a cumulative dose of 160 mSv [52]. An azoospermia lasting for 14–22 months has been reported for fractionated doses of 620–860 mSv [53]. The actually during LD-EBRT received testicular dose is about 100 times smaller than the lowest dose causing temporary changes in testicular tissues.

The dose to the testicles can be further reduced by utilizing a special testicular shielding. However, clinically meaningful dose reductions have been only measured in MV treatment of subdiaphragmatic/pelvine lymphatic regions or tumors [54, 55].

The mean lethal dose for human oocytes has been estimated at 2 Gy (2000 mSv) [56]. Permanent ovarian failure after radiotherapy is age dependent: in perimenopausal women, a dose of 6 Gy is sufficient [57], while in younger women up to 20 Gy are tolerated. The dose scattered to the ovaries during LD-EBRT for calcaneodynia cannot cause such sequelae (0.75 mSv).

Naturally, pregnancy has to be excluded in all premenopausal women before beginning with LD-EBRT, to avoid any risk to the fetus.

3.4. Induction of malignancies

So far, no studies with long-term observation periods have been published, describing a case of malignancy induced by LD-EBRT for calcaneodynia. However, induction of malignancies is a stochastic effect of ionizing radiation. This means that there is no threshold dose—in contrast for example to the above-mentioned reactions of the skin. A photon can accidentally trigger a mutation, which in turn leads to tumor formation many years later. The higher the radiation dose, the higher the probability of such an event occurring.

The best available data on tumor induction of full dose EBRT in oncology has been collected in patients treated with breast cancer. Almost 11,000 patients have been followed for over 20 years. The risk of a radiation-induced tumor was approx. 1% per decade after radiotherapy [58].

To estimate the risk associated with much lower doses of LD-EBRT, mathematical models on the basis of epidemiological long-term observations of atomic bomb victims have been developed by the ICRP [59].

Jansen et al. applied the ICRP model on LD-EBRT of a painful heel spur [46]. Assumed was a single field entering at the foot sole with a size of 8 × 10 cm, 200 kV photons, SSD 40 cm. For an LD-EBRT series with 6 × 1 Gy the average attributable lifetime risk for induction of a fatal tumor was calculated to be about 0.5 in a thousand patients. An important risk factor for radiogenic-induced cancer is the patient's age by the time the radiation exposure occurs. The risk is already reduced in the 3rd decade of the patient's life, it starts to decrease steadily from the age of 40 [60]. Applying these calculations, the estimated lifetime risk per one thousand patients for a fatal tumor accounts for the age of 25 0.6 (male)/0.8 (female), for the age of 50 0.2/0.3, for the age of 75 0.07/0.1 [46].

However, it must be critically noted that this mathematical model was developed for radiation protection and relates to the exposure of complete organ systems with approx. 1 Gy. Therefore, other groups argue that a significantly lower risk of radiogenic cancer induction—approx. ten times less—should be adopted [49, 61]. Furthermore, taken the new standard scheme with 6 × 0.5 Gy into account, these risks are additionally halved.

This risk (max. 1/1000, very likely much lower) must be seen in relation to the tumor risk of the not additionally radiotherapeutical-treated population. In 2008, the lifetime risk of a man in Germany to suffer from cancer was 50.7% (25.9% to die from malignancy), in women 42.8% and 20.2% respectively [62].

By limiting the application of LD-EBRT treatment to patients > 30 years of age, an exposure of the juvenile "relatively higher risk" patient population is avoided.

4. Future perspectives: Definition of questions in further randomized trials and future research

4.1. Target volume definition in LD-EBRT

Traditionally target volume definition has been quite large. Field sizes of 12 × 17cm were treated, including the entire dorsal and middle foot, and not just the calcaneus [37, 82] (**Figure 3A**).

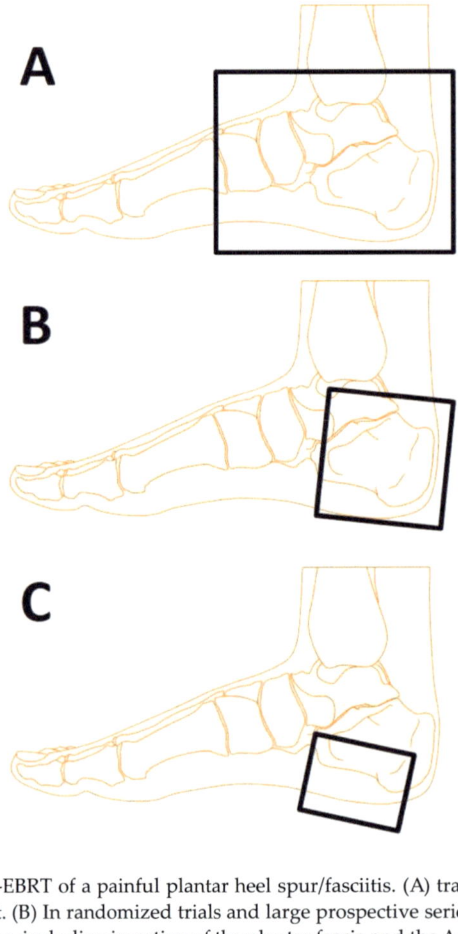

Figure 3. Field definitions in LD-EBRT of a painful plantar heel spur/fasciitis. (A) traditional field definition including the entire dorsal and middle foot. (B) In randomized trials and large prospective series commonly used field definition encompassing the entire calcaneus, including insertion of the plantar fascia and the Achilles tendon. (C) Proposed small field definition for localized painful plantar fasciitis/plantar spur, encompassing only the painful area with 2 cm margins extending into the neighboring areas (calcaneus, fascia, fat pad).

In the recent randomized trials and prospective observational studies target volume definition was more restricted and confined to the calcaneus (**Figure 3B**). "The target volume consisted of the calcaneus and the region of the plantar aponeurosis" [26]. "The ventral margin is corresponding to the ventral surface of the calcaneus, the plantar and dorsal margins are surrounding the soft-tissue border, and the cranial margin is below the ankle" [30]. "Target volume is the calcaneus, normally with a field size of 6 cm × 8 cm" [32]. "The calcaneus and the plantar aponeurosis were included in the target volume" [25].

In a German national survey 2001 on LD-EBRT of painful heel spurs the target volume definition "large" (dorsal and middle foot) vs. "small" (entire calcaneus) was not correlated with treatment outcome [83]. Consequently, very large field definitions should be regarded as obsolete.

However, as the pathophysiological cause of calcaneodynia is thought to be a localized inflammatory process (see Section 1), it is questionable, whether the entire calcaneus has to be irradiated (as long as there are not a plantar as well as a painful dorsal spurs). There are some clinical data that support a further restriction of target volume definition.

Field sizes have been given in the study by Miszczyk et al. on 327 patients treated with X-ray beams [39]. Target volume was "… the insertion of the plantar fascia with a calcaneal spur and a reasonable margin. The field size varied from 27 to 150 cm^2 (mean 47 cm^2)." However, although not explicitly stated, no correlation was found between field size and duration of pain relief after LD-EBRT. Treatment efficacy in itself was apparently not investigated.

In the above-mentioned series of 285 heels Hermann et al. analyzed treatment efficacy in dependence of field sizes, too [38]. The mean field size was 74 cm^2. No correlation between field size (smaller vs. larger than 74 cm^2) with treatment efficacy was found. Further analyses of small fields (< 6 × 6 cm), medium-sized fields (36–64 cm^2) and larger fields revealed no significant differences.

This is why it seems to suffice to encompass the painful region with 2 cm margins extending into the neighboring areas (calcaneus, fascia, fat pad; **Figure 3C**). However, this recommendation is deducted from pathophysiological considerations and the above-mentioned case series. A randomized trial is necessary to proof clinical equivalence of a field definition "entire calcaneus" (**Figure 3B**) vs. "insertion of the plantar fascia" (**Figure 3C**).

4.2. Fractionation of LD-EBRT

The optimal fractionation schedule has not been elucidated yet. All randomized trial used twice weekly treatments. Only one experimental arm was scheduled three times a week [25]. In a National Survey in Germany with 146 answering institutions, about 45% applied two fractions and 37.5% three fractions weekly [83].

Interestingly, in the landmark study by von Pannewitz a fractionation schedule of only once per week was established [34]. Until now, there is no proof of a higher efficacy applying LD-EBRT twice or three times per week.

In radiotherapy of another benign disease (endocrine orbitopathy) a 1 Gy per week over 20 weeks schedule was more effective than the standard schedules (10 × 2 Gy or 10 × 1 Gy every working day) [84]. Although other immunological mechanisms cause endocrine orbitopathy in comparison with plantar fasciitis, there is sufficient clinical evidence to test in a randomized trial different fractionation schedules (twice a week vs. once a week, possibly thrice a week).

4.3. Comparison of LD-EBRT with other therapies

Other therapies than LD-EBRT have been applied in painful heel spur. In the following, just a rough overview can be given.

Different kinds of insoles and foot orthoses have been developed. The goal was to reduce plantar contact pressure and to distribute the pressure uniformly over the whole rearfoot [63]. Magnetic insoles do not seem to provide additional benefit [64]. As a short-term treatment, low-Dye taping techniques are often used. However, in a randomized trial only a modest improvement in 'first-step' pain was seen in comparison with sham-intervention [65].

Manual stretching is often recommended. A systematic review of six studies found only statistically significant differences in comparison with the control in one study combining calf muscle and plantar fascia stretches [66].

Several trials have investigated acupuncture. A systematic review from 2010 showed (limited) evidence for the effectiveness [67]. A randomized trial published in 2014 recruited 84 patients [68]. The authors concluded, that "dry needling provided statistically significant reductions in plantar heel pain, but the magnitude of this effect should be considered against the frequency of minor transitory adverse events."

Ultrasound therapy has led to questionable results [69], but a randomized trial on cryo-ultrasound with about 100 patients published in 2014 showed good effectiveness [70].

Low-level laser light (635 nm), given twice a week for a total of six applications, reduced in a randomized trial VAS scores significantly after 8 weeks in comparison with placebo [71]. However, the study comprised of just 69 patients; other similar studies have not been reported so far.

Extracorporeal shock waves are widely applied. Three metaanalyses comprising at least five randomized trials found significant short-term pain relief and improved functional outcomes for this therapeutic option [72–74]. Another study compared the analgesic efficacy of ultrasound and shock wave therapy in 47 patients [75]. The results suggested that the shock wave therapy had greater analgesic efficacy.

Another basic approach is the oral administration of nonsteroidal anti-inflammatory drugs (NSAID) to achieve a symptomatic relief. Injections into the painful area are also recommended. A recent review summarized ten randomized trials on corticosteroid injections into the plantar fascia [76]. A significant effect of the steroids on the pain has been shown. However, it was usually short-term, lasting 4–12 weeks in duration. No advantage of ultrasound-guided injection techniques in comparison with palpation guidance was found, and no superiority of one type of corticosteroid over another was seen. A longer lasting pain relief has been suggested by a small randomized trial of botulinum toxin injections [77]. Another option is the injection of autologous platelet-rich plasma. A recent review identified three randomized trials, all showing promising results [78]. However, a very small trial challenged this method of plasma preparation, as the same clinical effectivity was observed after the injection of whole blood [79].

Different surgical approaches have been developed. Releases of the plantar fascia are done, in some studies combined with a spur resection [80]. Due to a probably faster recovery after surgery with comparable functional results endoscopic procedures are recommended nowadays [81]. Surgery is usually indicated after failure of conservative therapies as the ultimate "salvage-therapy."

There is only a limited amount of studies randomizing patients between LD-EBRT and the above-mentioned alternative therapies.

Canyilmaz et al. randomized 123 patients between LD-EBRT (6 × 1 Gy, three times a week) and 1 ml injection of 40 mg methylprednisolone and 0.5 ml 60 mg 1% lidocaine under the guidance of palpation [85]. After 3 and 6 months, VAS values and CS-scores were compared between both groups. After 3 months, the results in the radiotherapy arm were significantly superior compared with those after injections.

To corroborate these findings, similar studies should be conducted. Furthermore, more studies randomizing LD-EBRT against other therapies (e.g. extracorporeal shock waves) are needed. A minimum size of 50 patients per treatment arm should be assured to gain more statistically relevant results. Recruiting patients without prior excessive other therapies for these studies would be optimal.

The goal must be an evidence-based algorithm defining the therapeutic sequence of the different conservative treatment modalities for plantar fasciitis.

5. Conclusions

LD-EBRT for painful plantar fasciitis/heel spur is an effective and safe treatment option for patients over 30 years of age and after exclusion of pregnancy. A fractionation of 6 × 0.5 Gy twice weekly up to a total dose of 3 Gy is currently recommended. In the case of an insufficient response a second course can be offered to the patient.

Randomized trials on target volume definition and further optimization of LD-EBRT fractionation are currently in the process of planning. Further trials to compare the different conservative therapies for plantar fasciitis with each other are necessary to allow the development of an evidence-based treatment algorithm.

Acknowledgements

This chapter is dedicated to Professor Gisela Hermann-Brennecke on the occasion of her 70th birthday.

Abbreviations

AP	anterior-posterior
CI	confidence interval
CR	complete remission
CS	Calcaneodynia score
Cu	chemical element symbol for copper
EC	endothelial cells
GCG-BD	German Cooperative Group on Radiotherapy for Benign Diseases
Gy	Gray
ICRP	International Commission on Radiological Protection
IL	interleukin
iNOS	inducible nitric oxide synthases
KV	kilovoltage
LD-EBRT	low dose external beam radiotherapy
mA	milliampere
mRNA	messenger ribonuclein acid
mSv	milliSievert
MV	megavoltage
NC	no change
NF-κB	nuclear factor kappa B
NO	nitric oxide
NSAID	non-steroidal anti-inflammatory drug
PBMC	peripheral blood mononuclear cells
PR	partial remission
QOL	quality of life
ROS	reactive oxygen species
SSD	skin-to-source distance
TGF-β_1	transforming growth factor β_1
VAS	visual analogue scale

Author details

Robert Michael Hermann[1, 2]*, Frank Bruns[2] and Mirko Nitsche[1, 3]

*Address all correspondence to: hermann@strahlentherapie-westerstede.com

1 Center for Radiotherapy and Radiooncology, Bremen and Westerstede, Westerstede, Germany

2 Department of Radiotherapy and Special Oncology, Hannover Medical School, Hannover, Germany

3 Department of Radiotherapy, Karl-Lennert Cancer Center, University of Schleswig-Holstein, Kiel, Germany

References

[1] Yi TI, Lee GE, Seo IS, Huh WS, Yoon TH, Kim BR. Clinical characteristics of the causes of plantar heel pain. Ann Rehabil Med. 2011;**35**:507–513. DOI: 10.5535/arm.2011.35.4.507

[2] Irving DB, Cook JL, Young MA, Menz HB. Obesity and pronated foot type may increase the risk of chronic plantar heel pain: a matched case-control study. BMC Musculoskelet Disord. 2007;**8**:41. DOI: 10.1186/1471-2474-8-41

[3] Sahin N, Oztürk A, Atıcı T. Foot mobility and plantar fascia elasticity in patients with plantar fasciitis. Acta Orthop Traumatol Turc. 2010;**44**:385–91. DOI: 10.3944/AOTT.2010.2348

[4] Menz HB, Zammit GV, Landorf KB, Munteanu SE. Plantar calcaneal spurs in older people: longitudinal traction or vertical compression? J Foot Ankle Res. 2008;**1**:7. DOI: 10.1186/1757-1146-1-7

[5] McMillan AM, Landorf KB, Barrett JT, Menz HB, Bird AR. Diagnostic imaging for chronic plantar heel pain: a systematic review and meta-analysis. J Foot Ankle Res. 2009;**2**:32. DOI: 10.1186/1757-1146-2-32

[6] Kumai T, Benjamin M. Heel spur formation and the subcalcaneal enthesis of the plantar fascia. J Rheumatol. 2002;**29**:1957–1964. PMID:12233893

[7] Plettner P. [Exostoses of the calcaneus]. Jahresber Ges Natur Heilkunde. 1900.

[8] McGonagle D, Wakefield RJ, Tan AL, D'Agostino MA, Toumi H, Hayashi K, Emery P, Benjamin M. Distinct topography of erosion and new bone formation in achilles tendon enthesitis: implications for understanding the link between inflammation and bone formation in spondylarthritis. Arthritis Rheum. 2008;**58**:2694–2699. DOI: 10.1002/art.23755

[9] Thomas JL, Christensen JC, Kravitz SR, Mendicino RW, Schuberth JM, Vanore JV, Weil LS Sr, Zlotoff HJ, Bouché R, Baker J; American College of Foot and Ankle Surgeons heel pain committee. The diagnosis and treatment of heel pain: a clinical practice guideline-revision 2010. J Foot Ankle Surg. 2010;**49**(3 Suppl):S1–19. DOI: 10.1053/j.jfas.2010.01.001

[10] Trott KR. Therapeutic effects of low radiation doses. Strahlenther Onkol. 1994;**170**:1–12. PMID: 8303572

[11] Hermann RM, Wolff HA, Jarry H, Thelen P, Gruendker C, Rave-Fraenk M, Schmidberger H, Christiansen H. In vitro studies on the modification of low-dose hyper-radiosensitivity in prostate cancer cells by incubation with genistein and estradiol. Radiat Oncol. 2008;**3**:19. DOI: 10.1186/1748-717X-3-19

[12] Kern P, Keilholz L, Forster C, Seegenschmiedt MH, Sauer R, Herrmann M. In vitro apoptosis in peripheral blood mononuclear cells induced by low-dose radiotherapy displays a discontinuous dose-dependence. Int J Radiat Biol. 1999;**75**:995–1003. PMID: 10465365

[13] Kern PM, Keilholz L, Forster C, Hallmann R, Herrmann M, Seegenschmiedt MH. Low-dose radiotherapy selectively reduces adhesion of peripheral blood mononuclear cells to endothelium in vitro. Radiother Oncol. 2000;**54**:273–282. PMID: 10738086

[14] Roedel F, Kley N, Beuscher HU, Hildebrandt G, Keilholz L, Kern P, Voll R, Herrmann M, Sauer R. Anti-inflammatory effect of low-dose X-irradiation and the involvement of a TGF-beta1-induced down-regulation of leukocyte/endothelial cell adhesion. Int J Radiat Biol. 2002;**78**:711–719. DOI: 10.1080/09553000210137671

[15] Arenas M, Gil F, Gironella M, Hernández V, Jorcano S, Biete A, Piqué JM, Panés J. Anti-inflammatory effects of low-dose radiotherapy in an experimental model of systemic inflammation in mice. Int J Radiat Oncol Biol Phys. 2006;**66**:560–567. DOI: 10.1016/j.ijrobp.2006.06.004

[16] Roedel F, Hantschel M, Hildebrandt G, Schultze-Mosgau S, Rödel C, Herrmann M, Sauer R, Voll RE. Dose-dependent biphasic induction and transcriptional activity of nuclear factor kappa B (NF-kappaB) in EA.hy.926 endothelial cells after low-dose X-irradiation. Int J Radiat Biol. 2004;**8**:115–123. DOI: 10.1080/09553000310001654701

[17] Roedel F, Schaller U, Schultze-Mosgau S, Beuscher HU, Keilholz L, Herrmann M, Voll R, Sauer R, Hildebrandt G. The induction of TGF-beta(1) and NF-kappaB parallels a biphasic time course of leukocyte/endothelial cell adhesion following low-dose X-irradiation. Strahlenther Onkol. 2004;**180**:194–200. DOI: 10.1007/s00066-004-1237-y

[18] Hildebrandt G, Loppnow G, Jahns J, Hindemith M, Anderegg U, Saalbach A, Kamprad F. Inhibition of the iNOS pathway in inflammatory macrophages by low-dose X-irradiation in vitro. Is there a time dependence? Strahlenther Onkol. 2003;**179**:158–166. DOI: 10.1007/s00066-003-1044-x

[19] Schaue D, Marples B, Trott KR. The effects of low-dose X-irradiation on the oxidative burst in stimulated macrophages. Int J Radiat Biol. 2002;**78**:567–576. DOI: 10.1080/09553000210126457

[20] Roedel F, Keilholz L, Herrmann M, Sauer R, Hildebrandt G. Radiobiological mechanisms in inflammatory diseases of low-dose radiation therapy. Int J Radiat Biol. 2007;**83**:357–366. DOI: 10.1080/09553000210137671

[21] Pokorny, L.: [X-ray treatment of the calcaneal spur]. Fortschr. Röntgenstr. 1937;**56**:61–66.

[22] Muecke R, Micke O, Reichl B, Heyder R, Prott FJ, Seegenschmiedt MH, Glatzel M, Schneider O, Schäfer U, Kundt G. Demographic, clinical and treatment related predictors for event-free probability following low-dose radiotherapy for painful heel spurs—a retrospective multicenter study of 502 patients. Acta Oncol. 2007;**46**:239–246. DOI: 10.1080/02841860600731935

[23] Goldie I, Rosengren B, Moberg E, Hedelin F. Evaluation of the radiation treatment of painful conditions of the locomotor system. Acta Radiol Ther Phys Biol. 1970;**9**:311–322. DOI: 10.3109/02841867009129108

[24] Seegenschmiedt MH, Keilholz L, Katalinic A, Stecken A, Sauer R. Heel spur: radiation therapy for refractory pain—results with three treatment concepts. Radiology 1996;**200**:271–276. DOI: 10.1148/radiology.200.1.8657925

[25] Niewald M, Holtmann H, Prokein B, Hautmann MG, Rösler HP, Graebe S, Dzierma Y, Ruebe C, Fleckenstein J. Randomized multicenter follow-up trial on the effect of radiotherapy on painful heel spur (plantar fasciitis) comparing two fractionation schedules with uniform total dose: first results after three months' follow-up. Radiat Oncol. 2015;**10**:174. DOI: 10.1186/s13014-015-0471-z

[26] Niewald M, Seegenschmiedt MH, Micke O, Graeber S, Muecke R, Schaefer V, Scheid C, Fleckenstein J, Licht N, Ruebe C; German Cooperative Group on Radiotherapy for Benign Diseases (GCGBD) of the German Society for Radiation Oncology (DEGRO). Randomized,multicenter trial on the effect of radiation therapy on plantar fasciitis (painful heel spur) comparing a standard dose with a very low dose: mature results after 12 months' follow-up. Int J Radiat Oncol Biol Phys. 2012;**84**:e455–e462. DOI: 10.1016/j.ijrobp.2012.06.022

[27] Niewald M, Seegenschmiedt MH, Micke O, Gräber S; German Cooperative Group on the Radiotherapy for Benign Diseases of the DEGRO German Society for Radiation Oncology. Randomized multicenter trial on the effect of radiotherapy for plantar Fasciitis (painful heel spur) using very low doses—a study protocol. Radiat Oncol. 2008;**3**:27. DOI: 10.1186/1748-717X-3-27

[28] Gandek B, Ware JE, Aaronson NK, Apolone G, Bjorner JB, Brazier JE, Bullinger M, Kaasa S, Leplege A, Prieto L, Sullivan M. Cross-validation of item selection and scoring for the SF-12 Health Survey in nine countries: results from the IQOLA Project. International Quality of Life Assessment. J Clin Epidemiol. 1998;**51**: 1171–1178. DOI: 10.1016/S0895-4356(98)00109-7

[29] Benign news;2:24. [Internet] 2001. Available from: http://www.benign-news.de/Full_text_online__PDF_/full_text_online__pdf_.html [Accessed: 2016-07-29]

[30] Heyd R, Tselis N, Ackermann H, Röddiger SJ, Zamboglou N. Radiation therapy for painful heel spurs: results of a prospective randomized study. Strahlenther Onkol. 2007;**183**:3–9. DOI: 10.1007/s00066-007-1589-1

[31] Rowe CR, Sakellarides HT, Freeman PA, Sorbie C. Fractures of the os calcis: a long-term follow-up study of 146 patients. JAMA 1963;**184**:920–923. DOI: 10.1001/jama.1963.03700250056007

[32] Ott OJ, Jeremias C, Gaipl US, Frey B, Schmidt M, Fietkau R. Radiotherapy for benign calcaneodynia: long-term results of the Erlangen Dose Optimization (EDO) trial. Strahlenther Onkol. 2014;**190**:671–675. DOI: 10.1007/s00066-014-0618-0

[33] Ott OJ, Jeremias C, Gaipl US et al. Radiotherapy for calcaneodynia. Results of a single center prospective randomized dose optimization trial. Strahlenther Onkol. 2013;**189**:329–334. DOI: 10.1007/s00066-012-0256-3

[34] von Pannewitz G. [X-ray therapy of arthritis deformans]. In: Holfeder H, Holthausen H, Jüngling O, Martius H, Schinz HR, editors. Ergebnisse der medizinischen Strahlenforschung. Leipzig: Thieme Press; 1933. pp. 61–126.

[35] von Pannewitz G. [Degenerative diseases]. In: Zuppinger A, Ruckensteiner E, editors. Handbuch der Medizinischen Radiologie, Bd. XVII: Spezielle Strahlentherapie gutartiger Erkrankungen. Heidelberg: Springer; 1970. pp.73–107.DOI: 10.1007/978-3-642-95153-4

[36] Koeppen D, Bollmann G, Gademann G. [Dose dependant effects in X-ray therapy of heel spurs]. Strahlenther Onkol. 2000;**176**(S1):91.

[37] Schneider O, Stückle CA, Bosch E, Gott C, Adamietz IA. Effectiveness and prognostic factors of radiotherapy for painful plantar heel spurs. Strahlenther Onkol. 2004;**180**:502–509. DOI: 10.1007/s00066-004-1204-7

[38] Hermann RM, Meyer A, Becker A, Schneider M, Reible M, Carl UM, Christiansen H, Nitsche M. Effect of field size and length of plantar spur on treatment outcome in radiation therapy of plantar fasciitis: the bigger the better? Int J Radiat Oncol Biol Phys. 2013;**87**:1122–1128. DOI: 10.1016/j.ijrobp.2013.08.042

[39] Miszczyk L, Jochymek B, Wozniak G. Retrospective evaluation of radiotherapy in plantar fasciitis. Br J Radiol. 2007;**80**:829–834. DOI: 10.1259/bjr/79800547

[40] Glatzel M, Bäsecke S, Krauß A, Fröhlich D. Radiotherapy of the Painful Plantar Heel Spur. Benign News 2001;**2**: 18–19. [Internet] Available from: http://www.benign-news.de/Full_text_online__PDF_/full_text_online__pdf_.html [Accessed: 2016-07-29]

[41] Lindner H, Freislederer R. Long term results of radiotherapy of degenerative joint diseases. Strahlenther. 1982;**158**:217–223. PMID: 7101335

[42] Seegenschmiedt MH, Keilholz L. Epicondylopathia humeri (EPH) and peritendinitis humeroscapularis (PHS): evaluation of radiation therapy long-term results and literature review. Radiother Oncol. 1998;**47**:17–28. DOI: 10.1016/S0167-8140(97)00182-5

[43] Hautmann MG, Neumaier U, Koelbl O. Re-irradiation for painful heel spur syndrome. Retrospective analysis of 101 heels. Strahlenther Onkol. 2014;**190**:298–303. DOI: 10.1007/s00066-013-0462-7

[44] Kirkpatrick JP, van der Kogel AJ, Schultheiss TE. Radiation dose-volume effects in the spinal cord. Int J Radiat Oncol Biol Phys. 2010;**76**(3 Suppl):S42–49. DOI: 10.1016/j.ijrobp.2009.04.095

[45] Adamietz IA. [Radiation induced dermatitis]. Onkologe 2011;**17**:61–74. DOI: 10.1007/s00761-010-1982-8

[46] Jansen JT, Broerse JJ, Zoetelief J, Klein C, Seegenschmiedt HM. Estimation of the carcinogenic risk of radiotherapy of benign diseases from shoulder to heel. Radiother Oncol. 2005;**76**:270–277. DOI: 10.1016/j.radonc.2005.06.034

[47] Fuchs G. [Radiation dosage of the gonads in roentgen therapy]. Strahlenther. 1960;**111**:297–300.

[48] Schuhmann E, Lademann W. [Gonadal exposure to radiotherapy during therapy of non-malignant diseases]. Radiobiol Radiother. 1965;**6**:455–457.

[49] Trott KR, Kamprad F. Estimation of cancer risks from radiotherapy of benign diseases. Strahlenther Onkol. 2006;**182**:431–436. DOI: 10.1007/s00066-006-1542-8

[50] Hansen PV, Trykker H, Svennekjaer IL, et al. Long-term recovery of spermatogenesis after radiotherapy in patients with testicular cancer. Radiother Oncol. 1990;**18**:117–125. DOI: 10.1016/0167-8140(90)90137-L

[51] Pedrick TJ, Hoppe RT. Recovery of spermatogenesis following pelvic irradiation for Hodgkin's disease. Int J Radiat Oncol Biol Phys. 1986;**12**:117–121. DOI: 10.1016/0360-3016(86)90425-6

[52] Sandeman TF. The effects of X-irradiation on male human fertility. Brit J Radiol. 1966;**39**:901–907. DOI: 10.1259/0007-1285-39-468-901

[53] Greiner R. Spermatogenesis after fractionated, low-dose irradiation of the gonads. Strahlenther. 1982;**158**:342–355. PMID: 7123582

[54] Marcie S, Costa A, Lagrange JL. Protection of testes during radiation treatment by irregular and focused fields of 25 MV x-rays: in vivo evaluation of the absorbed dose. Med Dosim. 1995;**20**:269–273. DOI: 10.1016/0958-3947(95)02003-9

[55] Bieri S, Rouzaud M, Miralbell R. Seminoma of the testis: is scrotal shielding necessary when radiotherapy is limited to the para-aortic nodes? Radiother Oncol. 1999;**50**:349–353. DOI: 10.1016/S0167-8140(99)00023-7

[56] Wallace WH, Thomson AB, Kelsey TW. The radiosensitivity of the human oocyte. Hum Reprod. 2003;**18**:117–121. DOI: 10.1093/humrep/deg016

[57] Bianchi M. Cytotoxic insult to germinal tissue, part 2; the ovary. In: Potten CS, Hendry JH, editors. Cytotoxic Insult to Tissue: Effects on Cell Lineages. Edinburgh, UK: Churchill-Livingstone; 1983. pp. 309–328.

[58] Early Breast Cancer Trialists' Collaborative Group (EBCTCG). Effect of radiotherapy after breast-conserving surgery on 10-year recurrence and 15-year breast cancer death: meta-analysis of individual patient data for 10,801 women in 17 randomised trials. Lancet 2011;**378**:1707–1716. DOI: 10.1016/S0140-6736(11)61629-2

[59] International Commission on Radiological Protection (ICRP) 1990 Recommendations of the International Commission on Radiological Protection. ICRP Publication 60. Annals of the ICRP 21, 1–3, Oxford (UK): Pergamon Press; 1991.

[60] Broerse JJ, Snijders-Keilholz A, Jansen JT et al. Assessment of a carcinogenic risk for treatment of Graves' ophthalmopathy in dependence on age and irradiation geometry. Radiother Oncol. 1999;**53**:205–208. DOI: 10.1016/S0167-8140(99)00118-8

[61] McKeown SR, Hatfield P, Prestwich RJ, Shaffer RE, Taylor RE. Radiotherapy for benign disease; assessing the risk of radiation-induced cancer following exposure to intermediate dose radiation. Br J Radiol. 2015;**88**:20150405. DOI: 10.1259/bjr.20150405

[62] Robert Koch-Institut und die Gesellschaft der epidemiologischen Krebsregister in Deutschland e.V. [Cancer in Germany] 2007/2008. 8th ed. Berlin; 2012. DOI: 10.17886/rkipubl-2015-004

[63] Chia KK, Suresh S, Kuah A, Ong JL, Phua JM, Seah AL. Comparative trial of the foot pressure patterns between corrective orthotics, formthotics, bone spur pads and flat insoles in patients with chronic plantar fasciitis. Ann Acad Med Singapore. 2009;**38**:869–875. PMID: 19890578

[64] Winemiller MH, Billow RG, Laskowski ER, Harmsen WS. Effect of magnetic vs sham-magnetic insoles on plantar heel pain: a randomized controlled trial. JAMA. 2003;**290**:1474–1478. DOI: 10.1001/jama.290.11.1474

[65] Radford JA, Landorf KB, Buchbinder R, Cook C. Effectiveness of low-Dye taping for the short-term treatment of plantar heel pain: a randomised trial. BMC Musculoskelet Disord. 2006;**7**:64. DOI: 10.1186/1471-2474-7-64

[66] Sweeting D, Parish B, Hooper L, Chester R. The effectiveness of manual stretching in the treatment of plantar heel pain: a systematic review. J Foot Ankle Res. 2011;**4**:19. DOI: 10.1186/1757-1146-4-19

[67] Cotchett MP, Landorf KB, Munteanu SE. Effectiveness of dry needling and injections of myofascial trigger points associated with plantar heel pain: a systematic review. J Foot Ankle Res. 2010;**3**:18. DOI: 10.1186/1757-1146-3-18

[68] Cotchett MP, Munteanu SE, Landorf KB. Effectiveness of trigger point dry needling for plantar heel pain: a randomized controlled trial. Phys Ther. 2014;**94**:1083–1094. DOI: 10.2522/ptj.20130255

[69] Crawford F, Snaith M. How effective is therapeutic ultrasound in the treatment of heel pain? Ann Rheum Dis. 1996;**55**:265–267. DOI: 10.1136/ard.55.4.265

[70] Costantino C, Vulpiani MC, Romiti D, Vetrano M, Saraceni VM. Cryoultrasound therapy in the treatment of chronic plantar fasciitis with heel spurs. A randomized controlled clinical study. Eur J Phys Rehabil Med. 2014;**50**:39–47. PMID: 24172641

[71] Macias DM, Coughlin MJ, Zang K, Stevens FR, Jastifer JR, Doty JF. Low-Level laser therapy at 635 nm for treatment of chronic plantar fasciitis: a placebo-controlled, randomized study. J Foot Ankle Surg. 2015;**54**:768–72. DOI: 10.1053/j.jfas.2014.12.014

[72] Yin MC, Ye J, Yao M, Cui XJ, Xia Y, Shen QX, Tong ZY, Wu XQ, Ma JM, Mo W. Is extracorporeal shock wave therapy clinical efficacy for relief of chronic, recalcitrant plantar fasciitis? A systematic review and meta-analysis of randomized placebo or active-treatment controlled trials. Arch Phys Med Rehabil. 2014;**95**:1585–1593. DOI: 10.1016/j.apmr.2014.01.033

[73] Aqil A, Siddiqui MR, Solan M, Redfern DJ, Gulati V, Cobb JP. Extracorporeal shock wave therapy is effective in treating chronic plantar fasciitis: a meta-analysis of RCTs. Clin Orthop Relat Res. 2013;**471**:3645–3652. DOI: 10.1007/s11999-013-3132-2

[74] Zhiyun L, Tao J, Zengwu S. Meta-analysis of high-energy extracorporeal shock wave therapy in recalcitrant plantar fasciitis. Swiss Med Wkly. 2013;**143**:w13825. DOI: 10.4414/smw.2013.13825

[75] Krukowska J, Wrona J, Sienkiewicz M, Czernicki J. A comparative analysis of analgesic efficacy of ultrasound and shock wave therapy in the treatment of patients with inflammation of the attachment of the plantar fascia in the course of calcaneal spurs. Arch Orthop Trauma Surg. 2016. [Epub ahead of print] DOI: 10.1007/s00402-016-2503-z

[76] Ang TW. The effectiveness of corticosteroid injection in the treatment of plantar fasciitis. Singapore Med J. 2015;**56**:423–432. DOI: 10.11622/smedj.2015118

[77] Díaz-Llopis IV, Gómez-Gallego D, Mondéjar-Gómez FJ, López-García A, Climent-Barberá JM, Rodríguez-Ruiz CM. Botulinum toxin type A in chronic plantar fasciitis: clinical effects one year after injection. Clin Rehabil. 2013;**27**:681–685. DOI: 10.1177/0269215512469217

[78] Franceschi F, Papalia R, Franceschetti E, Paciotti M, Maffulli N, Denaro V. Platelet-rich plasma injections for chronic plantar fasciopathy: a systematic review. Br Med Bull. 2014;**112**:83–95. DOI: 10.1093/bmb/ldu025

[79] Vahdatpour B, Kianimehr L, Ahrar MH. Autologous platelet-rich plasma compared with whole blood for the treatment of chronic plantar fasciitis; a comparative clinical trial. Adv Biomed Res. 2016;**5**:84. DOI: 10.4103/2277-9175.182215

[80] Tomczak RL, Haverstock BD. A retrospective comparison of endoscopic plantar fasciotomy to open plantar fasciotomy with heel spur resection for chronic plantar fasciitis/heel spur syndrome. J Foot Ankle Surg. 1995;**34**:305–311. DOI: 10.1016/S1067-2516(09)80065-3

[81] Chou AC, Ng SY, Koo KO. Endoscopic plantar fasciotomy improves early postoperative results: a retrospective comparison of outcomes after endoscopic versus open plantar fasciotomy. J Foot Ankle Surg. 2016;**55**:9–15. DOI: 10.1053/j.jfas.2015.02.005

[82] Mantell BS. Radiotherapy for painful heel syndrome. Br Med J. 1978;**2**:90–91. PMID: 667574

[83] Micke O, Seegenschmiedt MH. Radiotherapy in painful heel spurs (plantar fasciitis): results of a national patterns of care study. Int J Radiat Oncol Biol Phys 2004;**58**:828–843. DOI: 10.1016/S0360-3016(03)01620-1

[84] Kahaly GJ, Rösler HP, Pitz S, Hommel G. Low- versus high-dose radiotherapy for Graves' ophthalmopathy: a randomized, single blind trial. J Clin Endocrinol Metab. 2000;**85**:102–108. DOI: 10.1210/jcem.85.1.6257

[85] Canyilmaz E, Canyilmaz F, Aynaci O, Colak F, Serdar L, Uslu GH, Aynaci O, Yoney A. Prospective randomized comparison of the effectiveness of radiation therapy and local steroid injection for the treatment of plantar fasciitis. Int J Radiat Oncol Biol Phys. 2015;**92**:659–666. DOI: 10.1016/j.ijrobp.2015.02.009

Section 2

Side Effects

Chapter 9

Predictive Solution for Radiation Toxicity Based on Big Data

Suk Lee, Kwang Hyeon Kim, Choi Suk Woo,
Jang Bo Shim, Yuan Jie Cao,
Kyung Hwan Chang and Chul Yong Kim

Additional information is available at the end of the chapter

http://dx.doi.org/10.5772/67059

Abstract

Radiotherapy is a treatment method using radiation for cancer treatment based on a patient treatment planning for each radiotherapy machine. At this time, the dose, volume, device setting information, complication, tumor control probability, etc. are considered as a single-patient treatment for each fraction during radiotherapy process. Thus, these filed-up big data for a long time and numerous patients' cases are inevitably suitable to produce optimal treatment and minimize the radiation toxicity and complication. Thus, we are going to handle up prostate, lung, head, and neck cancer cases using machine learning algorithm in radiation oncology. And, the promising algorithms as the support vector machine, decision tree, and neural network, etc. will be introduced in machine learning. In conclusion, we explain a predictive solution of radiation toxicity based on the big data as treatment planning decision support system.

Keywords: big data, machine learning, radiation toxicity, predictive solution, radiation treatment planning

1. Introduction

1.1. Definition of big data and each clinical application overview

Trifiletti et al. [1] describe the big data as follows: a lot of information and massive data sets or number of grains of sand in the earth for human analysis with 10^{12}–10^{18} bytes [1].

Murdoch listed that the big data are the inevitable application in healthcare field as four things [10]:

(a) Expanding capacity to create new knowledge

(b) Helping with knowledge dissemination

(c) Translating personalized medicine in clinical practice with EHR data

(d) Allowing for a transformation of health care by transferring information to patient [10]

This trend is called to be "big bang" to adapt and research for big data and machine learning in medicine. Especially, machine learning is widely used [4–6]. Radiotherapy is a treatment method using radiation for cancer treatment based on a patient treatment planning for each radiotherapy machine. At this time, the dose, volume, device setting information, complication, tumor control probability, etc. are considered as a single-patient treatment for each fraction during radiotherapy process. Thus, these filed-up big data for a long time and numerous patient cases are inevitably suitable to produce optimal treatment and minimize the radiation toxicity and complication. Thus, we describe various clinical cases and key machine learning algorithms in radiation oncology in this chapter.

First, what is the big data for a single patient in hospital? The data type and its size for each patient can be summarized in **Table 1**. In case of radiation oncology, imaging and treatment planning information could be a major treatable data [15].

Data type	Format	Approx. size
Clinical features	Text	10 MB
Blood tests	Numbers	1 MB
Administrative	ICD-10 codes	1 MB
Imaging data	DICOM	450 MB
Radiation oncology data (planning and onboard imaging)	DICOM, RT-DICOM	500 MB
Raw genomic data	BAM: position, base, quality	6 GB
Total		**7.9 GB**

Table 1. Data type and its size for each patient. In case of radiation oncology, imaging and treatment planning information could be the major treatable data [15].

Second, we would like to explain radiation treatment planning and decision support system in radiation oncology. When we set up treatment planning with parameters for patient cure in radiotherapy, it is based on the radiation treatment planning (RTP) system. The clinical target volume (CTV) and planning target volume (PTV) have to be targeted by maximum radiation, and critical organs have to be radiated by minimum. It is established based on the correlation between the dose and volume, also known as dose-volume histogram (DVH). At this process, considered parameters are the prescription dose (PD), dose distribution, dose fractionation, dose constraints at normal tissue, target volume, treatment machine setting values, etc. [2, 16].

Third, when the finish treatment planning has been completed, the DVH is acquired. The dose-volume distribution will be the basic information whether it could be use or not. But, these limited information do not give hot spot for target volume, conformity, homogeneity,

http://dx.doi.org/10.5772/67059

and so on. And, the tumor control probability (TCP) and normal tissue complication probability (NTCP) have to be analyzed in parallel. As the knowledge-based judgment, other rival plans could be generated again [32]. Thus, some decision support system is needed to select the best treatment plan for personalized patient care. These decision support systems (BIOPLAN, CERR, DRESS, Slicer RT, etc.) that provide different functions to analyze treatment efficiency. And these were being researched and studied as the software program since the early 2000s to up to date [3, 26–28].

But now, these decision support systems are needed to add to specific function using machine learning and historical treatment results and previously mentioned big data information to predict patient toxicity or complication after radiation treatment.

2. Clinical application using big data in radiation oncology

2.1. Prostate cancer

Çınar et al. [25] describe prostate cancer as follows:

a. Prostate cancer occurs most frequently in men over 50.

b. Prostate cancer is currently most common in men except lung cancer [25].

Thus, this clinical application is meaningful to deal with machine learning in big data. Coates et al. [4] studied the integrated big data research for prostate cancer in radiation oncology. The parameters are dose-volume metrics (EUD), clinical parameter [gastrointestinal (GI) toxicities or rectal bleeding and genitourinary (GU) toxicities or erectile dysfunction (ED)], spatial parameters (zDVH), biological variables (genetic variables), etc., and the risk quantification modeling of TCP and NTCP has performed. These modeling methods are various, and the neural network and kernel-based methods are widely used. **Figure 1** shows that the toxicity prediction results using principle component analysis (PCA) [4].

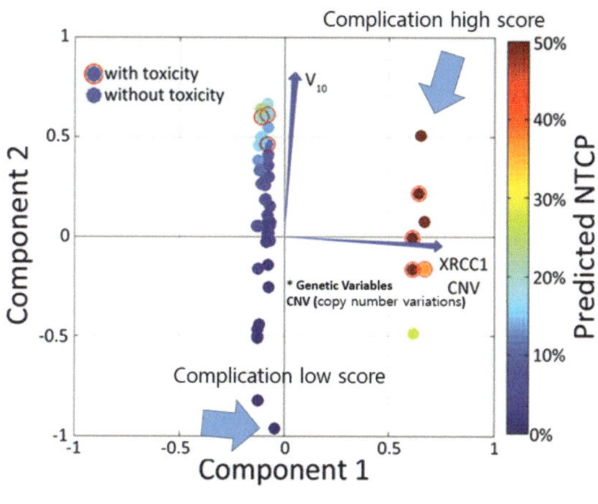

Figure 1. The predicted NTCP via principle component analysis (PCA) (reproduced from James Coates et al. [4]).

De Bari et al. [5] have done the pilot study for the prediction of pelvic nodal status using machine learning of prostate cancer. A 1555 cN0 and 50 cN+ prostate cancer patients enrolled, and decision tree and machine learning algorithm were used to study for performance results of Roach formula and Partin table. The accuracy, specificity, and sensitivity ranging between 48–86%, 35–91%, and 17–79%, respectively, were showed through this study (**Figure 2**).

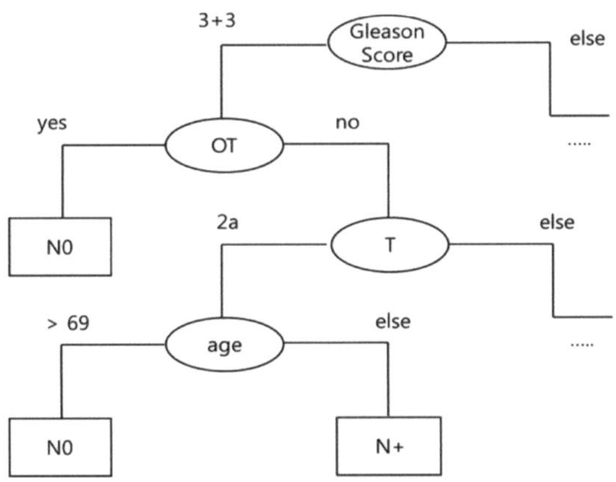

Figure 2. A decision tree example for prediction of pelvic nodal status in prostate cancer patients [5].

In addition, several analysis articles have been reported for prostate cancer with index results, which could be the example for adding above machine learning algorithm in the next step [30, 31].

2.2. Lung cancer

Das et al. [6] describe radiation-induced pneumonitis as a serious problem around thorax including the lung as follows:

a. Important problem for the incident radiation to the adjacent or surrounding normal lung.
b. Occurrence of high grade in 15–36% with retrospective studies.

Das et al. [6] conducted prediction modeling based on 234 lung cancer patients and Lyman normal tissue complication probability (LNTCP) by decision tree analysis. **Table 2** shows injury prediction by various settings for a male patient.

2.3. Head and neck cancer

Head and neck cancer patients undergo anatomical change during radiotherapy for a few weeks. Thus, kilovoltage cone-beam computed tomography (kV-CBCT) and mega-voltage computed tomography (MVCT) combined with a linear accelerator (LINAC) permit to control patient's daily anatomical change for treatment fractions in recent radiotherapy [7]. The adaptive radiotherapy (ART) could fix the anatomical variation for the patient through the dose distribution adjustment. Finally, reducing unexpected toxicity can be possible. But, This ART accompanies time and labor for daily setup about the variation fixing. At this time,

http://dx.doi.org/10.5772/67059

when replanning has to be done daily/weekly for numerous patients, then it is laborious and time-consuming for this process.

Plan name	Histological type	Chemotherapy before RT	Once/twice-daily treatment	LNTCP	Injury output (simplified model)	% Injured patients below	% Uninjured patients above
A1	Nonsquamous	No	Either	0.5	0.38	3	72
A2	Nonsquamous	No	Either	0.73	0.49	36	29
A1	Squamous	No	Either	0.5	0.5	37	28
A1	Any	Yes	Twice	0.5	0.51	43	24
A1	Any	Yes	Once	0.5	0.55	64	13
A2	Squamous	No	Either	0.73	0.61	88	4
A2	Any	Yes	Twice	0.73	0.62	91	3
A2	Any	Yes	Once	0.73	0.66	97	1

RT, radiotherapy; LNTCP, Lyman normal tissue complication probability.

Table 2. Comparison table of injury prediction for combinations of radiotherapy plan and various settings for a male patient [6].

Guidi et al. [7] studied the prediction of replanning benefit using unsupervised machine learning on retrospective data considering this process and patient characteristics. **Figure 3** is the algorithm architecture for this study. From the DVH input, clustering which classifies into data group, support vector machine (SVM) training which analyzes the parotid gland, and clinical acceptance level with test and output process are shown in **Figure 3** [7]. Thus, the results suggest that the replanning for 77% patients is needed because the significant morpho-dosimetric changes affect them when the fourth week of treatment starts.

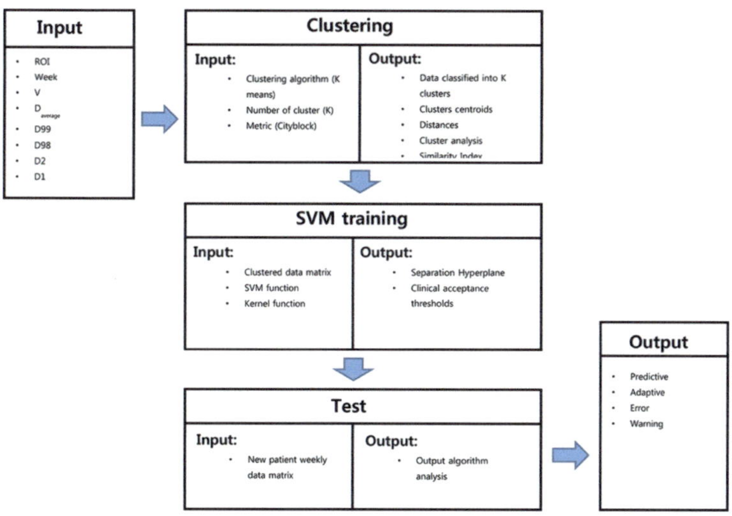

Figure 3. Algorithm architecture for prediction using clustering and support vector machine training [7].

3. Machine learning methodology

When the machine learning method has to be selected in radiation oncology, input and output variables are considered to predict expected analysis results by accuracy validation. Kang et al. [14] describe the principles of modeling as follows (**Figure 4**).

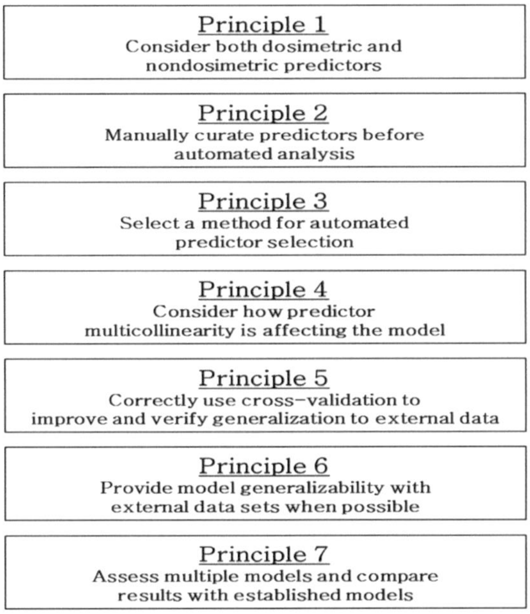

Figure 4. Core principles for modeling [14].

3.1. Machine learning introduction

Ethem Alpaydin [8] defines machine learning as the computer program for optimizing performance factor using data, and Mitchell also describes that a computer program can be said to be learned in experience (E), task (T), and performance (P) [9].

A machine learning algorithm can be divided into the unsupervised learning and supervised learning [8, 11]. For unsupervised and supervised learning process is little different as with training and test in **Figure 5**. A differentiation is the feedback loop for training and test difference between supervised and unsupervised learning in Figure 5(a) and (b).

3.2. Supervised learning

A supervised learning is a machine learning method to find a result from training data. For example, we know beforehand about the doughnut and bagel classification group. Doughnut is classified from the training. Then, we classify the group whether this doughnut belongs to doughnut group or bagel. This is the example of supervised learning.

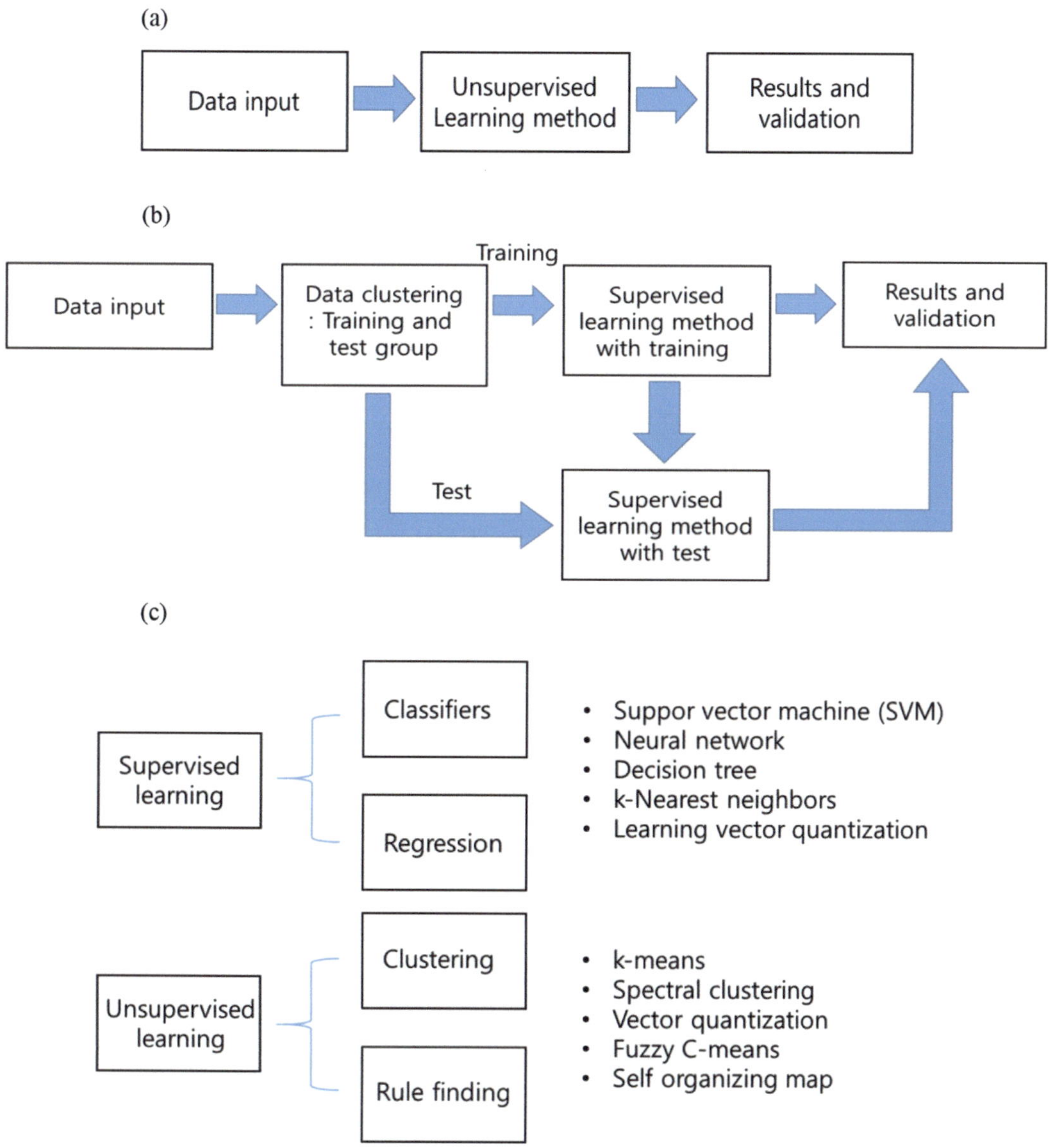

Figure 5. Unsupervised learning and supervised learning algorithm process and types. (a) Unsupervised learning process; (b) supervised learning process; and (c) Supervised and unsupervised learning algorithm types.

Generally, the training data include input characteristics with vector type; the vector presents wanted results. Thus, this continuous trial showing the result process is the regression. A classification is the division of input vector whether this value comes from several groups. When the supervised learner is executed, training data have to be measured by proper method to achieve final goal. The accuracy and validation for classification are needed to count numerically to measure its performance.

3.2.1. Decision tree

A decision tree consists of node and branch. If the nodes have more complicated hierarchy, leaf nodes and braches follow by certain decision. Thus, a diagram formed into the unknown condition at the nodes and the decision "yes" or "no" goes to a direction in a tree. This is beneficial to trace for a created hypothesis with the results. **Figure 6** shows that a decision tree and it is shown that its rules for their conditions whether patient characteristics about chemotherapy, cell, treatment, and sex for RT radiotherapy.

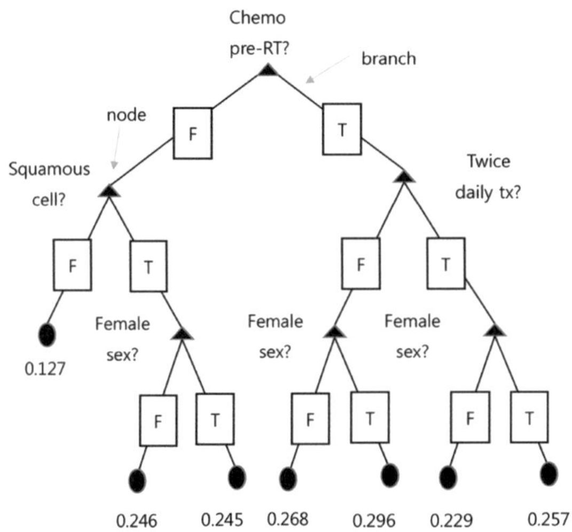

Figure 6. A decision tree and its rules for their conditions whether patient characteristics about chemotherapy, cell, treatment, and sex for RT radiotherapy (reproduced from Das et al. [7]).

A hyperplane h(x) defines Eq. (1) for the points x [12]:

$$h(x): w^T x + b = 0 \tag{1}$$

where w is the weight vector and b is the offset. The generic form of a separate point for a numeric attribute X_i is given in Eq. (2):

$$X_i \le v \tag{2}$$

where v = −b is the certain value in the domain of X_i. The decision point $X_i \le v$ thus divides R, the input data space into two regions R_{YY} and R_{NN}. Each split of R into R_{YY} and R_{NN} also induces a binary partition of the corresponding input data point D. That is, a split point of the form $X_i \le v$ induces the data partition in Eqs. (3) and (4):

$$D_{YY} = \{x \mid x \in D, x_i \le v\} \tag{3}$$

$$D_{NN} = \{x \mid x \in D, x_i > v\} \tag{4}$$

where D_{YY} is the subset of data points that lie in region R_{YY} and D_{NN} is the subset of input points that line in R_{NN} [12].

3.2.2. *Support vector machine*

A support vector machine (SVM) is a machine learning method for pattern recognition and information analysis. Generally, it is used for classification and regression analysis. The SVM makes the decision about input data to determine whether a given set of data belongs to any category. For understanding the SVM, data group and hyperplane terms have to be defined.

A hyperplane in d dimensions is given as the set of all points x ∈ Rd that satisfies the equation h(x) = 0, where h(x) is the hyperplane function, defined as follows in Eq. (5) [12]:

$$h(x) = w^T x + b \tag{5}$$

Here, w is the d dimensional weight vector and b is the scalar, called the bias. For points that lie on the hyperplane, it gives us Eq. (6):

$$h(x) = w^T x + b = 0 \tag{6}$$

The hyperplane is defined as the set of all points $w^T x = -b$. If the input data group is linearly able to classify, then a dividing hyperplane h(x) = 0 could be found for all points classified as yi = −1, h(xi) < 0 and for all points classified as yi = +1, thus h(xi) > 0:

$$y = \begin{cases} +1 \text{if } h(x) < 0 \\ -1 \text{if } h(x) < 0 \end{cases} \tag{7}$$

$$w^T(a1 - a2) = 0 \tag{8}$$

The weight vector w can be designated at the direction that is normal to the hyperplane, however, b; the bias fixes the offset of the hyperplane in the d-dimensional space. Because w and −w are normal to the hyperplane, the vagueness that h(xi) > 0 where yi = 1 and h(xi) < 0 where yi = −1 can be removed.

Thus, let **xp** be the orthogonal projection, x the hyperplane, and let $\mathbf{r_1} = \mathbf{x} - \mathbf{xp}$:

$$\mathbf{x} = \mathbf{x}_{p`} + \mathbf{r}_1 \tag{9}$$

$$\mathbf{x} = \mathbf{x}_p + \mathbf{r}_1 \frac{w}{\|w\|} \tag{10}$$

where r is the directed distance of x from $x_{p'}$, r_1 is the x from $x_{p'}$, $\frac{w}{\|w\|}$ is the unit weight vector.

r_1: + when r_1 is in the same direction as w; r_1 : − when r_1 is in an opposite direction to w (**Figure 7**) [12].

In case of nonlinear SVM, the classes are not separable by linear SVM. The shape is in **Figure 8**, and some kernels include polynomial, Gaussian, etc.

There is the library for various programming languages using the support vector machine in **Table 3**.

3.2.3. *Neural network*

A neural network example in radiation oncology is shown in **Figure 9**. A three-layer neural network defines as follows, and this would have the following model for the approximated function as [11]

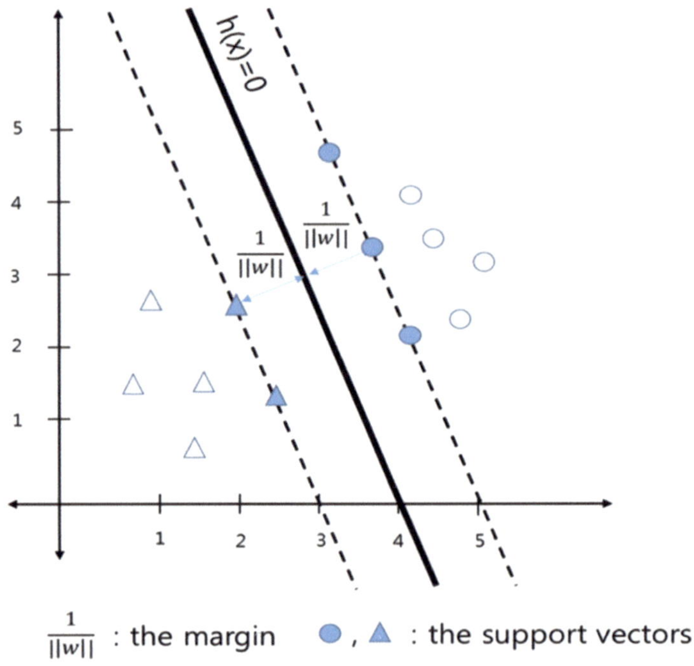

Figure 7. The support vectors and hyperplane (reproduced from Zaki and Wagner Meira [12]).

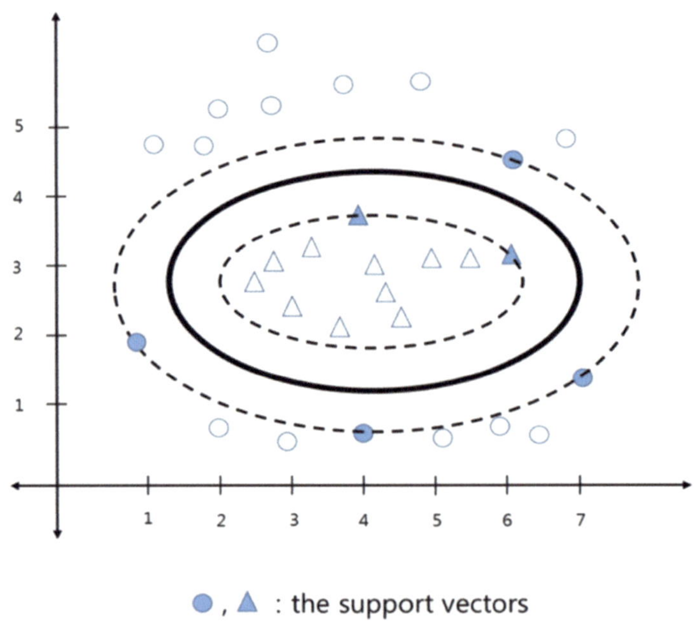

Figure 8. A nonlinear SVM (reproduced from Zaki and Wagner Meira[12]).

Programming language	Library name	Library diversity
MATLAB	MATLAB toolbox and open library	●
C/C++	Open library	●
JAVA	Open library	○
Python	Open library	●
LabVIEW	Machine learning toolkit	◑

Table 3. Various programming languages to implement SVM algorithm (Good, ○; Better, ◑; Best, ●).

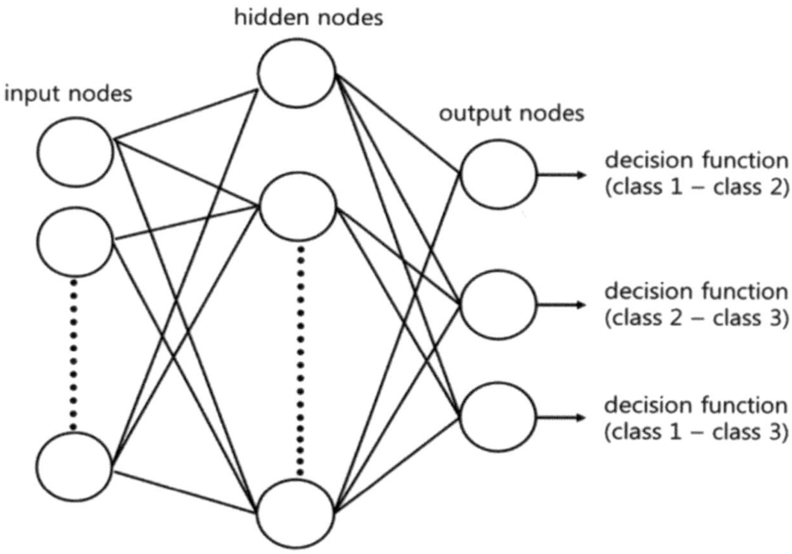

Figure 9. Neural network for head and neck cancer of 3-class classification example [17].

$$f(x)=y^T w^{(2)} + b^{(2)} \tag{11}$$

where the elements are the output of the neurons:

$$v=s\left(x^T w_i^{(1)} + b^{(1)}\right) \tag{12}$$

(where x: the input vector; $w^{(j)}$, $b^{(j)}$: the interconnect weight vector, and j: the bias of layer)

3.3. Unsupervised learning

Unsupervised learning, otherwise supervised learning, does not know the specific group information. But the learning algorithm infers the results such as doughnut and bagel example. That is, there is no target value in unsupervised learning. It is related to density estimation on statistics. This unsupervised learning is beneficial to data characteristics analysis and its explanation. Typical example is clustering. Another one is an independent component analysis.

3.3.1. Principal component analysis (PCA)

Zaki and Wagner Meira defined the PCA as follows:

a. Finding r-dimensional basis that take the data variance.

b. It is called that the largest projected variance direction is the first principal component.

c. In case of orthogonal direction, then it is the second principal component and so forth.

And also, the mean squared error can be minimized by maximizing the data variance [12].

Principal component analysis (PCA) is applied to the normalized X to identify a set of principal components (PCs) [11]:

$$\mathrm{PC} = \mathrm{U}^{\mathrm{T}}\mathrm{X} = \sum \mathrm{V}^{\mathrm{T}} \tag{13}$$

where $U\Sigma V^T$ is the singular value decomposition of X.

3.3.2. Clustering

Clustering is an unsupervised learning method, and that is finding the cluster without data label. The data and data label are required to classify. Thus, it needs different classification methods for unlabeled data. There are several ways to define cluster. One simple way is that we can define as "the data in same cluster inside" is close to each other, and the closest distance data could be selected. k-Means assume the data is close in same cluster. One center exists, and cost which is a distance between center and each data can be defined. Thus, k-means is an algorithm to reduce and minimize cost in cluster.

Given a clustering $C = \{C_1, C_2, \ldots, C_k\}$, the scoring function evaluates its quality. This sum of squared error scoring function is defined as [12]

$$SSE(C) = \sum_{i=0}^{k} \sum_{X_j \in C_i} \left|\left| X_j - u_i \right|\right|^2 \tag{14}$$

The goal is to find the clustering that minimizes the SSE score, thus,

$$C^{*}=\mathrm{argmin}_{c}\{SSE(C)\} \tag{15}$$

k-Means employs a greedy iterative approach to find a clustering that minimizes the SSE objective [12].

Here is the advantage and disadvantage of various machine learning algorithms in radiation oncology in **Table 4**.

Algorithm	Advantages	Limitations
Decision tree	Easy to understand	Classes must be mutually exclusive
	Fast	Results depend on the order of attribute selection
		Risk of overly complex decision trees
Naïve Bayesian	Easy to understand	Variables must be statistically independent
	Fast	Numeric attributes must follow a normal distribution
	No effect of order on training	Classes must be mutually exclusive
		Less accurate
k-Nearest neighbors	Fast and simple	Variables with similar attributes will be sorted in the same class
	Tolerant of noise and missing values in data	All attributes are equally relevant
	Can be used for nonlinear classification	Requires considerable computer power as the number of variables increases
	Can be used for both regression and classification	
Support vector machine	Robust model	Slow training
	Limits the risk of error	Risk of overfitting
	Can be used to model nonlinear relations	Output model is difficult to understand
Artificial neural network and deep learning	Tolerant of noise and missing values in data	Output model is difficult to understand (black box)
	Can be used for classification or regression	Risk of overfitting
	Can be easily updated with new data	Requires a lot of computer power
		Requires experimentation to find the optimal network structure

Table 4. The advantages and disadvantages by various machine learning algorithms in radiation oncology [15].

4. Conclusion

We summarized various clinical applications such as head, neck, lung, and prostate cancer using machine learning algorithm in radiation oncology [13, 18, 19]. And those machine learning algorithm introductions and several definitions were listed. For the precision medicine in radiation oncology, radiation toxicity and complication factors are inevitable parameters for patients after radiotherapy. The dose-volume distribution will be the basic information, but this limited information does not give the tumor control probability (TCP) and normal tissue complication probability (NTCP) and grade level. Thus, some decision support system is needed to select the best treatment plan for personalized patient care. But now, although this decision support system is needed to add specific function using machine learning and historical treatment results and previously mentioned big data information to predict patients toxicity or complication after radiation treatment [29].

Another current big data trend is the research for the medical imaging such as DICOM RT in radiotherapy. The images have a lot of information for current patient status and future undergoing information as prediction of patient's quality of life. Thus, lung cancer and breast cancer applications are good applications in case of using simple chest X-ray or low-cost imaging method for big data research in clinical application.

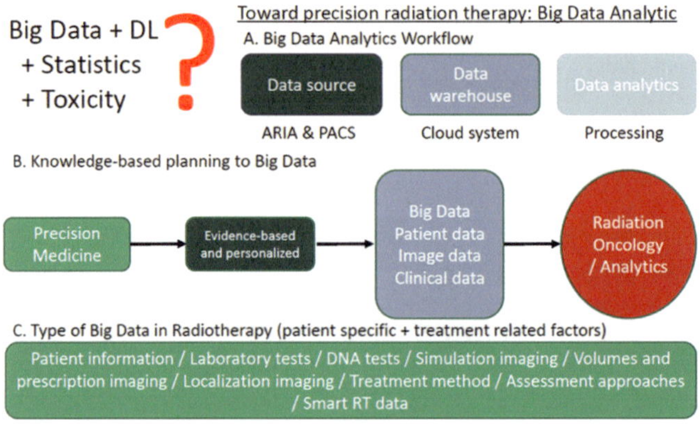

(a)

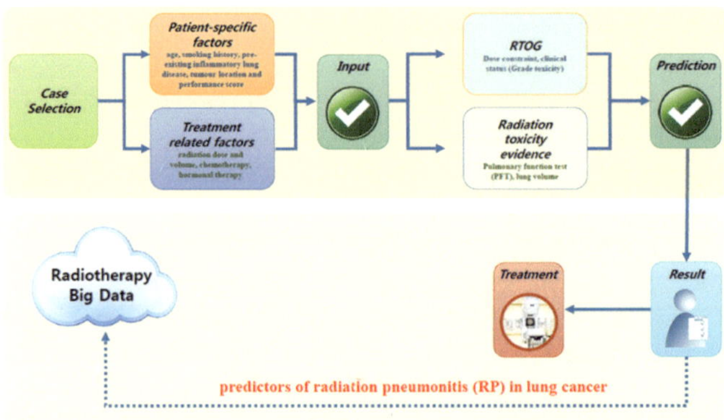

(b)

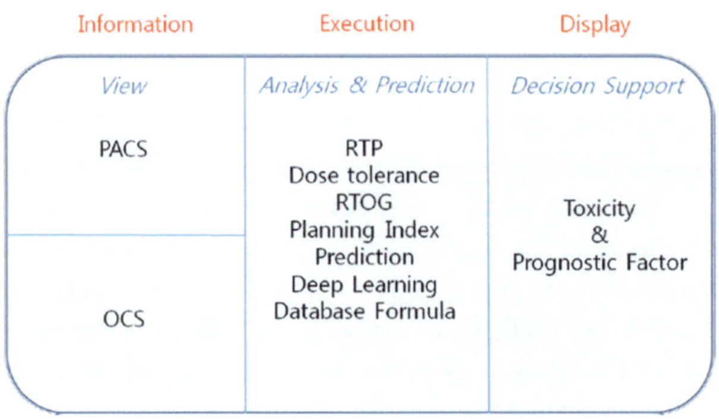

(c)

Figure 10. An example of the big data based on patient-specific treatment prediction in radiation oncology (a), its block diagram (b), and overview (c).

Thus, we explain a predictive solution of radiation toxicity based on the big data as treatment planning decision support system in **Figure 10**. From this block diagram, the input part gives treatment data (i.e., rival plans with DVH) through a radiation treatment planning system. After this process, the dosimetric and biological index analysis process is performed by program. The normal tissue complication probability (NTCP) model could be adaptable, and it is used to consider central lung distance (CLD) and maximal heart distance information to be measured such as two-dimensional radiation therapy indicators between the three-dimensional conformal radiation therapies in case of lung cancer. Dose-volume relationship and tolerance dose in organ-at-risk information are analyzed by some machine learning algorithm in decision support system. At this time, numerous patient treatment "big data" could be used to evaluate machine learning results and predict toxicity and normal tissue complication versus know-based approach. Thus, this will be the evidence-based decision to finalize treatment plan for customized patient cure [20–24].

Therefore, current decision support system can be modified and developed to predict complication and toxicity after radiotherapy by adding not only dosimetric index and biological index function but also clinical big data analysis with various machine learning algorithms. This is the fusion solution for customized patient cure method in big data era in radiation oncology.

Author details

Suk Lee[1]*, Kwang Hyeon Kim[1], Choi Suk Woo[2], Jang Bo Shim[1], Yuan Jie Cao[3], Kyung Hwan Chang[4] and Chul Yong Kim[1]

*Address all correspondence to: sukmp@korea.ac.kr

1 Department of Radiation Oncology, College of Medicine, Korea University, Seoul, Korea

2 CQURE Healthcare, Seoul, Korea

3 Department of Radiation Oncology, Tianjin Medical University Cancer Institute and Hospital, Tianjin, China

4 Department of Radiation Oncology, College of Medicine, Asan Medical Center, Seoul, Korea

References

[1] Trifiletti DM, Showalter TN. Big data and comparative effectiveness research in radiation oncology: synergy and accelerated discovery. Front Oncol. 2015; 5: 274

[2] Khan FM. Treatment planning in radiation oncology. 2nd ed. Philadelphia: Lippincott Williams & Wilkins; 2007.

[3] Lee S, Cao YJ and Kim CY. Physical and radiobiological evaluation of radiotherapy treatment plan, evolution of ionizing radiation research. Dr. Mitsuru N (Ed.), Croatia, InTech; 2015, DOI: 10.5772/60846.

[4] Coates J, Souhami L and El Naqa I. Big data analytics for prostate radiotherapy. Front Oncol. 2016;6:149.

[5] De Bari B, Vallati M, Gatta R, Simeone C, Girelli G, Ricardi U, Meattini I, Gabriele P, Bellavita R, Krengli M, Cafaro I, Cagna E, Bunkheila F, Borghesi S, Signor M, Di Marco A, Bertoni F, Stefanacci M, Pasinetti N, Buglione M, Magrini SM. Could machine learning improve the prediction of pelvic nodal status of prostate cancer patients? Preliminary results of a pilot study. Cancer Investig. 2015 Jul;33(6):232–40.

[6] Das SK, Zhou S, Zhang J, Yin FF, Dewhirst MW, Marks LB. Predicting lung radiotherapy-induced pneumonitis using a model combining parametric Lyman probit with nonparametric decision trees. Int J Radiat Oncol Biol Phys. 2007 Jul 15;68(4):1212–21.

[7] Guidi G, Maffei N, Vecchi C, Ciarmatori A, Mistretta GM, Gottardi G, Meduri B, Baldazzi G, Bertoni F, Costi T. A support vector machine tool for adaptive tomotherapy treatments: prediction of head and neck patients criticalities. Phys Med. 2015 Jul;31(5):442–51.

[8] Alpaydin E. Introduction to machine learning. 3rd ed. Cambridge, MA: The MIT Press; 2014.

[9] Mitchell TM. Machine learning. New York: McGraw-Hill; 1997.

[10] Murdoch TB, Detsky AS. The inevitable application of big data to health care. JAMA. 2013;309(13):1351–1352.

[11] El Naqa I, Li R, Murphy MJ. Machine learning in radiation oncology: theory and applications. Switzerland, Springer; 2015.

[12] Zaki MJ, Wagner Meira JR. Data mining and analysis. USA, Cambridge University Press; 2014.

[13] El Naqa I, Bradley JD, PE L, Hope AJ, Deasy JO. Predicting radiotherapy outcomes using statistical learning techniques. Phys Med Biol. 2009;54(18):S9.

[14] Kang J, Schwartz R, Flickinger J, Beriwal S. Machine learning approaches for predicting radiation therapy outcomes: a clinician's perspective. Int J Radiat Oncol Biol Phys. 2015 Dec 1;93(5):1127–35.

[15] Bibault JE, Giraud P, Burgun A. Big Data and machine learning in radiation oncology: state of the art and future prospects. Cancer Lett. 2016 May 27. pii: S0304-3835(16)30346–9.

[16] Videtic GMM, Woody N, Vassil AD. Handbook of treatment planning in radiation oncology. 2nd ed. New York: Demos Medical; 2015.

[17] Kang S, Cho S. Approximating support vector machine with artificial neural network for fast prediction. Expert Syst Appl. 2014;41:4989–95

[18] Dean JA, Wong KH, Welsh LC, Jones AB, Schick U, Newbold KL, Bhide SA, Harrington KJ, Nutting CM, Gulliford SL. Normal tissue complication probability (NTCP) modelling using spatial dose metrics and machine learning methods for severe acute oral mucositis resulting from head and neck radiotherapy. Radiother Oncol. 2016 Jul;120(1):21–7.

[19] Chen S, Zhou S, Yin FF, Marks LB, Das SK. Investigation of the support vector machine algorithm to predict lung radiation-induced pneumonitis. Med Phys. 2007 Oct;34(10):3808–14.

[20] Tiziana Rancati, et al. Factors predicting radiation pneumonitis in lung cancer patients: a retrospective study. Radiother Oncol. 2003;67:275–283

[21] George Rodrigues, et al. Prediction of radiation pneumonitis by dose–volume histogram parameters in lung cancer—a systematic review. Radiother Oncol. 2004;71:127–138

[22] Milano MT, et al. Normal tissue tolerance dose metrics for radiation therapy of major organs. Semin Radiat Oncol. 2007;17:131–140.

[23] Weytjens R, et al. Radiation pneumonitis: occurrence, prediction, prevention and treatment. Belg J Med Oncol. 2013;7(4):105–10

[24] Emami B, et al. Tolerance of normal tissue to therapeutic irradiation. Int J Radiation Oncol Biol Phys. 1991;21:109–22

[25] Çınar M, Engin M, Engin EZ, Ziya Ateşçi Y. Early prostate cancer diagnosis by using artificial neural networks and support vector machines. Expert Syst Appl. 2009;36:6357–6361.

[26] Sanchez-Nieto B, Nahum AE. BIOPLAN: software for the biological evaluation of radiation therapy. Med Dosim. 2000;25(2):71–6.

[27] Pinter C, Lasso A, Wang A, Jaffray D, Fichtinger G. SlicerRT: radiation therapy research toolkit for 3D Slicer. Med Phys. 2012;39(10):6332–8.

[28] Sanchez-Nieto B, Nahum AE. BIOPLAN: software for the biological evaluation of radiotherapy treatment plans. Med Dosim. 2000;25(2):71–6.

[29] Bentzen SM, Constine LS, Deasy JO, Eisbruch A, Jackson A, Marks LB, et al. Quantitative analyses of normal tissue effects in the clinic (QUANTEC): an introduction to the scientific issues. Int J Radiat Oncol Biol Phys. 2010;76(3 Suppl):S3–S9.

[30] Cao YJ, Lee S, Chang KH, Shim JB, Kim KH, et al. Patient performance-based plan parameter optimization for prostate cancer in tomotherapy. Med Dosim. 2015;40(4):285–9.

[31] Cao YJ, Lee S, Chang KH, Shim JB, Kim KH, et al. Optimized planning target volume margin in helical tomotherapy for prostate cancer: is there a preferred method? J Korean Phys Soc. 2015;67(1):26–32.

[32] Luxton G, Keall PJ, King CR. A new formula for normal tissue complication probability (NTCP) as a function of equivalent uniform dose (EUD). Phys Med Biol. 2007;53(1):23–36

Chapter 10

Radiation-Related Heart Disease: Up-to-Date Developments

Wenyong Tan, Xianming Li and Yong Dai

Additional information is available at the end of the chapter

http://dx.doi.org/10.5772/67325

Abstract

Approximately 25–30% of patients with cancer undergo thoracic radiation therapy (RT). RT might inadvertently induce heart injury and result in various forms of radiation-related heart disease (RRHD). The main endpoints of RRHD include cardiac death from RT, clinical heart disease (congestive heart disease, ischemic heart disease, and myocardial infarction), and subclinical heart disease (cardiac perfusion defects). Advanced RT techniques, such as breath control, intensity-modulated RT, and image-guided RT, as well as limited target volume definition might spare or avoid cardiac doses and/or volume, which may translate into decreased incidence of RRHD. The total delivered radiation dose to cardiac implantable electronic devices was strongly recommended not to exceed 2 Gy. The treatment strategies of RRHD were based on the various recommended consensus of related heart diseases in cardiology. However, the standardized definitions of the cardiac structures, dose-volume limits during radiation planning design, the optimal dose-volume parameters, and the dose-volume effects of various cardiac substructures warrant further investigation. The recognition, prediction, prevention, and management of RRHD require close collaboration between oncologists and cardiologists.

Keywords: radiation therapy, heart disease, prevention, treatment

1. Introduction

Cancer is a leading cause of death in both developed and less developed countries worldwide, and its health burden is expected to increase rapidly [1]. In 2012, an estimated 14.1 million new cancer cases and 8.2 million deaths occurred worldwide [1]. Currently, approximately 57% of cancer cases and 65% of cancer deaths occur in less developed countries [1]. Worldwide, the new cases or deaths from lung and breast cancer were at the top of the list [1]. In China, in 2015, an estimated 4,292,000 new cancer cases and 2,814,000 cancer deaths occurred [2]. Lung cancer is the most common incident cancer and the leading cause of cancer death in China, and esophageal cancer is also commonly diagnosed. Worldwide, lung, esophageal, and breast cancer account for approximately 27% of new cancer cases which means that more than 20% of patients will receive thoracic radiation therapy (RT). Many studies have proven that local RT improves local control and prolongs overall survival [3–11]. However, thoracic RT might inadvertently result in various forms of cardiac toxicity and manifest as clinical and subclinical cardiac disease, termed radiation-related heart disease (RRHD) [12, 13]. In this chapter, we will present the epidemiological data and discuss the possible pathophysiological mechanisms in brief. We will also address the cardiac avoidance techniques and the dose-volume-effect relationship. Although many cytotoxic and molecularly targeted drugs also result in various cardiac toxicities [14], consideration of these is outside the scope of this chapter.

2. Epidemiological data for radiation-related heart disease

Following the use of mantle field radiation for Hodgkin lymphoma in the 1960s, RRHD was recognized because substantial cardiac damage was observed to occur after the whole heart received doses of radiation higher than 30 Gy [12]. Traditionally, RRHD mainly included radiation-related pericarditis, pericardial and myocardial fibrosis, and coronary artery disease, as well as conduction system abnormalities. However, with improvements in RT techniques and refinements in RT delivery, radiation doses to the heart have decreased in the past three decades. For example, in lung and esophageal cancer, the mean heart dose might be >20 Gy [15], while in postoperative RT for breast cancer, it might be <10 Gy [16, 17]. As a reference point, the survivors of the atomic bombings of Japan received up to 4 Gy [18]. The endpoints of RRHD could be categorized as radiation-induced death from heart disease (mortality), clinical manifestations (clinical disease), and imaging or laboratory abnormalities (subclinical disease) [14] as shown in **Figure 1**.

Breast cancer is a curable disease. Therefore, minimization of anticancer therapy-induced toxicity is an important concern during treatment decision-making. In a study of breast cancer, mortality due to heart disease was increased by 27% (2p = 0.0001) in women who received surgery plus RT compared to the rate in those who did not receive postoperative RT. The proportional excess of vascular deaths was similar in the first decade and the period thereafter (ratio 1·32 vs. 1·27). However, the absolute rates were about three times higher in the second decade and the latter period for the patients with left-sided breast cancer [5]. Exposure to cardiac radiation in the treatment of breast cancer will increase the subsequent rate of ischemic heart disease for more than 10 years after completion of the therapy. In addition, women with cardiac risk factors experience greater increases in risk after thoracic RT. Darby et al. quantified the dose effect of ischemic heart disease in patients with breast cancer who received adjuvant thoracic RT. They found that the rate of major coronary events increased by 7.4% per Gy without an apparent threshold, and the major coronary events included myocardial infarction, coronary revascularization, and death from ischemic heart disease [13, 19]. Even in the era of modern RT, in comparison with patients with right-sided breast cancer, those with left-sided breast cancer experienced a small increase in the risk of percutaneous coronary intervention (PCI) following RT, and the 10-year cumulative incidences in patients with left-sided and right-sided disease were 5.5 and 4.5%, respectively [20].

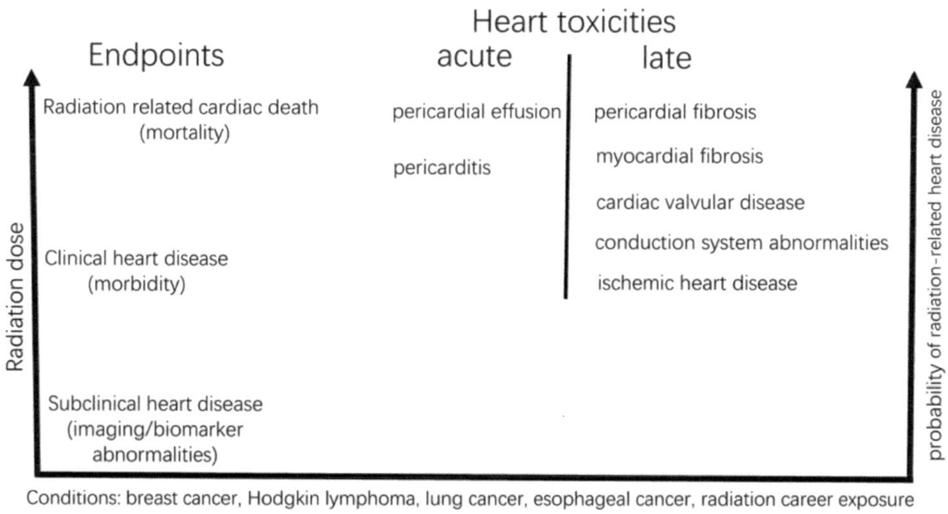

Figure 1. Radiation-related heart disease usually occurs with a certain latency from a few hours to several decades after the heart and its substructures receive direct or indirect irradiation. The endpoints of RRHD included its mortality and morbidity. According the occurrence timing of cardiac radiation response, RRHD includes acute and late cardiac toxicities. Generally, the probability of RRHD is positively related to the radiation dose that the heart received.

Hodgkin lymphoma usually occurs in young patients and is also one of the most curable cancers. Cytotoxic treatment with anthracyclines and vinca alkaloids and RT are the cornerstone choices for therapy of this cancer, and both are associated with the risk of cardiovascular disease. The cardiovascular risks after chemotherapy and RT have been well established [21, 22]. According to data from old cohort studies, Hodgkin lymphoma was usually treated with radiation doses of 35–45 Gy using extended field treatment such as mantle field radiation. The cumulative risks of heart disease among survivors of adult Hodgkin lymphoma are approximately 5–10% at 15 years, 16% at 20 years, and 34% at 30 years, and coronary artery disease, as the most common form, accounts for approximately 40–50% of adverse cardiac events [23]. A recent systemic analysis showed that among 6039 patients with a median length of follow-up of 9 years, 703 patients were recorded to have 1238 first cardiovascular events, which mostly included ischemic heart disease (19%), congestive heart failure (12%), arrhythmia (16%), and valvular disease (11%). The predictors of cardiovascular disease were the mean heart radiation dose per 1 Gy increase (HR 1015) and the dose of anthracyclines per 50 mg/m^2 increase in cumulative dose (HR 1077) [24]. In a Dutch study conducted to examine the relative and absolute excess risk of cardiovascular disease incidence, 1713 cardiovascular events were detected in 797 patients after a median follow-up of 20 years. Furthermore, 20% of patients with a cardiovascular disease developed multiple events. Mediastinal RT, anthracycline-containing chemotherapy, and smoking are appeared to be additive factors [25]. In addition, the data from both individuals exposed to radiation during a medical career [26, 27] and survivors of the atomic bombings in Japan [28] proved that radiation was the source of the risk for RRHD.

Cardiac valvular disease is less common, typically has a late onset (10 years after RT), and is related to higher doses (30 Gy) or young age at treatment. Treatment of a large cardiac volume with high doses can produce acute pericarditis, although this is uncommon. At times, this may lead to chronic or delayed reemergence of pericarditis with effusion.

Furthermore, due to the wide use of advanced imaging techniques, more subclinical manifestations are detected. With repeat nuclear imaging to assess changes in regional and global cardiac function after RT for left-sided breast cancer, a prospective clinical study found that volume-dependent perfusion defects occurred in approximately 40% of patients within the first 2 years after RT for left-sided breast cancer, and these perfusion defects were associated with cardiac wall motion abnormalities [29]. In addition, new perfusion defects usually occurred in the anterior left ventricle within 6 months after radiation [30]. The data from the Surveillance, Epidemiology, and End Results Medicare database showed that patients with left-sided breast cancer who had a history of cardiac disease had an increased risk of PCI after thoracic RT, and there was a lower survival rate in those who received PCI. The 10-year cumulative PCI incidence was 5.5% [95% confidence interval (CI) 4.9–6.2%] and 4.5% (95% CI 4.0–5.0%) for patients with left- and right-sided cancer, respectively [20].

For curable cancer types, such as breast cancer and Hodgkin lymphoma, both the radiation dose to the heart and its substructures and the risks and benefits of different regimens for individual patients should be well balanced during treatment decision-making.

3. Pathophysiological mechanisms of RRHD

The detailed pathogenesis of RRHD has been well reviewed [12, 31]. Overall, the endothelial system of blood vessels, particularly the arteries seem to be the critical target structures. After radiation, early functional alterations might include the pro-inflammatory responses and other changes, followed by slow progression [31, 32]. Although experimental animal models will help to elucidate the possible cellular and molecular mechanisms of RRHD, the results from various animals might be species-specific, and caution should be used in extrapolating to humans. In cancer patients, radiation induces macro- and microvascular injury. The former accelerates age-related atherosclerosis and leads to coronary artery disease after several years or decades due to reduced blood flow to the radiated myocardial territory. On the other hand, the latter reduces capillary density and results in decreased vascular reverse, which usually occurs within several months after RT and has only subclinical manifestations [12].

4. Dose-volume effect of RRHD

The dose-volume effect of RRHD is highly dependent on the definition of its endpoints. According to the length of its latency, RRHD could be divided into acute injury, which often manifests within a few months and is usually transient, and chronic toxicities, which often manifest as congestive heart failure and ischemic heart disease, among others, and occur with a long latency [33]. RRHD can have subclinical manifestations, such as localized cardiac imaging abnormalities on nuclear magnetic resonance imaging or regional wall motion abnormalities on cardiac ultrasonic examination, but manifestations could also be clinical, such as coronary artery disease or myocardial infarction [33].

The accurate definition of the heart and its substructures is critical to the estimation of the radiation dose-volume effect on RRHD. However, the imprecise definition of the heart in treatment planning computed tomography (CT) imaging poses a great challenge [33]. Feng et al. [34] developed a heart atlas to study cardiac exposure to radiation in the treatment of breast cancer. Using this consistent atlas for cardiac structure delineation, we could quantify the causative effects of RT on cardiac morbidity and mortality and study the dose-volume constraints on the heart and its substructures [34] (**Figure 2**).

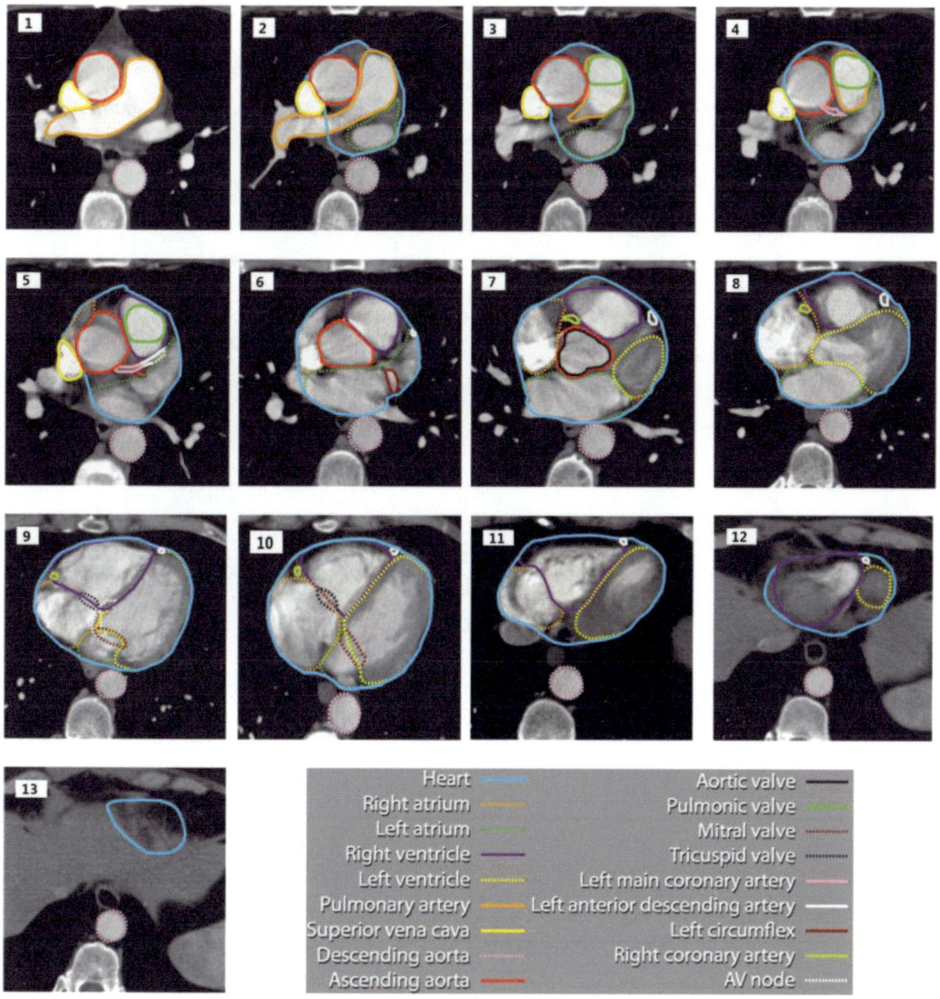

Figure 2. Cardiac atlas is illustrated in the CT images with intravenous contrast [34] (with permission).

In all of the published studies about the dose-volume response relationships of RRHD, mortality from pericarditis, ischemic heart disease, and decreased myocardial perfusion were three main clinical endpoints [33]. Gagliardi et al. [33] (**Figure 3**) summarized the dose-volume predictors and normal tissue complication probabilities of pericarditis/pericardial effusion, and the results showed that the mean doses to the pericardium (>30 Gy or >26.1 Gy) or mediastinum (>41 Gy) might be the predictors of radiation-induced pericarditis or pericardial effusion. The incidence of pericarditis was 7% (14/198) with a radiation dose of ≤6 Gy; 12% (5/42) with a dose of 6–15 Gy; 19% (23/123) with a dose of 15–30 Gy; and 50% (7/14) with a dose of >30 Gy. Regarding cardiac mortality from ischemic heart disease or myocardial infarction, radiation dose to the mediastinum >30 Gy; 35% of heart volume receiving a radiation dose > 38 Gy; mean dose to the whole heart volume > 2.5 Gy; and radiation to the internal mammary chain would be the predictive parameters [33]. When taking cardiac perfusion defects as the clinical endpoints, volume of the left ventricle receiving doses higher than 23 (V_{23Gy}) or 33 Gy (V_{33Gy}) could predict myocardial perfusion defects [35].

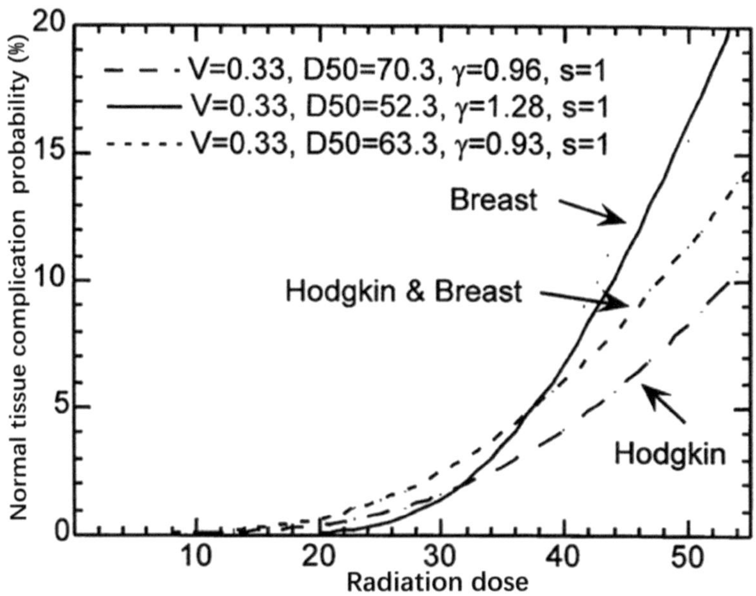

Figure 3. Dose-response curves of radiation-induced cardiac mortality. These data were estimated based on the breast cancer and Hodgkin lymphoma data sets [33] (with permission).

5. Cardiac dose sparing and avoidance techniques

For curable cancers, such as breast cancer and Hodgkin lymphoma, cardiac dose protection and/or avoidance techniques might be beneficial in minimizing RRHD. For breast cancer, several techniques have been utilized clinically. These techniques include the following: (1) RT delivery with breath control or holding techniques, (2) prone patient positioning, (3) new RT techniques such as intensity-modulated RT (IMRT), proton therapy, or partial breast irradiation techniques, and (4) single-fraction, intraoperative radiation [36] (**Figure 4**).

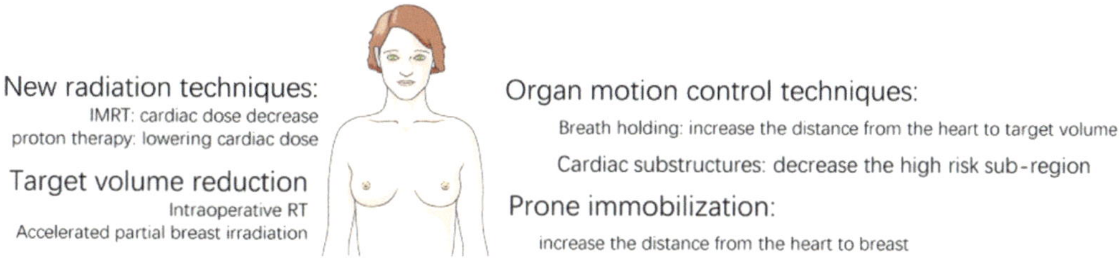

Figure 4. Cardiac sparing techniques is available nowadays. These techniques included radiation techniques improvement and patient or organ motion management.

With breath holding within inspiration, the distance from the chest wall to the heart will increase and the cardiac volume in the field will decrease, the mean or maximal dose to the heart or left anterior descending artery will be reduced [36], and the probability of cardiac mortality will also be reduced (4.8 vs. 0.1%) [37]. In the delivery of RT, patients are immobilized in the prone position so that the breast falls away from the chest wall and the distance from the heart to the RT beam increases. A few studies showed that with this technique, 75–85% of left-sided breast cancer patients had reduced cardiac volume in the field [38] and the mean cardiac dose decreased [39]. Although the main concerns of the prone position include its reproducibility and the potential increase in radiation to other normal tissues due to the poor setup, recent data showed that this technique could be well reproducible with daily cone-beam CT [40, 41].

For breast cancer patients, IMRT has been proven to have a cardiac dose sparing effect without compromising the dose homogeneity in the breast, especially for those with left-sided lesions [36, 42]. With the IMRT technique, the cardiac dose decreased with improved dose homogeneity in the breast [43]. A series of studies showed that, compared with breath holding in three-dimensional conformal RT and prone position techniques, IMRT has similar benefits and is more reproducible. The advantages of IMRT technique included the improvement of radiation dose homogeneity in target volume, the reduction of high cardiac dose volumes, and the decrease of normal tissue complication probability. In addition, IMRT technique showed its advantages in sparing the high-risk cardiac subregions such as the anterior part of the heart, the coronary arteries, and the left ventricle [16, 17, 44].

Partial breast irradiation, as an alternative method to reduce the cardiac dose, could decrease the irradiated breast volume and increase the distance from the target volume to the heart. Hypofractionation is required by partial breast irradiation, and two recent reviews suggest that hypofractionation has not resulted in increased cardiac morbidity [45, 46]. Dosimetric studies showed that interstitial brachytherapy could reduce cardiac doses with image-guided RT techniques [47, 48]. The mean cardiac dose decreased to 21% of the prescription dose in patients with left-sided breast cancer [48] and the cardiac volume receiving low doses (5 and 10 Gy) decreased significantly. In addition, the advantages of proton therapy including the rapid dose falloff and the Bragg peak make it possible to spare the radiation dose to the surrounding tissues including the heart. Several dosimetric studies showed that proton RT could reduce the maximal dose, V_{20Gy}, V_{5Gy}, etc [49–52]. However, because of the limited availability and high cost, at present, this technique is not advocated for cardiac dose sparing [36].

For Hodgkin lymphoma, the RT field has changed over the past decades. Previously, the majority of patients received mantle field radiation with/without upper abdomen field radiation, and a large volume of the heart had a prescribed dose irradiation. According to the anatomical sites of disease presence, the caudal border of the mantle field individually varied from the bottom border at the 8th–9th thoracic vertebrae (T8–T9) [53] to T10–T11 [54, 55], and the higher caudal border might spare most of the irradiated heart volume [53]. With advanced imaging modalities such as positron emission tomography–CT and improved RT delivery techniques such as IMRT, image-guided RT, and breath control techniques, among others, the previously applied extended field and involved field techniques have now been replaced by techniques using limited target volumes, such as involved node RT (INRT) and involved site RT (ISRT) [56]. With the optimal imaging during the course of treatment, both the INRT and ISRT techniques reduce the treated volume to a safe minimum [56]. In addition, with refinements of Hodgkin lymphoma, the prescription dose decreased to 20–36 Gy [57]. Due to more limited target volume and lower prescribed radiation doses, greater amounts of normal healthy tissues such as lung and heart could be spared.

Theoretically, for RT of non-small cell lung cancer, dose escalation to 74 Gy would be better than the standardized 60 Gy dose. However, the results of a randomized phase 3 study (RTOG 0617) showed that a higher dose did not translate to a better outcome and might even be potentially harmful [58]. One reasonable explanation is that patients receiving doses of 74 Gy usually had worse dose-volume effects on the heart. The dose volume parameters including V_{5Gy} and V_{30Gy} of the heart were the important predictors of patient survival [58]. The dose-volume effects on the heart substructures such as the pericardium, atria, and ventricles will be investigated and their dose-volume limitations will be included in future lung cancer trials. In addition, for early and locally advanced non-small cell lung cancer, proton RT will potentially be used for cardiac sparing [59].

6. Radiation for patients with cardiac implantable electronic devices

The numbers of patients with both cardiac implantable electronic devices (CIEDs) including pacemakers (PMs) and implantable cardiac defibrillators and cancer are expected to rise, and patients in these situations require RT. The potential interactions between high doses of radiation and the function, longevity, and integrity of the CIEDs, as well as the harm to the patients, remain unclear. The results of a recent review [60, 61] showed that the risk of device failure increases with increasing radiation doses, without a clear cutoff point. For patients with pacemakers, the delivered total radiation dose to the device was strongly recommended not to exceed 2 Gy and the dose in patients with implantable cardiac defibrillators should be within 1 Gy. The radiation energy should be less than 6 MV. Because of the potential dangers of device malfunction, the radiation oncologist should have all the measures designed to minimize the risk to patients. Furthermore, it is necessary for the cardiologist, oncologist, radiotherapist, and physicist to collaborate closely.

7. Treatment strategies of RRHD

Generally, the treatment strategies of various RRHDs are similar to those in normal population [62–64]. For example, radiation-induced left ventricular dysfunction or heart failure could be treated according to the recommended guidelines of heart failure [65]. And for those with anticancer drug-induced hypertension, antihypertensive agents should be individualized to the clinical circumstances of the patients [66]. Angiotensin-converting enzyme inhibitors or angiotensin II receptor blockers are usually considered for patients with proteinuria, metabolic syndrome, or high risk of chronic kidney disease [66]. Treatment with nondihydropyridine calcium channel blockers should be avoided in patients receiving cytochrome P450 inhibitors, while dihydropyridine calcium channel blockers are preferred in elderly patients [67, 68]. Low-molecular weight heparin for a minimum of 3–6 months is the recommended treatment for patients with newly diagnosed venous thromboembolism [69].

8. Unanswered questions regarding RRHD

Variability in certain risk factors may influence the development of a radiation-associated heart disease. These factors included patients themselves, RT techniques, the evaluable endpoints, and social-psychological variables [19]. The patient-related factors include age, personal alcohol and tobacco history, systemic anticancer drugs with potential cardiac toxicities such as anthracyclines, trastuzumab, taxanes, tamoxifen, and letrozole, among others, individual sensitivity to late heart morbidity, and hereditary heart disease [19]. The definitions of the heart and its substructures are shown in **Table 1**, and the standardized delineation consensus and atlas should be consulted by radiation oncologists. For the heart and cardiac substructures, further investigation should be conducted regarding which dose-volume limitations were used during the design of radiation planning and what optimal dosimetric parameters were reported to be necessary, such as maximal or mean heart dose, V_{5Gy}, V_{10Gy}, V_{20Gy}, etc. The clinical endpoints included cardiac mortality and radiation-associated clinical and subclinical heart diseases [33]. The optimal RT delivery techniques and reliable methods to evaluate these endpoints will require further studies. The designation of RRHD might unavoidably increase the psychological burden of patients. In addition, to find those patients who may develop late RRHD, health economic evaluations should be critically performed prior to the initiation of screening programs [19].

Substructure	Definition	Note
Heart [16, 34, 70]	Cranial: The whole heart starts just inferior to the left pulmonary artery Caudal: The heart blends with the diaphragm	If contrast is administered, the superior vena cava (SVC) can generally be separately contoured from the whole heart. In a noncontrast scan, the SVC can be included for simplification and consistency
Pericardium [34]	The whole heart	Cardiac vessels run in the fatty tissue within the pericardium and should be included in the contours
Left atrium [34]	Begins just inferior to the left pulmonary artery	–
Left ventricle [16, 34]	The visible heart according to both CT images and heart anatomy	Typically, anterior and to the left of the left atrium
Right atrium [34]	No	Starts to the right of the aortic root superiorly
Right ventricle [34]	No	Lies directly beneath the sternum and connects to the pulmonary trunk
Left main coronary artery [34, 70]	Defined from its origin in the aortic sinus to the first branches	Originates from the left side of the ascending aorta, inferior to the right pulmonary artery
Right coronary artery [34, 70]		Originates from the right side of the ascending aorta
Left anterior descending artery [34, 70]	Defined from where they branched at the left or right main coronary artery to the caudal edge of the endocardial surface of the left ventricle	Originates from the left coronary artery and runs in the interventricular groove between the right and left ventricles
Left circumflex artery [34, 70]		Originates from the left coronary artery and runs between the left atrium and ventricle
Right marginal artery [70]		–
Aortic valve [34]	No	Found within the ascending aorta and seen in cross section on axial CT
Pulmonic valve [34]	No	Found within the pulmonary trunk and seen in cross section on axial CT
Tricuspid valve [34]	No	Located between the right atrium and ventricle. It is difficult to see, but it is defined as the area where the blood pool between the atrium and ventricle is shared
Mitral valve [34]	No	Located between the left atrium and ventricle. It is difficult to see, but it is defined as the area where the blood pool between the atrium and ventricle is shared
Atrioventricular node [34]	No	Cannot be seen on CT. It is located on the basal portion of the interventricular septum and extends between the right atrium and ventricle
Anterior myocardial territory [16, 17, 70]	Comprises the myocardium from the anterior surface of the heart up to 1.0 cm posteriorly and the main branches of the coronary arteries at the anterior portion of the heart	It is an imaged subregion in the anterior port of the heart as a high-risk region for breast cancer radiation therapy

Table 1. Recommended delineations of the heart and substructures.

9. Conclusion

As a significant radiation-induced toxicity, RRHD should not be neglected during clinical decision-making, especially for patients who could be cured by modern anticancer modalities. RRHD includes radiation-induced death from heart diseases, as well as clinical and subclinical heart disease. Advanced RT techniques including breath control, IMRT, and imaging-guided RT might be used to avoid or spare cardiac doses and/or volume, which might translate into decreased incidence of RRHD. Furthermore, the significance and implications of RRHD differ depending on the clinical scenario; therefore, a consensus has not yet been reached regarding the recommended dose-volume limits. It is prudent to minimize the cardiac dose/volume and optimize the patient cardiovascular risk profiles. The recognition, prevention and prediction, and treatment of RRHD should be within the domain of oncocardiology, which requires close collaboration between oncologists and cardiologists [14, 63].

Acknowledgements

This work was granted by Shenzhen Scientific Innovation in basic research project JCYJ20160422162900408 and Shenzhen Sanming Project.

Author details

Wenyong Tan*, Xianming Li and Yong Dai

*Address all correspondence to: tanwyym@hotmail.com

Department of Oncology, The Second Clinical Medical College (Shenzhen People's Hospital), Ji'nan University, Shenzhen, China

References

[1] Torre LA, Bray F, Siegel RL, Ferlay J, Lortet-Tieulent J, Jemal A. Global cancer statistics, 2012. *CA: A Cancer Journal for Clinicians*. Mar 2015;65(2):87–108.

[2] Chen W, Zheng R, Baade PD, et al. Cancer statistics in China, 2015. *CA: A Cancer Journal for Clinicians*. Mar 2016;66(2):115–132.

[3] Early Breast Cancer Trialists' Collaborative G, Darby S, McGale P, et al. Effect of radiotherapy after breast-conserving surgery on 10-year recurrence and 15-year breast cancer death: meta-analysis of individual patient data for 10,801 women in 17 randomised trials. *Lancet*. Nov 12 2011;378(9804):1707–1716.

[4] Early Breast Cancer Trialists' Collaborative G. Effects of chemotherapy and hormonal therapy for early breast cancer on recurrence and 15-year survival: an overview of the randomised trials. *Lancet*. May 14–20 2005;365(9472):1687–1717.

[5] Group EBCTC. Favourable and unfavourable effects on long-term survival of radiotherapy for early breast cancer: an overview of the randomised trials. Early Breast Cancer Trialists' Collaborative Group. *Lancet*. May 20 2000;355(9217):1757–1770.

[6] Group EBCTC. Effect of radiotherapy after mastectomy and axillary surgery on 10-year recurrence and 20-year breast cancer mortality: meta-analysis of individual patient data for 8135 women in 22 randomised trials. *The Lancet*. 2014;383(9935):2127–2135.

[7] Albain KS, Swann RS, Rusch VW, et al. Radiotherapy plus chemotherapy with or without surgical resection for stage III non-small-cell lung cancer: a phase III randomised controlled trial. *Lancet*. Aug 1 2009;374(9687):379–386.

[8] Auperin A, Le Pechoux C, Rolland E, et al. Meta-analysis of concomitant versus sequential radiochemotherapy in locally advanced non-small-cell lung cancer. *Journal of Clinical Oncology*. May 1 2010;28(13):2181–2190.

[9] Rodrigues G, Choy H, Bradley J, et al. Definitive radiation therapy in locally advanced non-small cell lung cancer: executive summary of an American Society for Radiation Oncology (ASTRO) evidence-based clinical practice guideline. *Practical Radiation Oncology*. May-Jun 2015;5(3):141–148.

[10] Shapiro J, van Lanschot JJ, Hulshof MC, et al. Neoadjuvant chemoradiotherapy plus surgery versus surgery alone for oesophageal or junctional cancer (CROSS): long-term results of a randomised controlled trial. *The Lancet Oncology*. Sep 2015;16(9):1090–1098.

[11] Rustgi AK, El-Serag HB. Esophageal carcinoma. *The New England Journal of Medicine*. Dec 25 2014;371(26):2499–2509.

[12] Darby SC, Cutter DJ, Boerma M, et al. Radiation-related heart disease: current knowledge and future prospects. *International Journal of Radiation Oncology Biology Physics*. Mar 1 2010;76(3):656–665.

[13] Darby SC, Ewertz M, McGale P, et al. Risk of ischemic heart disease in women after radiotherapy for breast cancer. *The New England Journal of Medicine*. Mar 14 2013;368(11):987–998.

[14] Tan W, Wu X, Wei S. Chemoradiotherapy-associated cardiovascular toxicity: a need of cardio-oncology to improve. *Journal of Clinical & Experimental Cardiology*. J Clin Exp Cardiolog 5:320.

[15] Bezjak A, Temin S, Franklin G, et al. Definitive and adjuvant radiotherapy in locally advanced non-small-cell lung cancer: American Society of Clinical Oncology Clinical Practice Guideline Endorsement of the American Society for Radiation Oncology Evidence-Based Clinical Practice Guideline. *Journal of Clinical Oncology*. Jun 20 2015;33(18):2100–2105.

[16] Tan W, Wang X, Qiu D, et al. Dosimetric comparison of intensity-modulated radiotherapy plans, with or without anterior myocardial territory and left ventricle as organs at risk, in early-stage left-sided breast cancer patients. *International Journal of Radiation Oncology Biology Physics*. Dec 1 2011;81(5):1544–1551.

[17] Tan W, Liu D, Xue C, et al. Anterior myocardial territory may replace the heart as organ at risk in intensity-modulated radiotherapy for left-sided breast cancer. *International Journal of Radiation Oncology Biology Physics*. Apr 1 2012;82(5):1689–1697.

[18] Preston DL, Shimizu Y, Pierce DA, Suyama A, Mabuchi K. Studies of mortality of atomic bomb survivors. Report 13: Solid cancer and noncancer disease mortality: 1950–1997. *Radiation research*. Oct 2003;160(4):381–407.

[19] Offersen B, Hojris I, Overgaard M. Radiation-induced heart morbidity after adjuvant radiotherapy of early breast cancer—Is it still an issue? *Radiotherapy and oncology: Journal of the European Society for Therapeutic Radiology and Oncology*. Aug 2011;100(2):157–159.

[20] Boero IJ, Paravati AJ, Triplett DP, et al. Modern radiation therapy and cardiac outcomes in breast cancer. *International Journal of Radiation Oncology Biology Physics*. 2016;94(4):700–708.

[21] Aleman BM, van den Belt-Dusebout AW, De Bruin ML, et al. Late cardiotoxicity after treatment for Hodgkin lymphoma. *Blood*. Mar 1 2007;109(5):1878–1886.

[22] Swerdlow AJ, Higgins CD, Smith P, et al. Myocardial infarction mortality risk after treatment for Hodgkin disease: a collaborative British cohort study. *Journal of the National Cancer Institute*. Feb 7 2007;99(3):206–214.

[23] Hodgson DC. Late effects in the era of modern therapy for Hodgkin lymphoma. Hematology American Society of Hematology Education Program 2011;2011:323–9.

[24] Maraldo MV, Giusti F, Vogelius IR, et al. Cardiovascular disease after treatment for Hodgkin's lymphoma: an analysis of nine collaborative EORTC-LYSA trials. *Lancet Haematology*. Nov 2015;2(11):e492–502.

[25] van Nimwegen FA, Schaapveld M, Janus CP, et al. Cardiovascular disease after Hodgkin lymphoma treatment: 40-year disease risk. *JAMA Internal Medicine*. Jun 2015;175(6):1007–1017.

[26] Yan X, Sasi SP, Gee H, et al. Cardiovascular risks associated with low dose ionizing particle radiation. *PloS One*. 2014;9(10):e110269.

[27] Hauptmann M, Mohan AK, Doody MM, Linet MS, Mabuchi K. Mortality from diseases of the circulatory system in radiologic technologists in the United States. *American Journal of Epidemiology*. Feb 1 2003;157(3):239–248.

[28] Okubo T. Long-term epidemiological studies of atomic bomb survivors in Hiroshima and Nagasaki: study populations, dosimetry and summary of health effects. *Radiation Protection Dosimetry*. Oct 2012;151(4):671–673.

[29] Marks LB, Yu X, Prosnitz RG, et al. The incidence and functional consequences of RT-associated cardiac perfusion defects. *International Journal of Radiation Oncology Biology Physics*. Sep 1 2005;63(1):214–223.

[30] Prosnitz RG, Hubbs JL, Evans ES, et al. Prospective assessment of radiotherapy-associated cardiac toxicity in breast cancer patients: analysis of data 3 to 6 years after treatment. *Cancer*. Oct 15 2007;110(8):1840–1850.

[31] Schultz-Hector S, Trott KR. Radiation-induced cardiovascular diseases: is the epidemiologic evidence compatible with the radiobiologic data? *International Journal of Radiation Oncology Biology Physics*. Jan 1 2007;67(1):10–18.

[32] Lee MS, Finch W, Mahmud E. Cardiovascular complications of radiotherapy. *The American Journal of cardiology*. Nov 15 2013;112(10):1688–1696.

[33] Gagliardi G, Constine LS, Moiseenko V, et al. Radiation dose-volume effects in the heart. *International Journal of Radiation Oncology Biology Physics*. Mar 1 2010;76(3 Suppl):S77–85.

[34] Feng M, Moran JM, Koelling T, et al. Development and validation of a heart atlas to study cardiac exposure to radiation following treatment for breast cancer. *International Journal of Radiation Oncology Biology Physics*. Jan 1 2011;79(1):10–18.

[35] Das SK, Baydush AH, Zhou S, et al. Predicting radiotherapy-induced cardiac perfusion defects. *Medical Physics*. Jan 2005;32(1):19–27.

[36] Shah C, Badiyan S, Berry S, et al. Cardiac dose sparing and avoidance techniques in breast cancer radiotherapy. *Radiotherapy and Oncology: Journal of the European Society for Therapeutic Radiology and Oncology*. 2014;112:9–16.

[37] Korreman SS, Pedersen AN, Aarup LR, Nottrup TJ, Specht L, Nystrom H. Reduction of cardiac and pulmonary complication probabilities after breathing adapted radiotherapy for breast cancer. *International Journal of Radiation Oncology Biology Physics*. Aug 1 2006;65(5):1375–1380.

[38] Lymberis SC, deWyngaert JK, Parhar P, et al. Prospective assessment of optimal individual position (prone versus supine) for breast radiotherapy: volumetric and dosimetric correlations in 100 patients. *International Journal of Radiation Oncology Biology Physics*. Nov 15 2012;84(4):902–909.

[39] Fernandez-Lizarbe E, Montero A, Polo A, et al. Pilot study of feasibility and dosimetric comparison of prone versus supine breast radiotherapy. *Clinical & Translational Oncology*. Jun 2013;15(6):450–459.

[40] Jozsef G, DeWyngaert JK, Becker SJ, Lymberis S, Formenti SC. Prospective study of cone-beam computed tomography image-guided radiotherapy for prone accelerated partial breast irradiation. *International Journal of Radiation Oncology Biology Physics*. Oct 1 2011;81(2):568–574.

[41] De Puysseleyr A, Mulliez T, Gulyban A, et al. Improved cone-beam computed tomography in supine and prone breast radiotherapy. Surface reconstruction, radiation exposure, and clinical workflow. *Strahlentherapie und Onkologie: Organ der Deutschen Rontgengesellschaft ... [et al]*. Nov 2013;189(11):945–950.

[42] Arthur DW, Morris MM, Vicini FA. Breast cancer: new radiation treatment options. *Oncology (Williston Park)*. Nov 2004;18(13):1621–1629; discussion 1629–1630, 1636–1638.

[43] Li JG, Williams SS, Goffinet DR, Boyer AL, Xing L. Breast-conserving radiation therapy using combined electron and intensity-modulated radiotherapy technique. *Radiotherapy and Oncology: Journal of the European Society for Therapeutic Radiology and Oncology*. Jul 2000;56(1):65–71.

[44] Lohr F, El-Haddad M, Dobler B, et al. Potential effect of robust and simple IMRT approach for left-sided breast cancer on cardiac mortality. *International Journal of Radiation Oncology Biology Physics*. May 1 2009;74(1):73–80.

[45] Badiyan SN, Shah C, Arthur D, et al. Hypofractionated regional nodal irradiation for breast cancer: examining the data and potential for future studies. *Radiotherapy and Oncology: Journal of the European Society for Therapeutic Radiology and Oncology*. Jan 2014;110(1):39–44.

[46] Shaitelman SF, Khan AJ, Woodward WA, et al. Shortened radiation therapy schedules for early-stage breast cancer: a review of hypofractionated whole-breast irradiation and accelerated partial breast irradiation. *The Breast Journal*. Mar-Apr 2014;20(2):131–146.

[47] Major T, Polgar C, Lovey K, Frohlich G. Dosimetric characteristics of accelerated partial breast irradiation with CT image--based multicatheter interstitial brachytherapy: a single institution's experience. *Brachytherapy*. Sep-Oct 2011;10(5):421–426.

[48] Major T, Frohlich G, Lovey K, Fodor J, Polgar C. Dosimetric experience with accelerated partial breast irradiation using image-guided interstitial brachytherapy. *Radiotherapy and Oncology: Journal of the European Society for Therapeutic Radiology and Oncology*. Jan 2009;90(1):48–55.

[49] Lomax AJ, Cella L, Weber D, Kurtz JM, Miralbell R. Potential role of intensity-modulated photons and protons in the treatment of the breast and regional nodes. *International Journal of Radiation Oncology Biology Physics*. Mar 1 2003;55(3):785–792.

[50] Johansson J, Isacsson U, Lindman H, Montelius A, Glimelius B. Node-positive left-sided breast cancer patients after breast-conserving surgery: potential outcomes of radiotherapy modalities and techniques. *Radiotherapy and Oncology: Journal of the European Society for Therapeutic Radiology and Oncology*. Nov 2002;65(2):89–98.

[51] Ares C, Khan S, Macartain AM, et al. Postoperative proton radiotherapy for localized and locoregional breast cancer: potential for clinically relevant improvements? *International Journal of Radiation Oncology Biology Physics*. Mar 1 2010;76(3):685–697.

[52] Jimenez RB, Goma C, Nyamwanda J, et al. Intensity modulated proton therapy for post-mastectomy radiation of bilateral implant reconstructed breasts: a treatment planning study. *Radiotherapy and Oncology: Journal of the European Society for Therapeutic Radiology and Oncology*. May 2013;107(2):213–217.

[53] Ng AK, Li S, Neuberg D, et al. Long-term results of a prospective trial of mantle irradiation alone for early-stage Hodgkin's disease. *Annals of Oncology*. Nov 2006;17(11):1693–1697.

[54] Page V, Gardner A, Karzmark CJ. Physical and dosimetric aspects of the radiotherapy of malignant lymphomas. I. The mantle technique. *Radiology*. Sep 1970;96(3):609–618.

[55] Anderson H, Deakin DP, Wagstaff J, et al. A randomised study of adjuvant chemotherapy after mantle radiotherapy in supradiaphragmatic Hodgkin's disease PS IA-IIB: a report from the Manchester lymphoma group. *British Journal of Cancer*. Jun 1984;49(6):695–702.

[56] Specht L, Yahalom J, Illidge T, et al. Modern Radiation Therapy for Hodgkin Lymphoma: Field and Dose Guidelines From the International Lymphoma Radiation Oncology Group (ILROG). *International Journal of Radiation Oncology Biology Physics*. Jun 18 2013.

[57] Ansell SM. Hodgkin Lymphoma: Diagnosis and Treatment. Mayo Clinic proceedings 2015;90:1574–83.

[58] Bradley JD, Paulus R, Komaki R, et al. Standard-dose versus high-dose conformal radiotherapy with concurrent and consolidation carboplatin plus paclitaxel with or without cetuximab for patients with stage IIIA or IIIB non-small-cell lung cancer (RTOG 0617): a randomised, two-by-two factorial phase 3 study. *The Lancet Oncology*. 2015;16(2):187–199.

[59] Chang JY, Jabbour SK, De Ruysscher D, et al. Consensus statement on proton therapy in early-stage and locally advanced non-small cell lung cancer. *International Journal of Radiation Oncology Biology Physics*. May 1 2016;95(1):505–516.

[60] Tajstra M, Gadula-Gacek E, Buchta P, Blamek S, Gasior M, Kosiuk J. Effect of therapeutic ionizing radiation on implantable electronic devices: systematic review and practical guidance. *Journal of Cardiovascular Electrophysiology*. 2016;27:1247–51.

[61] Salerno F, Gomellini S, Caruso C, et al. Management of radiation therapy patients with cardiac defibrillator or pacemaker. *La Radiologia Medica*. Jun 2016;121(6):515–520.

[62] Shu J, Zhou J, Patel C, Yan GX. Pharmacotherapy of cardiac arrhythmias—basic science for clinicians. *Pacing and Clinical Electrophysiology: PACE*. Nov 2009;32(11):1454–1465.

[63] Curigliano G, Cardinale D, Dent S, et al. Cardiotoxicity of anticancer treatments: Epidemiology, detection, and management. *CA: A Cancer Journal for Clinicians*. Jul 2016;66(4):309–325.

[64] Curigliano G, Cardinale D, Suter T, et al. Cardiovascular toxicity induced by chemotherapy, targeted agents and radiotherapy: ESMO Clinical Practice Guidelines. *Annals of Oncology*. Oct 2012;23 Suppl 7:vii155–166.

[65] Yancy CW, Jessup M, Bozkurt B, et al. 2013 ACCF/AHA guideline for the management of heart failure: a report of the American College of Cardiology Foundation/American Heart Association Task Force on Practice Guidelines. *Journal of the American College of Cardiology*. Oct 15 2013;62(16):e147–239.

[66] James PA, Oparil S, Carter BL, et al. 2014 Evidence-Based Guideline for the Management of High Blood Pressure in Adults: Report From the Panel Members Appointed to the Eighth Joint National Committee (JNC 8). *JAMA: The Journal of the American Medical Association*. 2014;311:507–20.

[67] Izzedine H, Ederhy S, Goldwasser F, et al. Management of hypertension in angiogenesis inhibitor-treated patients. *Annals of Oncology*. May 2009;20(5):807–815.

[68] Lackland DT. Hypertension: Joint National Committee on Detection, Evaluation, and Treatment of High Blood Pressure guidelines. *Current Opinion in Neurology*. Feb 2013;26(1):8–12.

[69] Farge D, Bounameaux H, Brenner B, et al. International clinical practice guidelines including guidance for direct oral anticoagulants in the treatment and prophylaxis of venous thromboembolism in patients with cancer. *The Lancet Oncology*. 2016;17(10):e452–e466.

[70] Tan W, Xu L, Wang X, Qiu D, Han G, Hu D. Estimation of the displacement of cardiac substructures and the motion of the coronary arteries using electrocardiographic gating. *OncoTargets and Therapy*. 2013;6:1325–1332.

Section 3

Physical Parameters

Chapter 11

Radiotherapy Dose Optimization in Target Tissues Using Internal Radiation-Generating Devices and Microspheres

Joseph John Bevelacqua

Additional information is available at the end of the chapter

http://dx.doi.org/10.5772/67203

Abstract

Preferentially delivering ionizing radiation to target tissues during radiotherapy procedures is investigated using internal radiation-generating devices and microspheres loaded with radioactive material. This chapter presumes the existence of internal radiation-generating devices and develops their requisite characteristics to permit the selective irradiation of tumors. The feasibility of disrupting a tumor's vascular structure is also investigated. Calculated absorbed dose profiles for both approaches demonstrate that dose can be successfully localized in a target tissue while minimizing the delivery to healthy tissue.

Keywords: absorbed dose, internal radiation-generating devices, microspheres, radiation therapy, tumor vascular disruption

1. Introduction

A significant issue associated with existing radiotherapy approaches is that agents that deliver dose to tumor cells also irradiate healthy tissue [1–6]. Short-term as well as long-term detriments can appear following radiotherapy procedures. These effects occur when healthy tissue outside the target volume is irradiated and affect the patient's subsequent recovery and quality of life. For example, short-term detriments (e.g., incontinence and erectile dysfunction) occur following prostate cancer therapy [7]. Long-term effects include secondary cancers and cardiovascular disease [8]. In view of these detriments, alternative therapy approaches that preferentially deliver dose to the target tissue are of interest and should be investigated.

This chapter considers two approaches that have the potential to significantly minimize the dose to healthy tissue while maximizing the dose delivered to the target tissue. The first technique utilizes internal radiation-generating devices that are in their conceptual development phase, and the second is an enhancement of the ^{90}Y microsphere approach that has been successfully utilized to treat liver cancers by disrupting the tumor's vasculature.

Heavy ions, neutrons, protons, and other radiation types have numerous applications for treating a variety of cancers [1–3, 6, 9–14]. To date, these techniques have focused on beams originating outside the body. These external beams selectively irradiate the tumor mass, but still deliver some dose to healthy tissue. This chapter investigates the possibility of using radiation-generating devices that would be implanted within a tumor to preferentially irradiate its volume and develops their requisite characteristics to permit the selective irradiation of tumors. These devices are postulated to have a size on the order of 10^{-6} m [1–3, 6].

Microspheres offer a unique approach that has the potential to impact tumor cells by disrupting their vascular structure. A number of authors [15, 16] have proposed a therapy approach that prevents the development of the tumor's vascular supply. Vascular disruption agents incorporate both chemotherapy [17, 18] as well as radiotherapy [18–27]. Radiotherapy vascular disruption techniques utilizing ^{90}Y microspheres, including anti-angiogenic and radioembolization therapies, are used to treat liver cancers [18–23]. Other radionuclides (e.g., ^{32}P) are under investigation, but radiation types other than high-energy beta particles are not under active consideration [22].

2. Internal radiation-generating devices

The requisite technology to construct internal radiation-generating devices (IRGDs) is being developed (e.g., electron accelerators powered by lasers [28]). These devices are optical cavities [28] whose size depends on the laser's wavelength. The utilization of shorter wavelength lasers leads to devices of the size envisioned for IRGDs [1–3, 6].

Refs. [1–6] provide calculations for the range of heavy ions in water. By selecting appropriate ion and energy combinations, specific target irradiation locations are preferentially irradiated. The capability to localize dose in the target is a positive feature that makes heavy ions an attractive tool for external beam therapy and supports their potential use in an IRGD. By adjusting the beam energy and radiation type, an IRGD has the capability to selectively irradiate the tumor.

2.1. Candidate radiation types

Internal devices could incorporate pions, muons, photons, electrons, protons, and heavy ions to deposit energy into tumors. Ranges on the order of a centimeter are achieved using 10–20 MeV pions and muons, 30–40 MeV protons, 100–200 MeV alpha particles, and energies on the order of 90 MeV/nucleon for ^{12}C, ^{16}O, ^{20}Ne ions, and heavier ions [1–6].

2.2. IRGD characteristics and arrangement

The feasibility of using IRGDs for therapy applications is illustrated using a cubic Cartesian configuration. This configuration is repeated to irradiate various tumor sizes. A unit cell concept is arbitrary, but simplifies the calculation of absorbed dose to the tumor site.

The cubic Cartesian configuration utilizes 27 devices arranged in three planes with nine devices in each plane. The coordinates of the devices are written in terms of a scaled dimension ξ:

$$\xi = \frac{R}{d} \tag{1}$$

where d is the internal device grid spacing and R is the maximum ion range. This approach facilitates a general discussion and eliminates adjustments for specific ion-energy combinations.

The 27 devices reside at the locations (x, y, z): (0, 0, z), (ξ, 0, z), (ξ, − ξ, z), (0 − ξ, z), (−ξ, − ξ, z), (−ξ, 0, z), (−ξ, ξ, z), (0, ξ, z), and (ξ, ξ, z) for z = -ξ, 0, and ξ. Utilizing additional devices enhances the delivery of dose in a more uniform manner.

IRGDs should incorporate a number of characteristics to facilitate the dose delivery to the target volume. In general, the IRGDs should have the capability to (1) irradiate 4π steradians, (2) deliver various ion-energy combinations, (3) be controlled in real time, (4) rapidly change the radiation type, energy, and fluence, (5) produce a variable fluence to deliver a uniform dose, (6) position itself at a desired location, (7) monitor the delivered dose profile using positron emission tomography or other techniques to verify that it is preferentially irradiating the tumor volume, and (8) have the capability to be removed from the body.

Delivering a uniform absorbed dose (D) requires careful control of the fluence, ion type, and energy (E). These parameters are varied during the irradiation time (T) to deliver a uniform dose within the unit cell:

$$D=\sum_{i=1}^{N}\int_{-\xi}^{+\xi}\int_{-\xi}^{+\xi}\int_{-\xi}^{+\xi}\int_{0}^{T}\frac{1}{\rho(x_i,y_i,z_i)}\left(-\frac{dE(x_i,y_i,z_i,t)}{dr(x_i,y_i,z_i)}\right) \times \Phi(x_i,y_i,z_i,t)\,dx_i\,dy_i\,dz_i\,dt \tag{2}$$

where $r(x_i, y_i, z_i)$ is the distance measured from each device, $\Phi(x_i, y_i, z_i, t)$ is the time-dependent fluence rate, *N* is the number of implanted devices, and *i* labels the individual device [1–3, 6].

2.3. Absorbed dose calculations

Eq. (2) is used to calculate the absorbed dose from internal radiation-generating devices within a Cartesian lattice. Stopping powers are determined using the methodology outlined in Refs. [1–6], and energy-dependent cross sections are obtained from Shen et al's parameterization [29] or models [1–6].

As an initial example of the internal device concept, a spectrum of eight proton groups (i.e., 10, 20, 30, 40, 50, 60, 70, and 80 MeV) is selected to be the output of the device. A spectrum of energies facilitates the irradiation of the entire tumor volume. A uniform distribution of proton dose requires a continuous proton energy distribution. The 27 proton generating devices are distributed in a 10 × 10 × 10 cm volume of water. Each device is assumed to radiate isotropically. The results of irradiating this water volume with 27 internal devices generating an output of 10, 20, 30, 40, 50, 60, 70, and 80 MeV protons are illustrated in **Figure 1**. The fluence at each proton energy is selected to be the same.

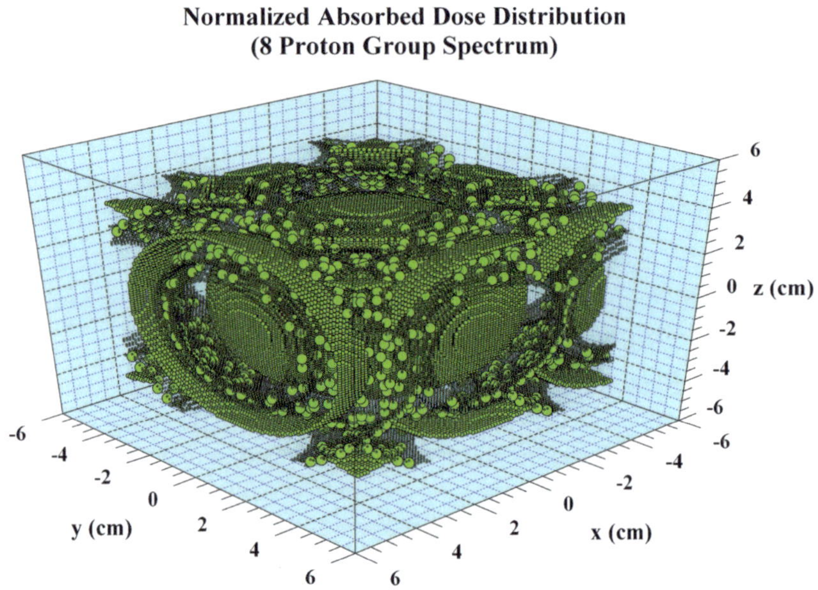

Figure 1. Normalized absorbed dose distribution from 27 internal radiation-generating devices producing a spectrum of eight proton groups (i.e., 10, 20, 30, 40, 50, 60, 70, and 80 MeV protons). The absorbed dose is proportional to the plotted circle radius.

Since the total absorbed dose of **Figure 1** is the superposition of a number of manifolds (i.e., the various isodose surfaces), the structure of the surface is governed by the proton output spectrum, fluence, attenuating medium characteristics, ion stopping power, and reaction cross section as noted in Eqs. (1) and (2). **Figure 1** represents the three-dimensional absorbed dose profile. In **Figure 1**, the dose at each point is proportional to the plotted circle radius.

Figure 1 illustrates the symmetry of the absorbed dose distribution associated with the 27 internal radiators. Although the distribution is not uniform, the IRGDs effectively irradiate the target volume. The average dose to the target 10 × 10 × 10 cm volume depends on the IRGD proton spectrum. For example, proton energy groups of 10 MeV; 10 and 20 MeV; 10, 20, 30, and 40 MeV; and 10, 20, 30, 40, 50, 60, 70, and 80 MeV produce to an average dose over the target volume of 5.89×10^{-6}, 5.75×10^{-4}, 3.00×10^{-2}, and 9.79×10^{-2} relative to the peak dose, respectively.

Increasing the number of proton energy groups between 10 and 80 MeV range will continue to increase the average absorbed dose to the tumor site. The discussion of the characteristics of the detailed three-dimensional absorbed dose profile illustrates the complexity of therapy planning when implementing a new technology.

http://dx.doi.org/10.5772/67203

3. Radionuclide vascular disruption therapy using microspheres

Conventional radiotherapy often involves the deposition of the radionuclide within a tumor mass. It is also feasible to attack the tumor by disrupting its blood supply. Vascular disruption agents have been developed and utilized in chemotherapy and radiotherapy.

3.1. Tumor vasculature

The vascular structure of normal tissue provides an efficient method to deliver nutrients. Growing tumors have a poorly developed vasculature that does not adequately nourish the cells [17]. The tumor's weak vascular structure can be degraded using a chemical or radioactive agent.

Vessels that are dilated and have elongated shapes, blind ends, bulges, leaky sprouts, and abrupt diameter changes are defects that occur in a tumor's vascular structure. These vessel defects create sluggish and irregular blood flow that poorly nourish cancer cells and result in hypoxic tumors. Hypoxic conditions limit the effectiveness of both chemotherapy and radiotherapy and provide a measure of radioresistance to tumor cells when compared to normal, oxygenated cells. Since a tumor's growth is dependent on sufficient nourishment, eliminating its blood supply provides an additional opportunity to facilitate its destruction [17].

3.2. Current radiological efforts

Radiological efforts at tumor vascular disruption have focused on ^{90}Y. ^{90}Y was a logical choice for anti-angiogenic therapy since the dose to destroy a tumor is ≥70 Gy. However, the 2.27 MeV ^{90}Y beta particles have a range in tissue of about 1.1 cm, which deposits dose to healthy tissue well beyond the target vasculature. Bremsstrahlung from the ^{90}Y beta particles provides additional dose to healthy tissue. The properties of ^{90}Y microspheres used in therapy applications are summarized by Kennedy et al. [22].

Medical reviews suggest that the ^{90}Y approach is a safe and effective therapy method for selected patients. However, a number of negative features are associated with ^{90}Y microsphere therapy [22]. First, ^{90}Y bremsstrahlung affects healthy tissue well beyond the vasculature. Second, resin microspheres may have trace ^{90}Y on their surface, which is excreted through urine. As the ^{90}Y is excreted, additional absorbed dose is delivered to healthy tissues. Third, the total dose delivered to the lung should not exceed 30 Gy to prevent radiation pneumonitis. Fourth, patients can exhibit abdominal pain, fatigue, and nausea within three days posttreatment. Fifth, dose delivered to healthy tissue causes acute damage that includes pancreatitis, gastrointestinal ulceration, and radiation pneumonitis. Radiation-induced liver disease is a possible late effect of ^{90}Y microsphere therapy.

3.3. Theoretical methodology

A tumor's blood supply is reduced by a vascular disruption agent that causes the vessel wall to become restricted or breached to increase leakage. IRGDs and microspheres using alpha-emitting radionuclides (MAs) preferentially deliver absorbed dose to the blood vessel wall to facilitate its disruption. The wall thicknesses for a variety of human blood vessel types [30] are summarized in **Table 1**.

Blood vessel type	Wall thickness	Lumen diameter
Aorta	2 mm	25 mm
Artery	1 mm	4 mm
Arteriole	20 μm	30 μm
Capillary	1 μm	8 μm
Venule	2 μm	20 μm
Vein	0.5 mm	5 mm
Vena Cava	1.5 mm	30 mm

[a]Barrett et al. [30].

Table 1. Characteristics of various blood vessel types[a].

Tumor vessel wall sizes, including arterioles, are usually <100 μm [17]. Although arterioles are used as the base case in this chapter, the vessel sizes summarized in **Table 1** suggest that a variety of blood vessel types could service a developing tumor [30].

3.4. Microsphere radionuclide selection and characteristics

An alternative to the use of ^{90}Y is provided by radionuclides that emit low-energy photons, low-energy beta particles, or alpha particles. These radionuclides would replace ^{90}Y as the radioactive material loading the microspheres.

Desirable characteristics for the radionuclide and candidate microsphere to facilitate tumor blood vessel disruption include the (1) nuclide has a short effective half-life, (2) range of the emitted radiation is <100 μm or the maximum vessel wall thickness, (3) arteriole wall dose is at least 100 Gy, (4) healthy tissue dose is minimized, (5) microsphere preferentially attaches to the wall of the tumor's arteriole, (6) candidate radionuclide is compatible with the microsphere, and (7) the microsphere can be removed from the body at a desired time.

Although these characteristics provide a basis for the calculations presented in this chapter, they have not been optimized to produce a viable alternative to the ^{90}Y microsphere approach. As noted in Refs. [4–6], both alpha-emitting and low-energy beta-gamma loaded microspheres can be utilized to disrupt a tumor's vasculature. However, the daughter radiation presents a problem, and this radiation can often irradiate healthy tissue that was an original concern associated with the ^{90}Y approach.

Production challenges and associated availability are impediments for the use of alpha-emitting radionuclides. Therefore, the availability of the selected radionuclide is an important consideration. ^{222}Rn is readily available and would be a candidate for microsphere use. The ^{222}Rn daughters yield additional dose to the tumor vasculature, which could enhance the approach if healthy dose is avoided.

3.4.1. *Selection of radionuclide*

In Refs. [4–6], a list of candidate alpha- and beta-gamma-emitting radionuclides was created. Unfortunately, most candidate radionuclides, including ^{149}Tb, ^{211}At, ^{212}Bi, ^{213}Bi, ^{223}Ra, ^{225}Ac, and ^{227}Th, have daughter gamma, beta, or bremsstrahlung radiation that irradiates healthy tissue well beyond the target volume, which does not meet the goal of minimizing the dose delivered beyond the arteriole wall. As part of that goal, ^{222}Rn was noted as an interesting possibility since it occurs naturally as part of the ^{238}U decay chain. Eq. (3) lists the ^{222}Rn decay daughters with the associated decay scheme:

$$\begin{aligned} &^{222}Rn \xrightarrow{\alpha} {}^{218}Po \xrightarrow{\alpha} {}^{214}Pb \xrightarrow{\beta^-} {}^{214}Bi \xrightarrow{\beta^-} {}^{214}Po \xrightarrow{\alpha} {}^{210}Pb \xrightarrow{\beta^-} \\ &^{210}Bi \xrightarrow{\beta^-} {}^{210}Po \xrightarrow{\alpha} {}^{206}Pb \end{aligned} \quad (3)$$

Although ^{222}Rn has a number of desirable characteristics, its daughters emit beta and gamma radiation that deliver absorbed dose well beyond the thickness of the arteriole wall. Therefore, ^{222}Rn is not a primary candidate to achieve selective dose delivery to the vascular wall. However, a review of the ^{222}Rn daughters suggests that ^{210}Po has the desired characteristics for vascular disruption without significantly irradiating healthy tissue. In particular, the ^{210}Po 5.3 MeV alpha particle irradiates the arteriole wall and limits the absorbed dose beyond the target tissue. In addition, the weak 803 keV ^{210}Po photon radiation with a yield $<1.0 \times 10^{-3}\%$ delivers minimal dose beyond the target tissue.

3.4.2. *Basic microsphere design*

The base case microsphere is loaded with 0.3 Bq of ^{210}Po uniformly distributed in a 1-μm-diameter ^{12}C sphere having a density of 2.0 g/cm^3. Subsequent discussion provides the basis for the 0.3 Bq activity.

Subsequent discussion is based on a single microsphere. However, treatment procedures will utilize many spheres with the actual number determined by the cancer type and its progression. Although microsphere delivery methods other than the usual catheter approach [2–6] may be feasible, initial efforts will likely focus on the traditional delivery method [17–23].

3.4.3. *Absorbed dose computational model*

A ^{210}Po activity of 0.3 Bq delivers an absorbed dose of about 100 Gy to the arteriole wall. Defining a more exact activity value is not necessary because the design has yet to be refined. The activity value also depends on the insertion and removal methods, fabrication details, and relative biological effectiveness values for the ^{210}Po alpha and gamma radiation.

3.4.3.1. Absorbed dose from alpha particles

The absorbed dose (*D*) delivered by ions of a specific energy as a function of penetration distance *x* into tissue is [1, 12]:

$$D(x) = \frac{1}{\rho}\left(-\frac{dE}{dx}\right)\Phi(x) \tag{4}$$

where ρ is the density of tissue attenuating the ion, −dE/dx is the stopping power, and Φ(x) is the alpha particle fluence at the location of interest. The particle fluence varies with tissue penetration depth according to the relationship:

$$\Phi(x) = \Phi(0)\, e^{-\Sigma x} \tag{5}$$

where Φ(0) is the entrance fluence and Σ is the macroscopic reaction cross section. Alpha particle stopping powers are derived from Bethe's formulation [31] and follow an approach similar to the SPAR code [32]. The energy-dependent cross sections are obtained from Shen et al's parameterization [29] or models [1–6].

3.4.3.2. Photon absorbed dose

The photon absorbed dose is derived from the standard point source relationships [4–6]:

$$D = \frac{S}{4\pi r^2}\frac{\mu_{en}}{\rho} E\, B(\mu x)\, e^{-\mu x} \tag{6}$$

where S is the total number of photons irradiating the arteriole wall, r is the distance from the microsphere, μ_{en}/ρ is the mass-energy absorption coefficient, E is the photon energy, B is a buildup factor, and μ is the attenuation coefficient. The gamma absorbed dose contribution is obtained from the ISO-PC computer code [33]. Requisite photon data for ^{210}Po are based on Rittman [33].

3.4.4. Relative biological effectiveness

In therapy applications, the absorbed dose is multiplied by the relative biological effectiveness (RBE) to reflect the cell killing efficiency of a radiation type. The RBE of radiation type x is defined as the ratio of the dose of a reference energy photon to produce an effect and the dose of radiation type x to produce the same biological effect. Although the RBE is a simple concept, its therapy application is complex [34], because the RBE depends on a number of factors. These include the radiation type and its energy, the delivered absorbed dose, the delivery method (e.g., dose fractionization sequence), and the irradiated cell and tissue types. No RBE is applied to the absorbed doses calculated in this chapter because the design of the ^{210}Po microsphere is being developed. However, the alpha particle RBE is greater than unity. Therefore, the calculated absorbed doses for tumor disruption represent a lower bound for the dose delivered by the ^{210}Po microsphere.

3.4.5. Microsphere results and discussion

In subsequent discussion, the ^{210}Po microsphere resides at the inner wall of an arteriole. **Figures 2** and **3** illustrate absorbed dose profiles for water thicknesses ≤100 μm. Following previous work, the vessel wall is assumed to be water that is a good approximation for tissue [1–6, 12].

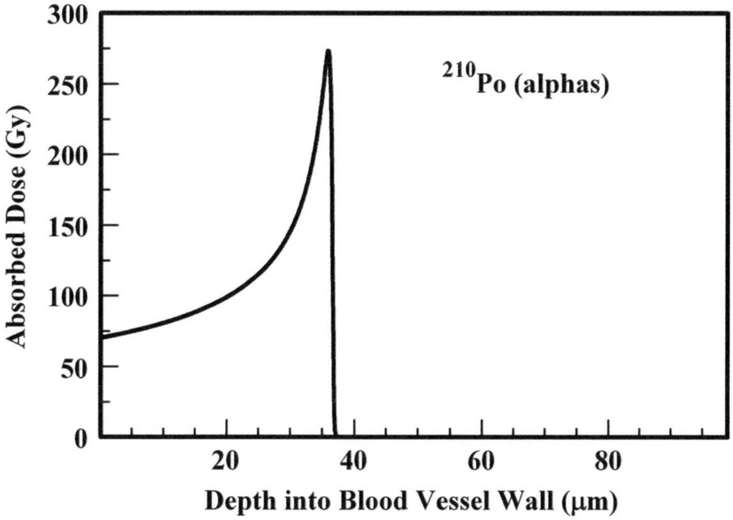

Figure 2. Absorbed dose profile for ^{210}Po alpha particles in a water medium. The absorbed dose is delivered by 0.3 Bq of ^{210}Po uniformly deposited within a 1-μm-diameter microsphere following the total decay of the radioactive material.

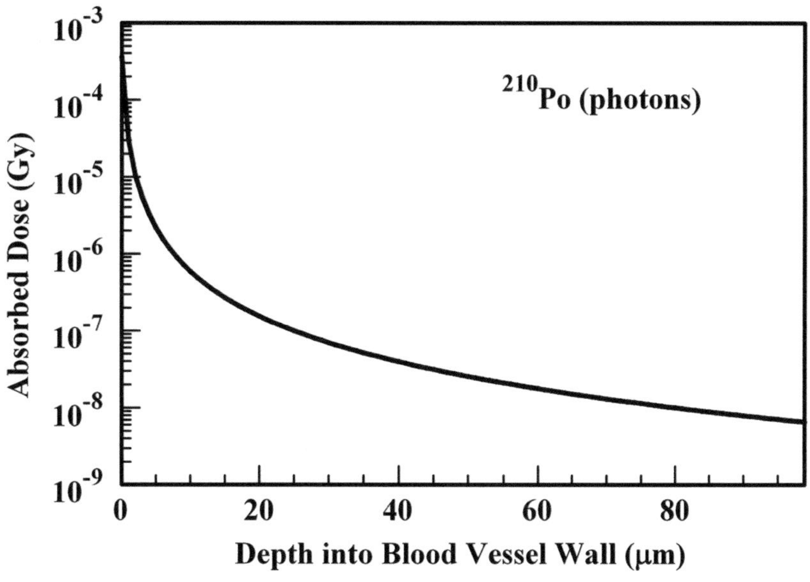

Figure 3. Absorbed dose profile for ^{210}Po photons in a water medium. The absorbed dose is delivered by 0.3 Bq of ^{210}Po uniformly deposited within a 1-μm-diameter microsphere following the total decay of the radioactive material.

Figures 2 and **3** provide the results of alpha and gamma contributions to the absorbed dose from a ^{210}Po microsphere, respectively. Since the gamma absorbed dose is significantly less than the alpha absorbed dose, **Figure 2** represents the total absorbed dose delivered by the ^{210}Po MA.

Since the peak dose is delivered at 35.9 μm, the 100 μm dose localization value is achieved. At the Bragg peak, the alpha to gamma dose ratio is 1.7×10^{10}. Beyond the Bragg peak, ^{210}Po photons deliver less than 0.1 μGy. Although ^{210}Po MAs achieve the desired dose localization, its longer half life (138 d) relative to ^{32}P (14.28 days) and ^{90}Y (2.669 days) [35] must be addressed.

The time (t)-dependent dose rate to the arteriole wall is given by the relationship:

$$\dot{D}(t) = \dot{D}(0)\, e^{-\lambda t} \tag{7}$$

where λ is the physical decay constant of the radionuclide. Integrating Eq. 7 yields the total dose at time T:

$$D(T) = \frac{\dot{D}(0)}{\lambda}\,(1 - e^{-\lambda T}) = D(\infty)\,(1 - e^{-\lambda T}) \tag{8}$$

Since the activity is proportional to the delivered dose, early removal of the microsphere at time T requires an increase in the initial activity loading by a factor (F), which is the ratio of $D(\infty)/D(T)$ [5]:

$$F = \frac{1}{(1 - e^{-\lambda T})} \tag{9}$$

This activity increase delivers the required dose to disrupt the microsphere as noted in **Figures 2** and **3**. For example, an activity of about 2 Bq (0.3 Bq × 7.19) is the requisite ^{210}Po activity loading to produce the doses summarized in **Figures 2** and **3** if the microspheres are removed at 30 days (F(30 days) = 7.19).

3.4.6. Microsphere delivery methods

In initial studies, a catheter will introduce the MA into the tumor vasculature. Following the methodology developed in ^{90}Y microsphere liver cancer therapy, the catheter enters through the femoral artery into the liver and deposits the microspheres into the tumor's blood vessels. Image-guided radiation therapy [26, 36] facilitates guiding the catheter to specifically target the tumor vasculature.

The catheter delivery method could be utilized in the treatment of a number of tumors. Specific catheter paths for the various tumor types will be refined and developed in a manner that was similar to the evolution of the ^{90}Y microsphere treatment of liver cancers [17–23]. For example, renal artery access would facilitate ^{210}Po MA deposition into the vasculature of kidney tumors.

Developing a method for preferentially depositing the MA into the desired blood vessel requires additional research and development. The microsphere research and design effort should investigate a number of chemical and physical approaches. These approaches include the use of electric charge, heat, pH, and electromagnetic fields to achieve the desired attachment of the MA to the tumor's vascular wall. The specific design options that require experimental effort include the MAs (1) electric charge and its spatial distribution, (2) dielectric and diamagnetic characteristics, (3) physical size and shape, and (4) material composition. Activating agents could be used to optimize the MA design. Electromagnetic fields heat, lasers, and a spectrum of electromagnetic radiation are possible activating agents.

3.4.7. Microsphere removal methods

Eqs. (7)–(9) suggest that extraction of MAs at a specified time requires the development of removal mechanisms. Removal could be accomplished by reversing the delivery methods discussed previously. For example, deposition and removal could be achieved by incorporating a magnetic material in the MA. The magnetic particles facilitate placement in the desired location using an active, localized magnetic field. Eliminating the magnetic field would facilitate microsphere removal. The protocol for microsphere implantation and removal requires additional research and development.

3.4.8. Effective half-life

As noted previously, the ^{210}Po physical half-life (T_p) must be addressed before the MA therapy application becomes a reality. The physical half-lives of ^{210}Po and ^{90}Y are 138 and 2.7 days, respectively. A ^{90}Y delivery approach will not be successful for ^{210}Po if the MA design does not shorten the biological half-life of the device.

In the case of the shorter half-life ^{90}Y, some microspheres are transported via blood into the lung and irradiate healthy tissue. Since the physical half-life of ^{90}Y is short, this deposition yields a relatively insignificant dose. Assuming the same transfer characteristics, ^{210}Po produces a larger lung dose and could create a significant biological detriment. This concern is eliminated if the ^{210}Po MA design produces a shorter biological half-life in the lung.

In view of these considerations, constructing ^{210}Po MAs with a short effective half-life is a design requirement. For example, the ^{210}Po MAs could be constructed using a material having ICRP 30 [37] Class D lung retention characteristics. Following the ICRP 30 methodology, Class D materials have a biological half-life <10 days. Part of ^{210}Po MA development is the use of a material with a short biological half-life. The ^{210}Po MA effective half-life in the lung is [38]:

$$T_e = \frac{T_p\ T_b}{T_p + T_b} \tag{10}$$

Following Eq. (10), the effective half-life (T_e) of a radionuclide depends on its biological and physical half-lives. Therefore, a long physical half-life is not a limiting factor if the biological half-life (T_b) is short. For example, the ^{210}Po effective half-life for a material with 2- and 10-day biological half-lives is 1.97 and 9.32 days, respectively. A MA design requirement for a Class D biological half-life eliminates the longer ^{210}Po physical half-life concern.

3.4.9. ^{210}Po toxicity and patient safety

^{210}Po has a specific activity of 1.7×10^{14} Bq/g, and its inhalation (ingestion) effective dose coefficient (EDC) is 3.0×10^{-6} Sv/Bq (2.4×10^{-7} Sv/Bq) [39]. The intake pathway caused by MA leaching has not been evaluated. In view of the inhalation and ingestion EDCs, the leaching EDC is probably in the range of the established conventional intake pathway values. For an initial scooping assessment, the leaching EDC is approximately 10^{-6} Sv/Bq. Considering the proposed 0.3 Bq ^{210}Po MA, complete ^{210}Po leaching from a single microsphere produces to an effective dose of about 0.3 μSv.

The effective dose from complete MA leakage is mitigated if the microspheres have good retention characteristics. With good ^{210}Po retention characteristics, the radiological hazard to the patient is not significant. For example, if 10^6 0.3 Bq MAs were administered with a ^{210}Po retention of 90%, the patient's 50-year effective dose commitment is only 30 mSv.

4. Vascular disruption using internal radiation-generating devices

Vascular disruption can also be achieved using internal radiation-generating devices. These devices meet the desired characteristics to maximize dose to the tumor's vascular walls while minimizing the dose to healthy tissue. For a tissue volume irradiated by a beam of ions of a given energy, the absorbed dose (D) as a function of penetration distance into tissue is given by Eqs. (4) and (5). Arteriole vascular disruption is outlined for beams of protons, alpha particles, and ^{12}C, ^{20}Ne, and ^{40}Ca ions. All beams were assumed to be fully ionized (e.g., ^{12}C ions have a +6 e charge).

The photon absorbed dose is derived from Eq. (6). Because higher energy photons have poor dose localization, low-energy photons are investigated as a possible vascular disruption agent.

4.1. Internal radiation-generating device results and discussion

The base case considered in this chapter is the 20 μm arteriole wall thickness. With this emphasis, the dose delivered to the arteriole wall and blood vessel wall thicknesses ≤100 μm [17] is calculated. The target dose, which is about of 100 Gy, is sufficient to disrupt the vessel wall. Dose delivery has not been optimized, and ion fluences to reach the 100 Gy dose level are 5×10^9, 5×10^8, 1×10^8, 5×10^7, and 1×10^7 ions/cm^2 for protons, alpha particles, ^{12}C, ^{20}Ne, and ^{40}Ca, respectively. 1×10^{10} photons are utilized in the calculations using Eq. (6).

In subsequent absorbed dose calculations, the internal radiation-generating device is assumed to reside at the inner arteriole wall. **Table 2** summarizes the calculations for photons, protons, alpha particles, and ^{12}C, ^{20}Ne, and ^{40}Ca ions and compares these results with beta-emitting nuclides currently used in therapy applications. To further illustrate the internal radiation-generating device concept, **Figure 4** illustrates the ^{12}C absorbed dose profiles for blood vessel wall depths ≤100 μm. The ^{12}C energies included in **Figure 4** are 10, 20, 25, 30, 40, and 50 MeV. Water is assumed to be the medium comprising the vessel wall.

http://dx.doi.org/10.5772/67203

Radionuclide or radiation delivery approach	Radiation type emitted	Range (μm)	E (MeV)
^{90}Y	β^-	1.1×10^4	2.281[a]
^{32}P	β^-	7.9×10^3	1.709[a]
^{33}P	β^-	5.9×10^2	0.249[a]
^{35}S	β^-	3.2×10^2	0.1674[a]
IRGD[b]	p	10–95	0.5–2.3
IRGD[b]	α	15–75	3.0–8.0
IRGD[b]	^{12}C	5–90	10.0–50.0
IRGD[b]	^{20}Ne	10–85	30.0–110.0
IRGD[b]	^{40}Ca	10–75	100.0–300.0
IRGD[b]	γ	0–20[c]	0.015–0.050
IRGD[b]	γ	0–70[d]	0.015–0.050

[a]Maximum beta energy.
[b]Internal radiation-generating device (IRGD).
[c]The dose decreases by a factor of about 10^3 over the listed depths.
[d]The dose decreases by a factor of about 10^4 over the listed depths.

Table 2. Dose localization for candidate radionuclides and radiation types.

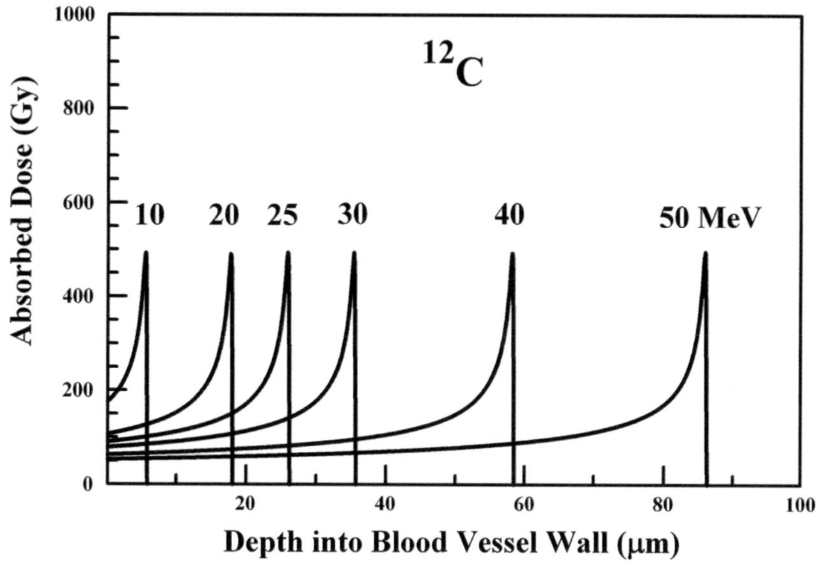

Figure 4. Absorbed dose profiles for ^{12}C ions in water. The absorbed dose curves peak at a greater depth with increasing ^{12}C ion energy. The total ion fluence for all energies is 1.0×10^8 ^{12}C ions/cm^2. The ions are delivered by an internal radiation-generating device.

Dose localization within an arteriole wall could be achieved using 1.0–1.5 MeV proton beams. Alpha particles with energies below 3 MeV will not penetrate the arteriole wall. The arteriole wall is disrupted, with minimal dose to surrounding tissue, by alpha particles in the 4–5 MeV energy range. Sufficient absorbed dose to disrupt vessels with wall thicknesses between 20 and 100 μm can be delivered by alpha particles having energies below 8 MeV.

^{12}C ions with energies below about 20 MeV do not penetrate the arteriole wall, and 20–50 MeV ions will deposit sufficient energy into a range of vessel wall thicknesses in the 20–100 μm range to produce vascular disruption. Selective arteriole wall disruption is achieved using 25–30 MeV ^{12}C ions. However, the generation of ^{12}C, ^{20}Ne, and ^{40}Ca ions is a more significant technical challenge than producing lighter ions in a first generation IRGD.

^{20}Ne ions below 30 MeV do not penetrate the arteriole wall. ^{20}Ne ions in the range of 50–110 MeV will be sufficient to reach the range of vessel wall thicknesses addressed in this chapter. Arteriole wall disruption with minimal dose to surrounding tissue is achieved using 50–70 MeV ^{20}Ne ions. In a similar manner, ^{40}Ca ions require 150–200 MeV to selectively disrupt the arteriole wall and 100–300 MeV ^{40}Ca ions penetrate vessel wall thicknesses of 10–75 μm.

Table 2 illustrates that photon energies in the range of 15–50 keV can deposit the requisite absorbed dose to disrupt an arteriole wall. Significant dose is also deposited in the 20–100 μm range by the 15–50 keV photons. However, protons and ^{4}He, ^{12}C, ^{20}Ne, and ^{40}Ca ions achieve better dose localization.

Internal radiation-generating devices can also be developed to emit low-energy electrons. Electrons present a concern because their bremsstrahlung radiation can irradiate healthy tissue beyond the target volume. However, low-energy electrons preferentially irradiate the arteriole wall with minimal bremsstrahlung. **Table 3** summarizes the range and bremsstrahlung production for 20–85 keV electrons impinging on the arteriole wall.

Electron energy (keV)	Range in water (μm)	Fraction of electron energy converted into bremsstrahlung
20	6.79	5.26×10^{-5}
25	10.6	6.57×10^{-5}
30	15.1	7.89×10^{-5}
35	20.3	9.20×10^{-5}
40	26.1	1.05×10^{-4}
50	39.6	1.31×10^{-4}
60	55.1	1.58×10^{-4}
70	72.6	1.84×10^{-4}
80	91.8	2.10×10^{-4}
85	102	2.23×10^{-4}

Table 3. Vascular disruption by low-energy electrons from an internal radiation-generating device.

The results summarized in **Table 3** suggest that 35–40 keV electrons also offer the potential to selectively disrupt an arteriole servicing a tumor. Dose localization is achieved with minimal bremsstrahlung production that permits vascular disruption without delivering absorbed dose to healthy tissue. **Table 3** also illustrates that electrons below 85 keV also selectively irradiate vessel wall thicknesses below 100 μm.

5. Conclusions

Internal radiation-generating devices and microspheres loaded with alpha-emitting radionuclides preferentially deposit dose in the target tissues while minimizing the dose delivered to healthy tissue. This selective deposition minimizes stray dose and limits the side effects that often accompany radiotherapy procedures. The microsphere approach can be realized in the near term, but an internal radiation-generating device relies on technology that is not currently available. Additional research is required to develop the techniques proposed in this chapter into practical radiotherapy protocols.

Author details

Joseph John Bevelacqua

Address all correspondence to: bevelresou@aol.com

Bevelacqua Resources, Richland, WA, USA

References

[1] Bevelacqua JJ. Systematics of heavy ion radiotherapy. Radiation Protection Management. 2005;**22(6)**:4–13.

[2] Bevelacqua JJ. Feasibility of using internal radiation-generating devices in radiotherapy. Health Physics. 2010;**98**:614–620. doi:10.1097/HP.0b013e3181c8f6ac

[3] Bevelacqua JJ. Angular absorbed dose dependence of internal radiation-generating devices in radiotherapy. Health Physics. 2012;**102**:2–7. doi:10.1097/HP.0b013e318227e80d

[4] Bevelacqua JJ. Tumor vascular disruption using various radiation types. PeerJ. 2014;**2**:e320. doi:10.7717/peerj.320

[5] Bevelacqua JJ. ^{210}Po microsphere radiological design for tumor vascular disruption. PeerJ. 2015;**3**:e1143. doi:10.7717/peerj.1143

[6] Bevelacqua JJ. Health physics: radiation-generating devices, characteristics, and hazards. Weinheim: Wiley-VCH; 2016. 800 p.

[7] Martinez AA, Gonzalez JA, Chung AK, Kestin LL, Balasubramaniam M, Diokno AC, Ziaja EL, Brabbins DS, Vicini FA. A comparison of external beam radiation therapy versus radical prostatectomy for patients with low risk prostate carcinoma diagnosed, staged and treated at a single institution. Cancer. 2000;**88**:425–432. doi:10.1002/(SICI)1097-0142(20000115)88:2<425::AID-CNCR25>3.0.CO;2-Z

[8] NCRP Report No. 170. Second primary cancers and cardiovascular disease after radiation therapy. 2012; Bethesda: NCRP Publications.

[9] Johns HE, Cunningham JR. The physics of radiology, 4th ed. Springfield, IL: Charles C. Thomas Publisher; 1983. 796 p.

[10] Hirao Y, Ogawa H, Yamada S, Sato Y, Yamada T, Sato K, Itano A, Kanazawa M, Noda K, Kawachi K, Endo M, Kanai T, Kohno T, Sudou M, Minohara S, Kitagawa A, Soga F, Takada E, Watanabe S, Endo K, Kumada M, Matsumoto S. Heavy ion synchrotron for medical use—HIMAC project at NIRS-Japan. Nuclear Physics. 1992;**A538**:541c–550c.

[11] Scheidenberger C, Geissel H. Penetration of relativistic heavy ions through matter. Nuclear Instruments and Methods in Physics Research Section B: Beam Interactions with Materials and Atoms. 1998;**135**:25–34.

[12] Kraft G. Tumor therapy with heavy charged particles. Progress in Particle and Nuclear Physics. 2000;**45**:S473–S544. doi:10.1016/S0146-6410(00)00112-5

[13] Akabani G, Kennel SJ, Zalutsky MR. Microdosimetric analysis of particle-emitting targeted radiotherapeutics using histological images. Journal of Nuclear Medicine. 2003;**44**:792–805.

[14] Li Q, Furusawa Y, Kanazawa M, Kanai T, Kitagawa A, Aoki M, Urakabe E, Sate S, Wei Z. Enhanced biological effect induced by a radioactive ^{9}C-ion beam at the depths around its Bragg peak. Nuclear Instruments and Methods in Physics Research Section B: Beam Interactions with Materials and Atoms. 2006; **245**:302–305.

[15] Folkman J. Tumor angiogenesis: therapeutic implications. New England Journal of Medicine. 1971;**285**:1182–1186. doi:10.1056/NEJM197108122850711

[16] Burke PA, DeNardo SJ. Antiangiogenic agents and their promising potential in combined therapy. Critical Reviews in Oncology/Hematology. 2001;**39**:155–171. doi:10.1016/S1040-8428(01)00115-9

[17] Carmeliet P, Jain RK. Angiogenesis in cancer and other diseases. Nature. 2000;**407**:249–257. doi:10.1038/35025220

[18] Rajput MS, Agrawal P. Microspheres in cancer therapy. Indian Journal of Cancer. 2010;**47**:458–468. doi:10.4103/0019-509X.73547

[19] Kennedy AS, Salem R. Comparison of two ^{90}Yttrium microsphere agents for hepatic artery brachytherapy. In: Proceedings of the 14th International Congress on Anti-cancer Treatment; 5–7 February 2013; ICACT, Paris: International Congress on Anti-Cancer Treatment; 2013. pp. 1–156.

[20] Carr BI. Hepatic arterial ^{90}Y glass microspheres (Therasphere) for unresectable hepatocellular carcinoma: interim safety and survival data on 65 patients. Liver Transplantation. 2004;**10**:S107–S110. doi:10.1002/lt.20036

[21] Murthy R, Nunez R, Szklaruk F, Erwin W, Madoff DC, Gupta S, Ahrar K, Wallace MF, Coehn A, Coldwell DM, Kennedy AS, Hicks ME. Yttrium-90 microsphere therapy for hepatic malignancy: devices, indications, technical considerations, and potential complications. RadioGraphics. 2005;**25**:S41–S55. doi:10.1148/rg.25si055515

[22] Kennedy A, Nag S, Salem R, Murthy R, McEwan AJ, Nutting C, Benson A, Espat J, Bilbao JI, Sharma RA, Thomas JP, Caldwell D. Recommendations for radioembolization of hepatic malignancies using Yttrium-90 microsphere brachytherapy: a consensus panel report from the radioembolization brachytherapy oncology consortium. International Journal of Radiation Oncology, Biology, Physics. 2007;**68**(1):13–23. doi:10.1016/j.ijrobp.2006.11.060

[23] Chaudhury PK, Hassanain M, Bouteaud JM, Alcindor T, Nudo CG, Valenti D, Cabrera T, Kavan P, Feteih I, Metrakos P. Complete response of heptocellular carcinoma with sorafenib and ^{90}Y radioembolization. Current Oncology. 2010;**17**(3):67–69.

[24] Dezarn WA, Cessna JT, DeWerd LA, Feng W, Gates VL, Halama J, Kennedy AS, Nag S, Sarfaraz M, Sehgal V, Selwyn R, Stabin MG, Thomadsen BR, Williams LE, Salem R. Recommendations of the American Association of Physicists in Medicine on dosimetry, imaging, and quality assurance procedures for ^{90}Y microsphere brachytherapy in the treatment of hepatic malignancies. Medical Physics. 2011;**38**(8):4824–4845. doi:10.1118/1.3608909

[25] Lau WY, Lai EC, Leung TW. Current role of selective internal irradiation with yttrium-90 microspheres in the management of hepatocellular carcinoma: a systematic review. International Journal of Radiation Oncology, Biology, Physics. 2011;**81**(2):460–467. doi:10.1016/j.ijrobp.2010.06.010

[26] Lee IK, Seong J. The optimal selection of radiotherapy treatment for hepatocellular carcinoma. Gut and Liver. 2012;**6**(2):139–148. doi:10.5009/gnl.2012.6.2.139

[27] Amor-Coarasa A, Milera A, Carvajal D, Gulec S, McGoron AJ. ^{90}Y-DOTA-CHS microspheres for live radiomicrosphere therapy: preliminary in vivo lung radiochemical stability studies. Journal of Radiotherapy. 2014;**2014**:1–6. doi:10.1155/2014/941072

[28] Travish G, Yoder RB. Laser-powered dielectric-structures for the production of high-brightness electron and x-ray beams. Proceedings of SPIE. 2011;**8079**:80790K–80790L. doi:10.1117/12.890263

[29] Shen WQ,Wang B, Feng J, Zhan WL, Zhu YT, Feng EP. Total reaction cross section for heavy-ion collisions and its relation to the neutron excess degree of freedom. Nuclear Physics A. 1989;**491**:130–146. doi:10.1016/0375-9474(89)90209-1

[30] Barrett KE, Barman SM, Boitano S, Brooks H. Ganong's review of medical physiology. 24th ed. New York: McGraw-Hill Medical; 2012. 752 p.

[31] Bethe H. Zur theorie des durchgangs schneller korpuskularstrahlung durch materie (The theory of the passage of fast corpuscular radiation through matter). Annalen der Physik (Annals of Physics). 1930;**5**:325–400. doi:10.1002/andp.19303970303

[32] Radiation Safety Information Computational Center. Computer code collection: code package CCC-228, SPAR. Calculation of stopping powers and ranges for muons, charged pions, protons, and heavy ions. 1985; Oak Ridge: Oak Ridge National Laboratory.

[33] Rittmann PD. ISO-PC version 2.2-user's guide. 2004; Richland: Fluor Government Group.

[34] IAEA. Relative biological effectiveness in ion beam therapy, International Atomic Energy Agency, IAEA Technical Reports Series, No. 461. 2008; Vienna: IAEA.

[35] Baum EM, Ernesti MC, Knox HD, Miller TR, Watson AM. Nuclides and isotopes chart of the nuclides. 17th ed. 2010; Schnectady: Knowles Atomic Power Laboratory.

[36] National Cancer Action Team. National radiotherapy implementation group report. Image guided radiotherapy (IGRT): Guidance for implementation and use. 2012; London: NCAT.

[37] ICRP Publication 30. Limits for intakes of radionuclides by workers. 1979; Oxford: Pergamon.

[38] Bevelacqua JJ. Basic health physics: problems and solutions. 2nd ed. 2010; Weinheim: Wiley-VCH. 743 p.

[39] ICRP Publication 119. Compendium of dose coefficients based on ICRP publication 60. 2012; Amsterdam: Elsevier.

Chapter 12

Application of pMOS Dosimeters in Radiotherapy

Momčilo M. Pejović and Milić M. Pejović

Additional information is available at the end of the chapter

http://dx.doi.org/10.5772/67456

Abstract

The results of a study on pMOS dosimeters manufactured by Tyndall National Institute, Cork, Ireland and their sensitivity on radiation doses used in radiotherapy are presented. Firstly, we deal with analysis of defect precursors created by ionizing radiation, responsible for increase in fixed and switching traps, which are further responsible for threshold voltage shift as a dosimetric parameter. Secondly, influence of some parameters, such as gate bias during irradiation, gate oxide thickness and photons energies, on threshold voltage shift is presented. Fading of irradiated pMOS dosimeters and possible application of commercial MOSFETs in ionizing radiation dosimetry are also presented.

Keywords: fading, MOSFET, pMOS dosimeter, radiation dose, threshold voltage shift

1. Introduction

External radiotherapy is a well-accepted and established therapeutic modality for cancer treatment [1]. In this technique, radiation beams, generated by either radiation source or linear accelerator, are specifically optimized to cause the death of the tumor cells without having a greater impact on the healthy tissues. It is estimated that dose precision in radiotherapy is approximately ±5%. However, in order to ensure proper dose delivery to the designated area and appropriate intensity, a sophisticated radiation oncology Quality Assurance (QA) program is required [1, 2]. Also, the verification of the final dose delivered to the patient, which can only be carried out by in vivo dosimeters, is very important and should basically be used for all patients undergoing radiation treatment [3].

In vivo dosimetry can be measured by thermoluminescent dosimeters (TLDs) [4, 5], diode dosimeters [6, 7] and MOSFET (Metal-Oxide-Semiconductor Field Effect Transistor) dosimeters [8, 9]. TLDs characteristics include the following: cable-free, accurate, small volume and tissue-equivalence. However, an important drawback of TLDs is the reading procedure because information is lost during the reading. Currently, TLDs are most popular dosimeters for QA radiotherapy despite the relatively high cost of the readout equipment and the requirement of a highly trained operator.

Diode dosimeters provide instantaneous readout; however, diodes must be connected to cable for applied voltage during radiation. Even though diode dosimeters are sensitive to the temperature and dependent on the radiation beam, the correction and calibration factors are generally well known.

The concept of radiation sensitive MOSFETs as dosimeter is based on converting the threshold voltage shift as a dosimetric parameter into radiation dose. Ionizing radiation creates positive charge in the MOSFETs oxide and interface trap at silicon dioxide-silicon interface leading to a transistors threshold voltage shift. In p-channel MOSFETs, both the positive charge in the oxide and interface traps contributes to threshold voltage shift in the same direction. This is reason why p-channel MOSFETs instead n-channel MOSFETs are usually used as dosimeters. p-channel MOSFETs can be application in low-field mode (without gate bias during irradiation) and in high-field mode (with gate bias during irradiation). High-field mode leads to the sensitivity increase in MOSFET dosimeters.

The p-channel MOSFET as integrating dosimeters has been proposed in 1970 [10] and results being verified in 1974 [11]. This further leads to the production of radiation sensitive p-channel MOSFETs, also known as RADiation-sensitive Field Effect Transistor (RADFET) or pMOS dosimeter [12]. Besides, radiotherapy pMOS dosimeters could be used for radiation space monitoring [13, 14], irradiation of food plants [15] and in personal dosimetry [16].

A major advantage of the MOSFET as a radiation sensor is that the radiation-sensitive region, the oxide film, is very small [11]. The sensing volume is much smaller than competing integral dose measuring devices, such as the ionization chamber or TLD. The MOSFETs sensitive volume is typically 1 μm x 200 μm x 200 μm [17] implying that it could be used in vivo dosimetry [18]. This MOSFETs property also makes them attractive for measurements in the gradient radiation field where the gradient mostly depends on a single space coordinate, like resolving dose of X-ray micro beams or dept dose distribution [19]. The advantages of MOSFETs as dosimeters also include real time or delayed reading, non-destructive and immediate dosimetric information readout, wide dose range, accuracy, competitive price and possible integration with other sensors and/or electronics [20]. Moreover, another field where it is possible to explore their advantages is hadron therapy, which is one of the promising radiation modalities in radiotherapy [21]. On the other hand, an important disadvantage of MOSFETs as radiation sensors is the need to separate calibration in fields of different modalities and energies. Furthermore, MOSFET's total accumulated dose range depends on the dosimeter sensitivity and type. The MOSFET needs to be replaced when the upper limit of linearity is achieved. Although, recently, the possibility of MOSFET reuse after recovering for a certain period of time at room or elevated temperature [22] or by current annealing [23] has been studied.

In radiotherapy, the radiation oncologist determines the radiation dose depending on many factors such as the type and size of tumor, location in the body, how close the tumor is to other radiation sensitive tissues, how deep into the body the radiation need to penetrate, the patient general health and medical history, whether the patient will have other type of cancer treatments (e.g., chemotherapy) and other factors such as patient age and medical conditions. Cumulative dose range used in radiotherapy ranges from 20 to 70 Gy [24], while typical radiation dose for one fraction is from 1 up to 5 Gy.

This chapter presents some of the results obtained in our laboratory, which considers the influence of some parameters to pMOS dosimeters sensitivity and fading. Dosimeters were manufactured in Tyndall National Institute, Cork, Ireland. Sensitivity results are also presented for commercial MOSFETs in order to investigate their possible application in radiotherapy.

2. Mechanisms responsible for threshold voltage shift during irradiation

The dosimetry of ionizing radiation using radiation-sensitive MOSFETs is based on the threshold voltage shift, conversion into absorbed radiation dose *D* [25, 26]. This shift originates in the radiation-induced electron-hole pairs formed during irradiation. Namely, gamma and X-rays interact with the electrons in SiO_2 molecules releasing secondary electrons and holes, that is, photons break $\equiv Si_o - ihSi_o \equiv$ and $\equiv Si_o - Si_o \equiv$ covalent bonds in the oxide [27] (the index $_o$ is used to denote silicon atom in the oxide). The released secondary electrons, which are highly energetic, may be recombined by holes at the place of production or may escape recombination. The secondary electrons that escape recombination pass through the oxide bulk, break covalent bonds and create $\equiv Si_o - O^{\bullet +} - Si_o \equiv$ complexes, where $^{\bullet}$ denotes the unpaired electron. This complex is energetically very shallow and trapped holes can easily escape it. It is obvious that secondary electrons play a more important role in the bond breaking than highly energetic photons, due to the difference in their effective masses, that is, in their effective cross section.

The $\equiv Si_o - O - Si_o \equiv$ mainly distributed near the Si/SiO_2 interface, can also the broken by passing secondary electrons, usually created by non-bridging oxygen (NBO) centers $\equiv Si_o - O$ and positively charged E' centers, $\equiv Si_o^+$ [28]. The main precursor of the traps in the oxide bulk and in interface regions is the NBO center, as an energetically deeper centre, and represents a more likely negative than positively charged amphoteric defect. Also, a secondary electron can also break $\equiv Si_o - Si_o \equiv$ bonds and create E'_γ centers, $\equiv Si_o^{\bullet}$ [27] by knocking out an electron.

Positive charge is formed in oxide by holes trapping, while electrons trapping lead to creation of negative charge. The concentration of positive charge in oxide is much higher since the hole trapping centers are more numerous compared to electron trapping centers. Moreover, trapped electrons and holes near Si/SiO_2 interface have the strongest impact on channel carriers, hence on MOSFET characteristics.

Amphoteric defects $Si_3 \equiv Si_s^{\bullet}$ (index $_s$ is used to indicate a silicon atom in substrate) are marked as true interface traps and represent defects at the Si/SiO_2 interface. At Si/SiO_2 interface, a silicon atom $\equiv Si_s^\bullet$ back bonds with three silicon atoms from the substrate $\equiv Si_s$ and is mostly marked as $\equiv Si_s^\bullet$ or $Si_s^\bullet$. Their creation can also originate from incident photons when they pass through the gate or substrate [27]; however, the amount can be neglected. Hydrogen released in the oxide (hydrogen-released species model H-model) [29, 30] is the main creator of interface traps. This model proposed that H ions released in the oxide by trapped holes at $\equiv Si_o - H$ and $\equiv Si_o - OH$ defects in the oxide drift toward the Si/SiO_2 interface under the positive electric field. When H^+ ions arrive at the interface, it picks up an electron from the substrate, becoming a highly reactive atom H^0 [31]. This atom reacts at the interface producing $Si_s^\bullet$ [32]. Dimerization of hydrogen atoms also exists near the Si/SiO_2 interface, what further leads to creation of H_2 molecule [31]. The increase in $Si_s^\bullet$ continues during annealing of irradiated MOSFETs for a long period of time [33].

Positive trapped charge in the oxide is called fixed traps (FT), and positive trapped charge near Si/SiO_2 interface is called switching traps (ST) [27], where FT represents traps in the oxide that without the ability to exchange the charge with the channel within the MOSFET transfer/subthreshold characteristic measurement time frame. On the other hand, ST represents traps created near and at Si/SiO_2 interface, and they do capture (communicate with) the carrier from the channel within the transfer/subthreshold characteristic measurement time frame. Furthermore, one can differentiate between slow switching traps (SST) created in the oxide near Si/SiO_2 interface and fast switching traps (FST) created at Si/SiO_2 interface also known as true interface traps ($Si_s^\bullet$).

Threshold voltage shift ΔV_T during irradiation is a consequence of the increase in concentration of FT, Q_{FT}, and the increase in the concentration ST, Q_{ST}. The threshold voltage V_T can be expressed as follows [33]

$$V_T = V_{T0} - \frac{Q_{FT} + Q_{ST}}{C_{ox}} = V_{T0} + \Delta V_T, \quad (1)$$

where V_{T0} is the value of V_T before irradiation and C_{ox} is the gate capacitance. In p-channel MOSFETs, both FT and ST are positive and they contribute to the threshold voltage shift in the same direction, i. e. both V_T and V_{T0} are negative. Also, the so-called rebound effect [34] is absent in p-channel MOSFETs: This phenomenon is due to the competitive effect of positive charge in the oxide and negative interface traps generated in n-channel MOSFETs leading to a positive or negative ΔV_T value dependence on the relative values of Q_{FT} and Q_{ST}. This is the reason why p-channel MOSFETs instead of n-channel MOSFETs are usually used in dosimetry of ionizing radiation.

3. Response of pMOS dosimeters to gamma and X-ray radiation

3.1. Important pMOS dosimetric parameters

The most important parameters that characterize the pMOS dosimetric radiation response are sensitivity, dose linearity and room temperature long-term stability [35, 36]. Sensitivity represents threshold voltage shift ΔV_T and radiation dose D ratio ($\Delta V_T/D$) and could be controlled by the gate bias during irradiation. It is well known [37, 38] that an increase in sensitivity could be achieved with increase in gate bias during irradiation. In the case of positive gate bias, the sensitivity is higher, than in the case of negative gate bias and the lowest sensitivity being for zero gate bias [20]. Moreover, sensitivity increase can be achieved by increasing the gate oxide thickness [36–39] and by processing conditions which determine the FT density, their capture cross section and their location as well as the ST density [40].

In practical applications, it is most convenient for pMOS dosimeters to have a linear response of threshold voltage shift ΔV_T regarding observed radiation dose D. In this case, the sensitivity is the same for considered dose interval. It was shown that the response is linear for low doses and progressively saturates at a maximum values which respect to gate bias [40]. The linear dependence is given by [36]

$$\Delta V_T = A \cdot D^n, \tag{2}$$

where A is the constant and n is the degree of linearity. For $n = 1$, the constant A represents sensitivity S:

$$S = \Delta V_T/D. \tag{3}$$

Positive gate bias during irradiation reduces the recombination of produced electron-hole pairs in SiO_2 and as a consequence the pMOS dosimeters response becomes more linear and sensitive [33, 41].

Room-temperature long-tem stability of irradiated pMOS dosimeters can be observed by calculating fading F. The percent of fading can be calculated as follows [27]:

$$F = \frac{V_T(0) - V_T(t)}{V_T(0) - V_{T0}} = \frac{V_T(0) - V_T(t)}{\Delta V_T(0)}, \tag{4}$$

where $V_T(0)$ is the threshold voltage immediately after irradiation, V_{T0} is the pre-irradiation threshold voltage, $V_T(t)$ is the threshold voltage after annealing time, t and $\Delta V_T(0)$ is the threshold voltage shift immediately after irradiation.

3.2. Influence of gate bias on threshold voltage shift during irradiation

Figures 1 and **2** show the threshold voltage shift ΔV_T of pMOS dosimeters with gate oxide thickness of 1 μm for X-ray (energy of 140 keV) as a function of radiation dose D in the range from 0 to 1 0 cGy and from 0 to 1 Gy, while gate bias during irradiation was 0 and 5 V [35], respectively. Experimental data fitting with Eq. (2) for $n = 1$ shows an almost linear response between ΔV_T and D. Namely, for gate bias during irradiation of $V_{irr} = 0$ V, correlation coefficient is $r^2 = 0.98$, whereas for $V_{irr} = 5$ V, correlation coefficient is $r^2 = 0.99$.

Figure 3 shows the threshold voltage shift ΔV_T of pMOS dosimeters with gate oxide thickness of 1 μm as a function of gamma-ray radiation dose D (gamma radiation originate from 60Co) in range from 0 to 1 Gy for gate bias during irradiation $V_{irr} = 0$ V and $V_{irr} = 5$ V [38]. The same dependence for gamma-ray radiation dose in range from 0 to 5 Gy is given in **Figure 4** [38].

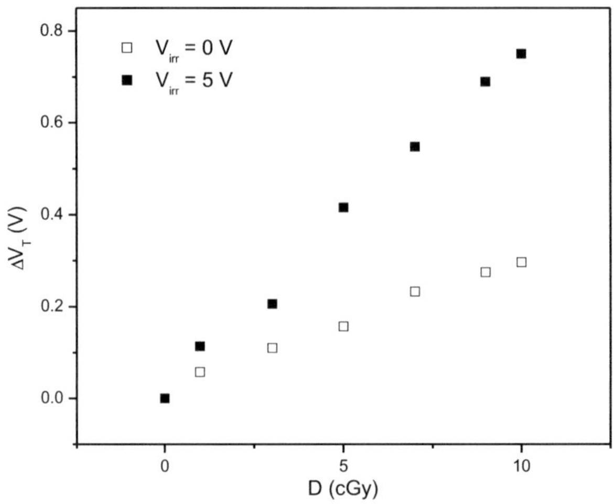

Figure 1. Threshold voltage shift ΔV_T in pMOS dosimeters with 1-μm-thick gate oxide as a function of X-ray radiation dose D in the 0–10 cGy range. Gate bias during irradiation V_{irr} was 0 or 5 V.

Experimental data fitting presented in these figures using Eq. (2) for $n = 1$ gives correlation coefficient $r^2 = 0.99$, so it is assumed that the linearity between ΔV_T and D is satisfactory for practical application.

Figure 5 shows the $\Delta V_T = f(D)$ dependence of pMOS dosimeters with gate oxide thickness of 1 μm for gamma-ray radiation dose in the range from 0 to 50 Gy [36]. During the irradiation, the gate biases V_{irr} were 0, 1.25, 2.50, 3.75 and 5 V. It can be seen that the threshold voltage shift for the same radiation dose increases with gate bias increase. The radiation dose up to 50 Gy did not significantly degrade the linearity of the pMOS dosimeters. Experimental data fitting

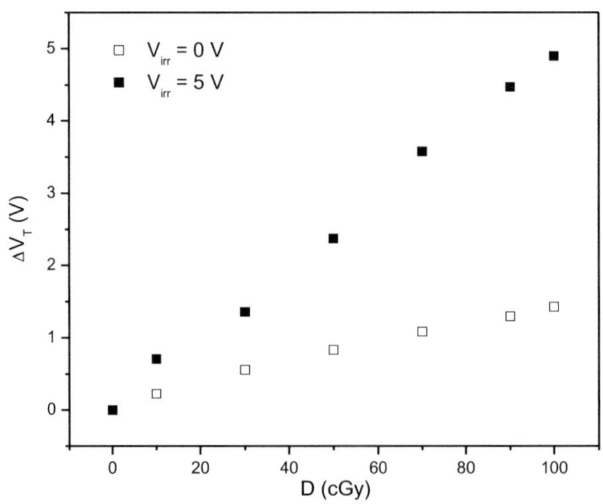

Figure 2. Threshold voltage shift ΔV_T in pMOS dosimeters with 1-μm-thick gate oxide as a function of X-ray radiation dose D in the 0–1 Gy range. Gate bias during irradiation V_{irr} was 0 or 5 V.

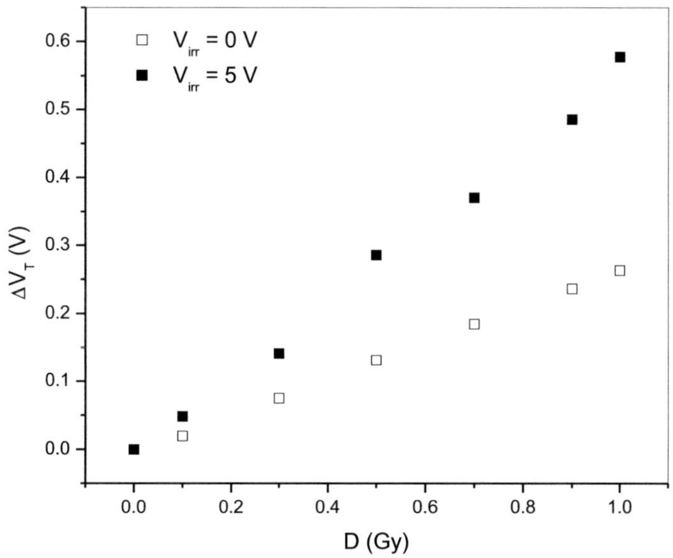

Figure 3. Threshold voltage shift ΔV_T in pMOS dosimeter with 1-μm-thick gate oxide as a function of gamma-ray radiation dose D in the 0–1 Gy range. Gate bias during irradiation V_{irr} was 0 or 5 V.

using Eq. (2) for $n = 1$ gives correlation coefficient, $r^2 = 0.98$. Having that r^2 are very close to one, it can be assumed that there is a linear dependence between ΔV_T and D and that the sensitivity of these devices for a given value of V_{irr} is the same in the range from 0 to 50 Gy.

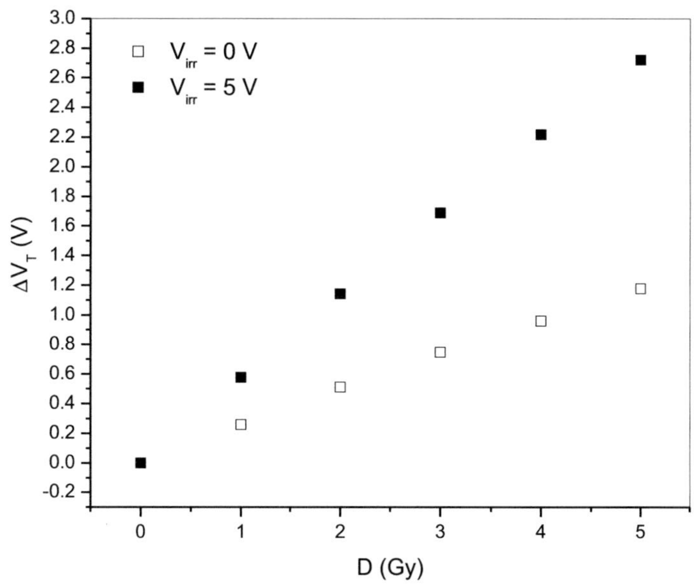

Figure 4. Threshold voltage shift ΔV_T in pMOS dosimeter with 1-μm-thick gate oxide as a function of gamma-ray radiation dose D in the 1–5 Gy range. Gate bias during irradiation V_{irr} was 0 or 5 V.

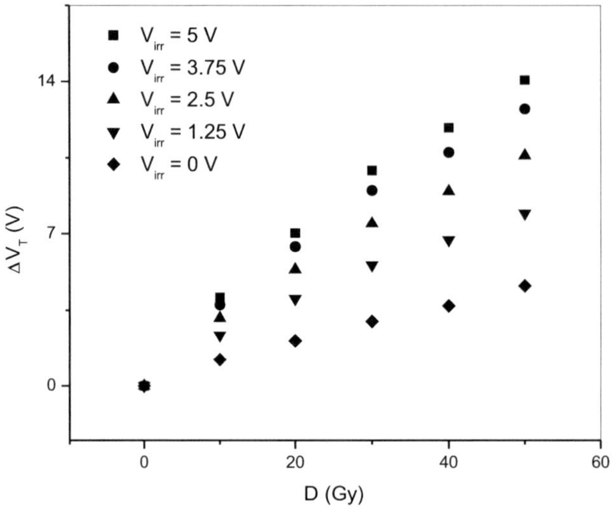

Figure 5. Threshold voltage shift ΔV_T in pMOS dosimeter with 1-μm-thick gate oxide as a function of gamma-ray radiation dose D in the 0–50 Gy range. Gate bias during irradiation V_{irr} was ranging from 0 to 5 V.

Figure 6 shows the sensitivity S as a function of gate bias V_{irr} during gamma-ray irradiation to 50 Gy of pMOS dosimeters with gate oxide thickness of 1 μm [36]. The symbols stand for experimental data, whereas the solid lines represent fits, which are exponential.

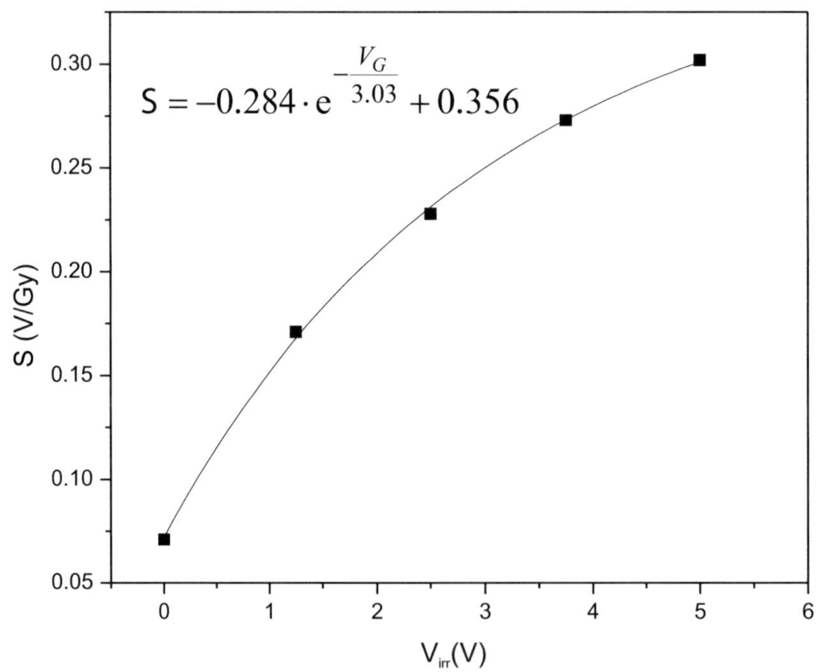

Figure 6. Sensitivity of pMOS dosimeter with 1-μm-thick gate oxide as a function of gate bias V_{irr} for 50 Gy gamma-ray irradiation.

The increase in ΔV_T with the increase in V_{irr} is due to the increase in FT and ST. It is well known that with the number of holes which have avoided the recombination with electrons, the number of created FT and ST increases. When V_{irr} = 0 V the electric field in the oxide is only due to work function difference between the gate and the substrate (zero bias conditions or dosimeter passive mode), so the probability for electron-hole recombination is higher than in the case when V_{irr} > 0 V. For higher value of V_{irr}, the large number of holes will escape the initial recombination, which further increase the probability for their capture at E', E'_γ and NBO centers and increase FT and SST which leads to increase in ΔV_T. Such conclusion is in agreement with results shown in **Figures 1–6**. It should be emphasized that during irradiation, the FT concentration is several times larger than ST concentration. This proves that the increase in ΔV_T value during irradiation is mainly due to increase in FT [42].

3.3. Influence of gate oxide thickness on threshold voltage shift during irradiation

Figure 7 shows the threshold voltage shift ΔV_T as a function of radiation dose D for pMOS dosimeters with gate oxide thicknesses of 400 nm and 1 μm [43]. Irradiation of these devices was performed with gamma-ray irradiation in the dose range from 0 to 5 Gy when gate bias during irradiation was V_{irr} = 5 V. It was shown that sensitivity $\Delta V_T/D$ increases with gate oxide thickness increase and that there is a linear dependence between ΔV_T and D (correlation coefficient r^2 = 0.99).

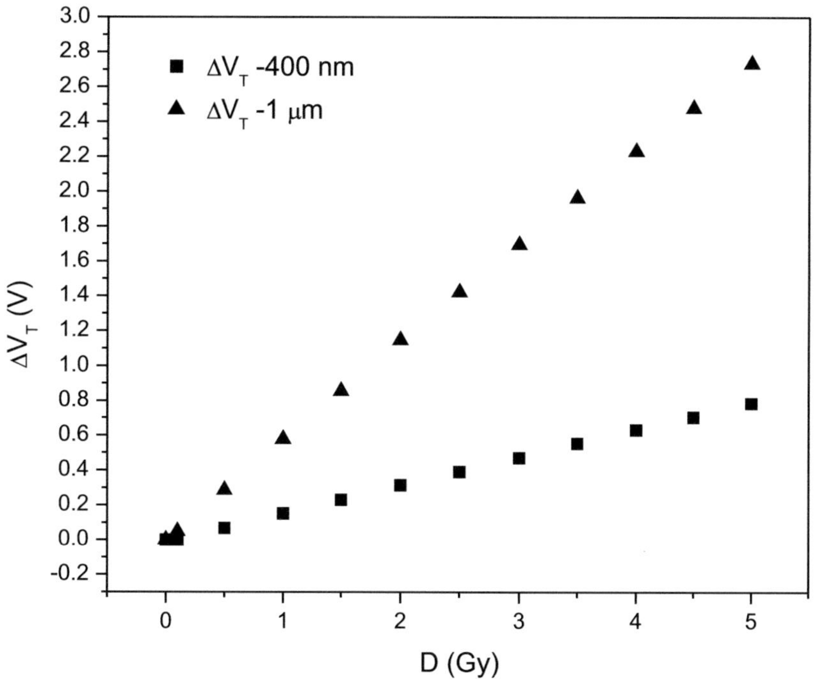

Figure 7. pMOS dosimeters threshold voltage shift ΔV_T as a function of gamma-ray dose in 0–5 Gy range. Gate bias during irradiation was V_{irr} = 5 V. Gate oxide thickness was 400 nm and 1 μm.

The $\Delta V_T = f(D)$ dependence for pMOS dosimeters with gate oxide layer thicknesses of 100 nm, 400 nm and 1 μm is shown in **Figure 8** [36]. The gamma-ray irradiation of these devices was performed in the dose range from 0 to 50 Gy, while the gate bias $V_{irr} = 5$ V. It can be seen that the increase in gate thickness leads to the increase in ΔV_T for the same radiation dose. It is mainly due to the increase in FT concentration [42]. Experimental data fitting using Eq. (2) for $n = 1$, gives the correlation coefficient values, for pMOS dosimeters with 100 nm, 400 nm and 1 μm gate oxide thickness 0.99, 0.99 and 0.98, respectively, what proves linear dependence between ΔV_T and D.

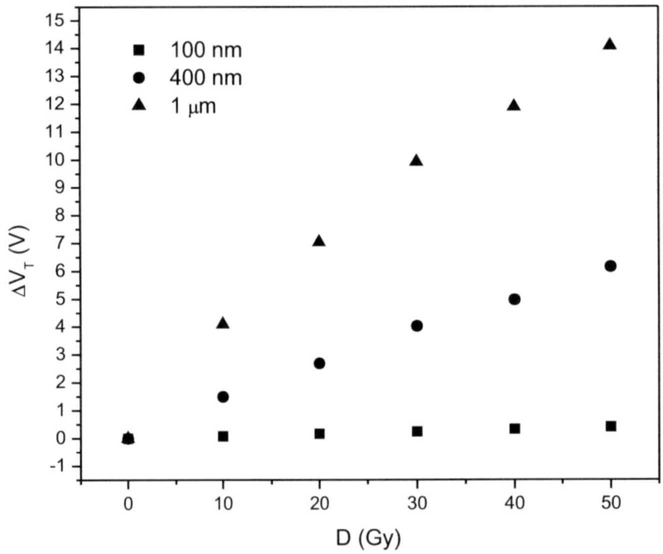

Figure 8. pMOS dosimeters threshold voltage shift ΔV_T as a function of gamma-ray dose in 0–50 Gy range. Gate bias during irradiation was $V_{irr} = 5$ V. Gate oxide thickness was 100 nm, 400 nm and 1 μm.

3.4. Influence of photon energy on pMOS dosimetry sensitivity

Figure 9 shows the threshold voltage shift ΔV_T as a function of radiation dose D for 1 μm gate oxide thickness pMOS dosimeters irradiated with gamma-rays which originates from 60Co and X-ray with energy 140 keV in dose range from 0 to 1 Gy for gate bias during irradiation $V_{irr} = 5$ V [35, 38]. Experimental results fitting using Eq. (2) for $n = 1$ gives the value of correlation coefficient $r^2 = 0.99$ assuming that there is linear dependence between ΔV_T and D, that is, sensitivity is the same for considered dose interval. It can be also seen from the figure that the sensitivity is much higher for X than for gamma radiation.

The $\Delta V_T = f(D)$ dependence for gamma and X-rays for pMOS dosimeters with gate oxide thickness of 1 μm in dose range from 0 to 5 Gy and $V_{irr} = 5$ V is shown in **Figure 10** [38]. Experimental results fitting using Eq. (2) for $n = 1$, gives correlation coefficient for gamma and X-rays 0.99 and 0.96, respectively. On the basis of these values, it can be concluded that for X-rays, there is no linear dependence between ΔV_T and D.

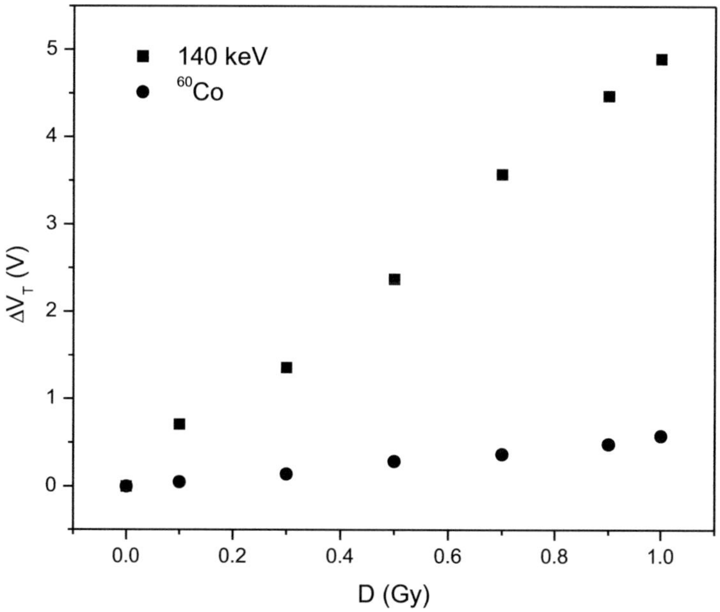

Figure 9. Threshold voltage shift ΔV_T in pMOS dosimeter with 1-μm-thick gate oxide as a function of gamma and X-ray radiation dose D in the 0–1 Gy range. Gate bias during irradiation V_{irr} was ranging from 0 to 5 V.

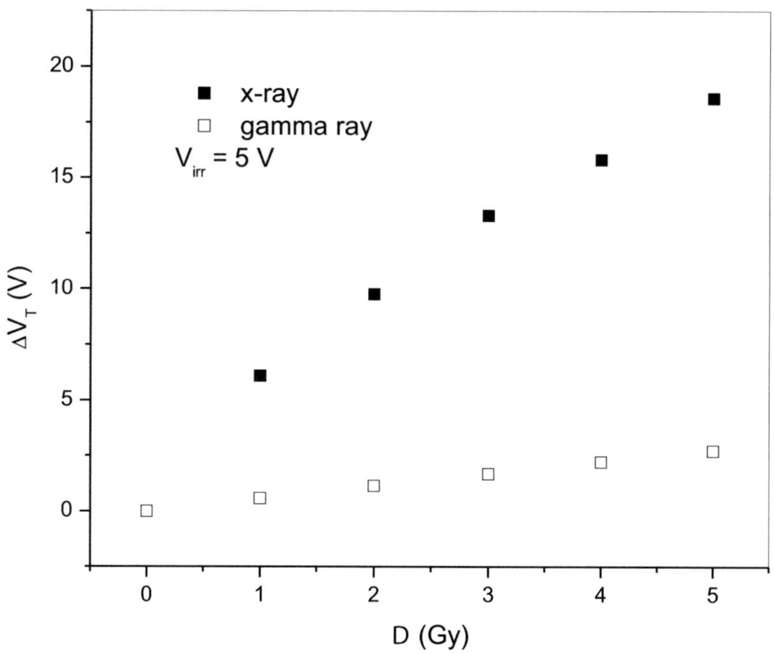

Figure 10. Threshold voltage shift ΔV_T in pMOS dosimeters as a function of gamma and X-ray radiation dose D in the 0–5 Gy range. Gate bias during irradiation was $V_{irr} = 5$ V.

From **Figures 9** and **10**, it can be seen that increasing in Δ V_T is much higher in the case when pMOS dosimeters are irradiated with X-rays (140 keV photon energy) than in the case of gamma-rays originating from ^{60}Co (energies of photons of 1.17 and 1.33 MeV). This is a consequence of different photon energies which lead to ionization of SiO_2 molecules. Namely, X-ray photons energy of 140 keV lead to molecule ionization by both photo effect and Compton's effect, while gamma-ray photons with energies of 1.17 and 1.33 MeV lead to SiO_2 molecules ionization only by Compton's effect [38]. A direct change in Δ V_T values is caused by a larger number of FT and ST, which are formed during X-ray irradiation compared to gamma-ray irradiation, the reason being the probability for molecule ionization by photoeffect is significantly higher than by Compton's effect.

4. Fading of irradiated pMOS dosimeters

As a dosimeter radiation sensitive MOSFET must satisfy a crucial demand, which implies compromising between sensitivity to irradiation and stability with time after irradiation. Stability represent insignificant change in ΔV_T of an irradiated MOSFET at room temperature for a long-time period (saved dosimetric information) [43]. Having that immediate dose readout is not always possible, also the exact moment of irradiation is often unknown as in the case of individual monitoring the radiation dose measurements must be performed periodically. Room temperature stability of irradiated pMOS dosimeters can be determined by calculating fading using Eq. (4).

Fading results for pMOS dosimeters with gate oxide thickness of 400 nm and 1 μm, at room temperature previously irradiated with X-ray (energy 140 keV) up to 1 Gy for V_{irr} = 0 V and V_{irr} = 5 V are presented in **Figures 11** and **12**, respectively [35]. It can be seen that fading of pMOS dosimeters with gate oxide thickness of 400 nm (**Figure 11**), which were irradiated with gate bias V_{irr} = 5 V, is about 40% in the first 7 days, whereas those of pMOS dosimeters irradiated without gate bias during irradiation have 22% fading also in the first 7 days. For the time period between 7 and 28 days, fading of pMOS dosimeters irradiated with gate bias 5 V increased for about 3%, whereas fading of pMOS dosimeters irradiated without gate bias during irradiation had a nearly constant value. Fading of 1 μm thick gate oxide pMOS dosimeter (**Figure 12**), which were irradiated up to 1 Gy with gate bias V_{irr} = 5 V, in the first 7 days was 14%, whereas for the time period between 7 and 28 days, it increases about 1%. pMOS dosimeters with the same gate oxide thickness, which were irradiated without gate bias the first 7 days, have fading increase for about 1%, and this value is kept up to 28 days. From **Figures 11** and **12**, it can be concluded that fading is lower when the gate oxide of pMOS dosimeters is thicker which in accordance with early study [44] showed that fading decreases with the increase in gate oxide thickness.

The decrease in the positive trapped charge causes fading of pMOS dosimeters. This decrease originates from electron tunneling from Si into SiO_2; once captured at positive oxide trapped charge, which lead to their neutralization/compensation and change in threshold voltage shift [45].

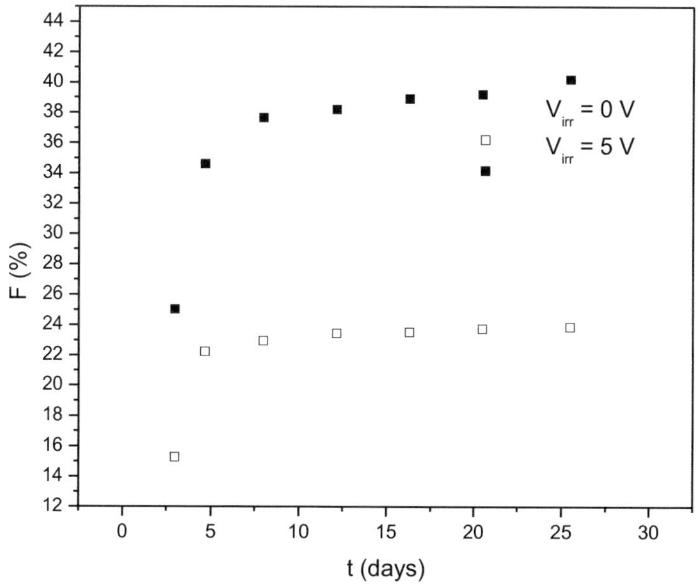

Figure 11. Fading F at room temperature for 30 days of pMOS dosimeter with 400 nm gate oxide thickness previously irradiated with X-ray (140 keV) radiation dose of 1 Gy. Gate bias during irradiation was $V_{irr} = 0$ V and $V_{irr} = 5$ V.

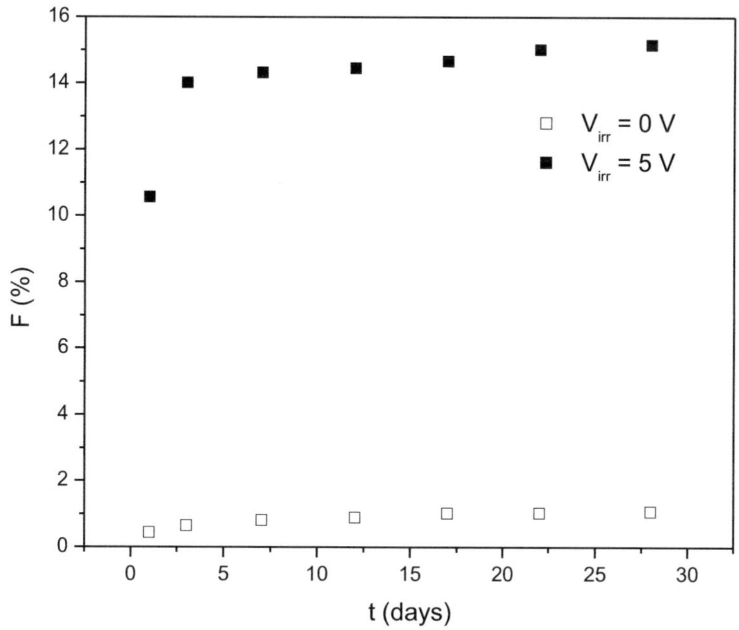

Figure 12. Fading F at room temperature for 30 days of pMOS dosimeter with 1 μm gate oxide thickness previously irradiated with X-ray (140 keV) radiation dose of 1 Gy. Gate bias during irradiation was $V_{irr} = 0$ V and $V_{irr} = 5$ V.

5. pMOS dosimeter reuse

For a while, it was widely thought that pMOS dosimeters could not be used for subsequent determination of radiation dose. They were, namely, just used to determine the maximum radiation dose, after which they would be replaced. However, studies on the pMOS dosimeter reuse are given in [46] for radiation dose 400 Gy. Recent work has shown that irradiated pMOS dosimeters manufactured in Tyndall National Institute, Cork, Ireland, could be annealed at room and elevated temperature and reused for ionizing radiation measurements. **Figures 13** and **14** show the threshold voltage shift ΔV_T as a function of gamma radiation dose D for gate bias V_{irr} = 5 V and V_{irr} = 0 V, respectively, for both the first and second irradiation [47, 48]. After the first irradiation, the pMOS dosimeters were annealed at room temperature for 5232 h without gate bias. Latter, the annealing process was continued at 120° C without gate bias for 432 h. The pMOS dosimeters were then irradiated under the same conditions. It can be seen from **Figure 13** that the values of ΔV_T during the first and second irradiation are very close. For pMOS dosimeters irradiated with the gate bias V_{irr} = 0 V (**Figure 14**), the values of ΔV_T are higher for the second than for first irradiation. Such results are contradictory with earlier results [46] for pMOS dosimeters irradiated up to 400 Gy where it was shown that the values of ΔV_T during the first irradiation (for V_{irr} = 5 V and V_{irr} = 0 V) were higher than the values obtained during the second irradiation.

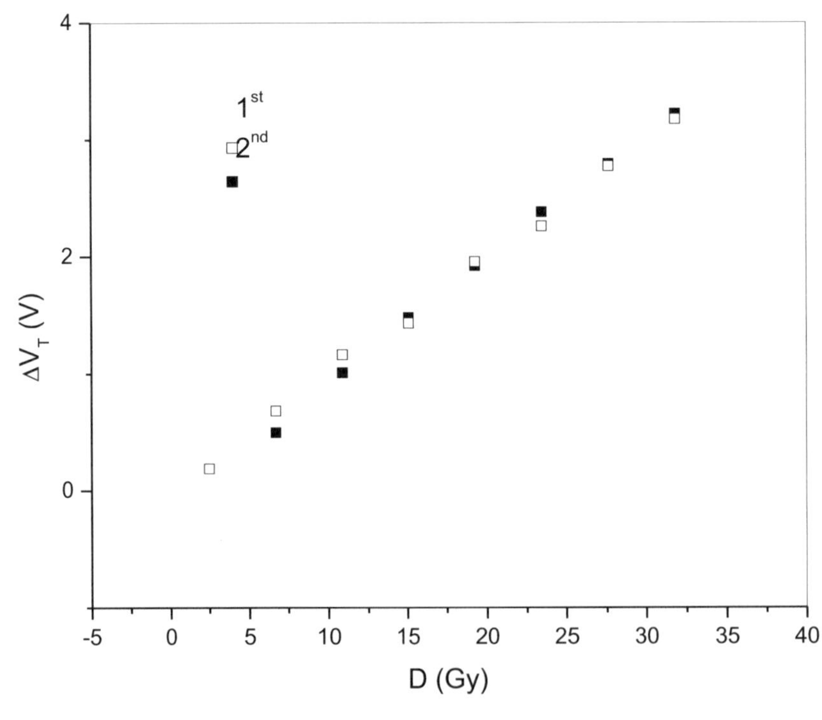

Figure 13. Dependence of the threshold voltage shift ΔV_T in pMOS dosimeters with 400 nm gate oxide thickness on the gamma-ray radiation dose D in the 0–35 Gy range during the first and second irradiation with gate bias V_{irr} = 5 V.

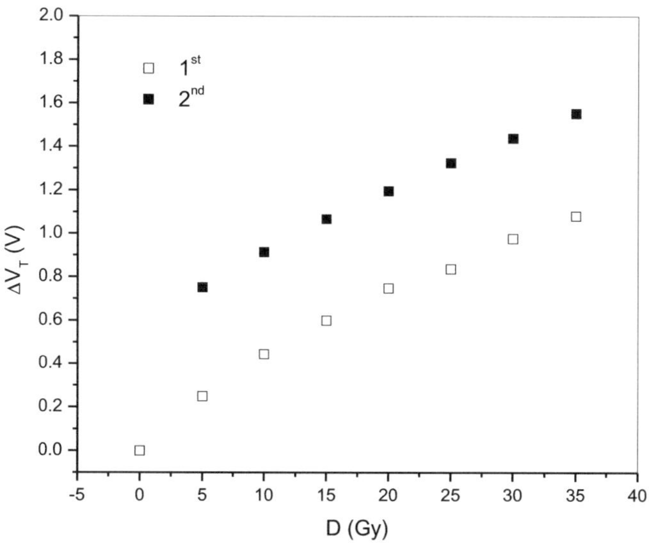

Figure 14. Dependence of the threshold voltage shift ΔV_T in pMOS dosimeters with 400 nm gate oxide thickness on the gamma-ray radiation dose D in the 0–35 Gy range during the first and second irradiation with gate bias V_{irr} = 0 V.

6. Low-cost commercial p-channel MOSFETs as pMOS dosimeters

In recent years, many investigations were driven toward application of low-cost commercial p-channel MOSFETs as a dosimeter in radiotherapy [49]. Asensio et al. [50] show results of some most important dosimetric parameters (sensitivity, linearity, reproducibility and angular dependence) for power p-channel MOSFETs 3N163. These transistors were irradiated by gamma-rays originating from ^{60}Co up to 55 Gy. These devices were irradiated without gate bias (V_{irr} = 0 V). **Figure 15** shows the $\Delta V_T = f(D)$ dependence for 15 devices. The data showed excellent linearity with a mean sensitivity value of 29.2 mV/Gy and reasonable good reproducibility. Moreover, the angular and dose rate dependencies are similar to those of other, more specialized pMOS dosimeters. The authors of this paper concluded that power p-channel MOSFET 3N163 would be an excellent candidate for low-cost system capable of measuring gamma-radiation dose.

The possibility of vertical diffusion MOS also called double-diffusion MOS transistor or simple DMOS as a sensor of electron beam was also investigated [51] These devices were DMOS BS250F, ZVP3306 and ZVP4525, manufactured by Diodes Incorporated (Plano, USA). The irradiation was performed by an electron beam of 6 MeV energy without gate bias. The same authors investigated the behavior of p-channel MOS transistors from integrated circuit CD4007 (Texas Instruments, Dallas, USA and NXP Semiconductor Eindhowen, Netherlands) under 6 MeV energy electron beam. In **Figure 16**, the ΔV_T versus D is plotted four samples of the ZVP3306 DMOS transistors. The results for other type DMOS transistors are similar. As it can be seen, there is a linear dependence between ΔV_T and D to radiation dose of 25 Gy. Values of sensitivity for BS250F, ZVP4525 and ZVP3306 are 3.1, 3.4 and 3.7 mV/Gy, respectively. It was also shown [51] that p-channel MOS

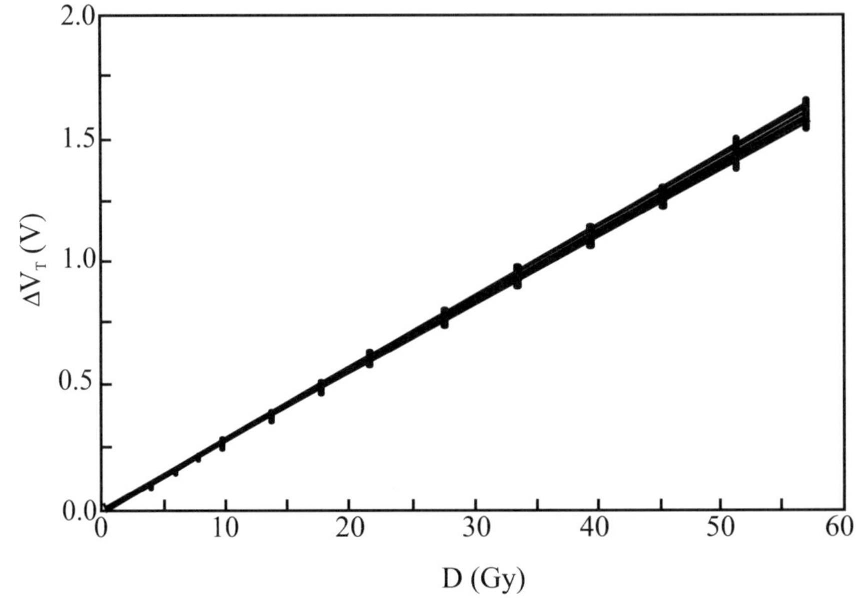

Figure 15. Threshold voltage shift ΔV_T in p-channel MOSFETs 3N163 as a function of gamma-ray radiation dose D in the 0–58 Gy range. Gate bias during irradiation was $V_{irr} = 0$ V.

transistors from integrating circuits CD4007 during irradiation without gate bias ($V_{irr} = 0$ V) presented the sensitivity 4.6 mV/Gy with a very good linear behavior of the threshold voltage shift compared to the radiation dose. Moreover, with the possibility of applying thermal compensation, this transistor may be a promising candidate in radiotherapy.

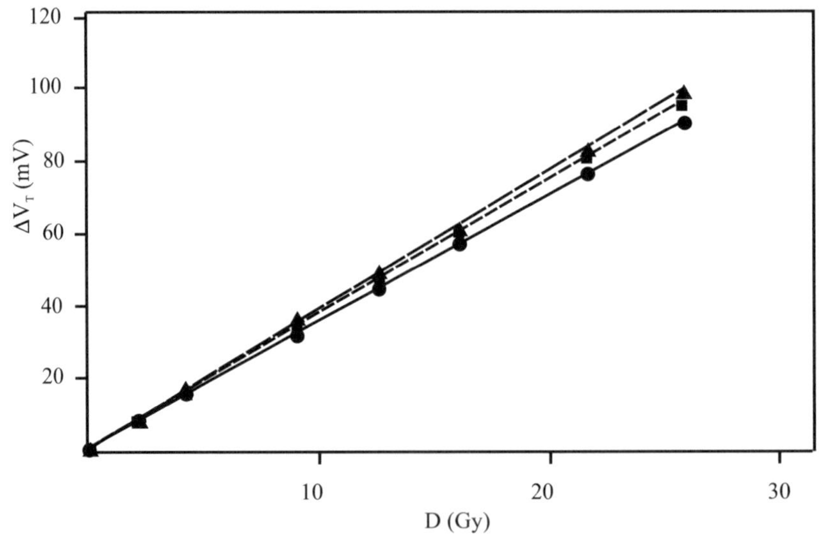

Figure 16. Threshold voltage shift ΔV_T in DMOS ZVP3306 as a function of 6 MeV electron beam radiation dose D in the 0–25 Gy range.

7. Conclusion

The sensitivity of pMOS dosimeters manufactured in Tyndall National Institute, Cork, Ireland, with 100 nm, 400 nm and 1 μm thick gate oxide to gamma and X-ray irradiation, for radiation doses used in radiotherapy, has been investigated. It is shown that their sensitivity can be increased either by increase in gate bias during irradiation or by increasing the gate oxide thickness. The sensitivity increases with the decrease in ionizing radiation photon energy. Sensitivity of pMOS dosimeters with 1 μm thick gate oxide is satisfactory even for 1 cGy doses in low-field mode. Unfortunately, their major disadvantage is large fading immediately after irradiation. Investigations in a past few years have shown that some low-cost commercial p-channel MOSFETs could be good candidates for radiation dose measurements used in radiotherapy.

Acknowledgements

The Ministry of Education, Science and Technological Development of the Republic of Serbia supported this work under contract no. 171007.

Author details

Momčilo M. Pejović* and Milić M. Pejović

*Address all correspondence to: momcilo.pejovic@elfak.ni.ac.rs

Faculty of Electronic Engineering, University of Niš, Niš, Serbia

References

[1] Siebel OF, Pereira JG, Souza RS, Ramirez-Fernandez FJ, Schneider MC and Galup-Montoro CA. A very-low-cost dosimeter based on the off-the-shelf CD4007 MOSFET array for in vivo radiotherapy applications. Radiat. Meas. 2015; **75**:53–63.

[2] Purdy JA, Klein E, Vijayakumar S, Perez CA and Levitt SH. Quality assurance in radiation oncology. In: Perez CA, Levitt SH, Purdy JA, Vijayakumar S (Eds). Technical Basis of Radiation Therapy: Practical Clinical Applications, Springer-Verlag, Berlin 2005:395–422.

[3] Rosenfeld AB. Electronic dosimetry in radiation therapy. Radiat. Meas. 2006; **41**:5134–5153.

[4] Kron T, Butson M, Hunt F and Denham J. TLD extrapolation for skin dose determination in vivo. Radiother. Oncol. 1996; **41**:119–123.

[5] Das R, Toye W, Kron T, Williams S and Duchesne G. Thermoluminescence dosimetry for in-vivo verification of high dose rate brachytherapy for prostate cancer. Australas. Phys. Eng. Sci. Med. 2007; **30**:178–184.

[6] Lancaster CM, Cosbe JC and Devis SR. In vivo dosimetry from total body irradiation patients (2000–2006); results and analysis. Australas. Phys. Eng. Sci. Med. 2008; **31**:191–195.

[7] Saini AS and Zhu TC. Energy dependence of commercially available diode detectors for in vivo dosimetry. Med. Phys. 2007; **34**:1704–1711.

[8] Scalchi P and Francescon P. Calculation of MOSFET detection system for 6-MV in vivo dosimetry. Int. J. Radiat. Oncol. Biol. Phys. 1988; **40**:987–993.

[9] Jornet N, Carrisio P, Jurada D, Ruis A, Eudaldo T and Ribas M. Comparison study of MOSFET detectros and diodes for entrace in vivo dosimetry in 18 MV x-ray beam. Med. Phys. 2004; **31**:2534–2542.

[10] Poch W and Holmes-Siedle AG. The mosmeter-a new instrument for measuring radiation dose. RCA Eng. 1970; **16**:56–59.

[11] Holmes-Siedle AG. The space charge dosimeter-general principles of a new method of radiation dosimetry. Nucl. Instr. Methods. 1974; **121**:169–171.

[12] Adams L and Holmes-Siedle A. The development of MOS dosimetry unit for use in space. IEEE Trans. Nucl. Sci. 1978; **18**:1607–1612.

[13] Kay K, Mullen E, Stopar W, Circle R and McDonald P. GRREs dosimetry results and comparison using the space radiation dosimeter and p-channel MOS dosimeter. IEEE Trans. Nucl. Sci. 1992; **39**:1846–1850.

[14] Scheik LZ, McNulty FJ and Roth DR. Dosimeter based on the ensure of floating gate in natural radiation environments. IEEE Trans. Nucl. Sci. 1998; **45**:2681–2688.

[15] Faigon A, Lipovetzky J, Redin E and Kruscenski G. Expression of measurement range of MOS dosimeters using radiation induce charge neutralization. IEEE Trans. Nucl. Sci. 2008; **55**:2141–2147.

[16] Sarrabayrouse G, Buchdahl D, Poliscuk V and Siscos S. Stacked-MOS ionizing radiation dosimeters: potentials and limitations. Rad. Phys. Chem. 2004; **71**:737–739.

[17] Rosenfeld AB, Kaplan GI, Kron T, Allen BJ, Dilmanian A, Orion I, Ren B, Lerch MLF and Holmes-Siedle A. MOSFET dosimetry of an X-ray microbeam. IEEE Trans. Nucl. Sci. 1999; **46**:1774–1780.

[18] Gladstone DJ, Lu XQ, Humm JL, Bowman HF and Chin LM. A miniature MOSFET radiation probe. Med. Phys. 1994; **21**:1721–1728.

[19] Kaplan GI, Rosemfeld AB, Allen BJ, Booth JT, Carolan MG and Holmes-Siedle. A special resolution by MOFET dosimetry of an x-ray microbeam. Med. Phys. 2000; **27**:239–244.

[20] Jaksic A, Ristic G, Pejovic M, Mohammadzadeh A, Sudre C and Lane W. Gamma ray irradiation and post-irradiation response of high dose range RADFETs. IEEE Trans. Nucl. Sci. 2002; **49**:1356–1363.

[21] Price RA. Towards an optimum design of a P-MOS radiation detector for use in high-energy medical phantom beam and neutron facilities: analysis of activation materials. Radiat. Prot. Dosimetry. 2005; **115**:386–390.

[22] Pejovic MM, Pejovic MM and Jaksic AB. Response of pMOS dosimeters on gamma ray irradiation during its re-use. Radiat. Prot. Dosimetry. 2013; **155**:394–403.

[23] Alchaikh S, Carolan M, Petasecca M, Lerch M and Metealfe AB. Direct and pulsed current annealing of p-MOSFET based dosimeter, the MOSkin. Australas Phys. Eng. Sci. Med. 2014; **37**:311–319.

[24] RCR. Available on www.rcr.uk. The royal college of radiologists, radiotherapy dose fractions. 2006.

[25] Lipovetzky J, Redin EG and Fajgon A. Electrically erasable metal-oxide-semiconductor dosimeters. IEEE Trans. Nucl. Sci. 2007; **54**:1244–1250.

[26] Moreno E, Picos R, Isern E, Roca M, Bota S and Suenoga K. Radiation sensor compatible with standard CMOS technology. IEEE Trans. Nucl. Sci. 2009; **56**:2910–2915.

[27] Pejovic M, Osmokrovic, P, Pejovic M.M and Stankovic K. Influence of ionizing radiation ant hot carrier injection on metal-oxide-semiconductor transistors, In Nenoi M. (Ed), Current Topics in Radiation Research. INTECH, Institute for New Technologies, Maastricht (NT), 2012, Chapter 33, OCLC: 846871029 (accessed 0.6.06.15)

[28] Griscom DL. Optical properties and structure of defects in silica glass. J. Ceram. Soc. Japan. 1991; **99**:923–941.

[29] McLean FB. A framework for understanding radiation-induced interface states in SiO_2 MOS structure. IEEE Trans. Nucl. Sci. 1980; **54**:1651–1657.

[30] Saks NS and Brown DB. Interface trap formation via the two-stage H^+ process. IEEE Trans. Nucl. Sci. 1989; **36**:1848–1857.

[31] Griscom DL. Diffusion of radiolytic molecular hydrogen as a mechanism for the post-irradiation buildup of interface states in SiO_2-on Si structures. J. Appl. Phys. 1985; **58**:2524–2533.

[32] Poindexter EH. Chemical reactions of hydrogen species in the Si-SiO_2 system. J. Non-Cryst. Solids. 1995; **187**:257–263.

[33] Pejovic MM. Processes in radiation sensitive MOSFETs during and post irradiation annealing responsible for threshold voltage shift. Radiat. Phys. Chem. 2017; **130**:221–228.

[34] Ma TP and Drensserdorfer PV, Ionizing Radiation Effects in MOS Devices and Circuits. J. Wiley; New-York USA: 1989.

[35] Pejovic SM, Pejovic MM, Stojanov D and Ciraj-Bjelac O. Sensitivity and fading of pMOS dosimeters irradiated with X-ray radiation doses from 1 to 100 cGy. Radiat. Prot. Dosimetry. 2016; **168**:33–39.

[36] Pejovic MM. Dose response, radiation sensitivity and signal fading of p-channel MOSFETs (RADFETs) irradiated up to 50 Gy with ^{60}Co. Appl. Radiat. Isot. 2015; **104**:100–105.

[37] Pejovic MM, Pejovic MM and Jaksic B. Radiation-sensitive field effect transistor response to gamma-ray irradiation. Nucl. Technol. Radiat. Protect. 2011; **26**:25–31.

[38] Pejovic MM, Pejovic SM, Stojanov D and Ciraj-Bjelac O. Sensitivity of RADFET for gamma and X-ray doses used in medicine. Nucl. Technol. and Radiat. Protect. 2014; **29**:179–185.

[39] Pejovic S, Bosnjakovic P, Ciraj-Bjelac O and Pejovic MM. Characteristics of PMOSFET suitable for use in radiotherapy. Appl. Radiat. Isot. 2013; **77**:44–49.

[40] Sarrabayrouse G and Gessinn FG. Thick oxide MOS transistors for ionizing radiation dose measurement. Radioprotection. 1994; **29**:557–572.

[41] Rosenfeld AB. MOSFET dosimetry an modern radiation oncology modalites. Radiat. Prot. Dosimetry. 2002; **101**:393–398.

[42] Pejovic MM, Pejovic MM and Jaksic AB. Contribution of fixed oxide traps to sensitivity of pMOS dosimeters during gamma ray irradiation and annealing at room and elevate temperature. Sens. Actuators A. 2012; **174**:341–345.

[43] Pejovic MM. The gamma-ray irradiation sensitivity and dosimetric information instability of RADFET dosimeter. Nucl. Technol. Radiat. Protect. 2013; **28**:415–421.

[44] Ristic G, Jaksic A and Pejovic M. pMOS dosimeter transistors with two-layer gate oxide. Sens. Actuators A. 1997; **63**:129–134.

[45] McWhorter PJ, Miller SL and Miller WM. Modeling the anneal of radiation-induced traps holes in a varying thermal environment. IEEE Trans. Nucl. Sci. 1990; **37**:1682–1689.

[46] Kelleher A, McDonnell N, O'Neill B, Lane W and Adams L. Investigation into the re-use of pMOS dosimeters. IEEE Trans. Nucl. Sci. 1994; **41**:445–449.

[47] Pejovic MM, Pejovic MM, Jaksic AB, Stankovic KDj and Markovic A. Successive gamma ray irradiation and corresponding post-irradiation annealing of pMOS dosimeters. Nucl. Technol. Radiat. Protect. 2012; **27**:341–345.

[48] Pejovic MM, Pejovic MM and Jaksic AB. Response of pMOS dosimeters on gamma-ray irradiation during its re-use. Radiat. Prot. Dosimetry. 2013; **155**:394–403.

[49] Aristru J, Calvo F, Martinez R,, Dubois M, Fisher S and Azinovic I. Lung cancer. In EBRT with or without IORT. From: Current Oncology: Intraoperative Irradiation: Techniques and Results, Ed. by Gunderson F. et al, Humana Press, Inc, Totowa, NJ., 1999

[50] Asensio LJ, Carvaial MA, Lopez-Villaneva JA, Vilches M, Lallena AM and Palma AJ. Evaluation of a low-cost commercial mosfet as radiation dosimeter. Sens. Actuators A. 2006; **125**:288–295.

[51] Martines-Garcia MS, Simancos F, Palma AJ, Lallena AM, Banqueri J and Carvajal MA. General purpose MOSFETs for the dosimetry of electron beams used in intra-operative radiotherapy. Sens. Actuators A. 2014; **210**:175–181.

Chapter 13

A Comparison of Physical vs. Nonphysical Wedge Modalities in Radiotherapy

Hiroaki Akasaka, Naritoshi Mukumoto,
Masao Nakayama, Tianyuan Wang, Ryuichi Yada,
Yasuyuki Shimizu, Saki Osuga, Yuki Wakahara and
Ryohei Sasaki

Additional information is available at the end of the chapter

http://dx.doi.org/10.5772/67057

Abstract

This chapter discusses the clinical application and implementation of wedge techniques in radiation therapy. Coverage of the target region with a curative dose is critical for treating several cancer types; to that end, wedge filters are commonly used to improve dose uniformity to the target volume. Initially, wedges designed for this purpose were physical and were made of high-density materials such as lead or steel. Subsequently, nonphysical wedges were introduced; these improved the dose uniformity using computer systems in lieu of physical materials. As wedge systems evolve, however, they each continue to have their advantages and disadvantages. When using physical wedges, it is difficult to control the generation of secondary radiation resulting from the collision of the radiation beam with the wedge body; conversely, nonphysical wedges do not create any secondary radiation because there is no physical interference with the beam. On the other hand, nonphysical wedges are less suitable for treating moving tumors, such as those in the lung, and physical wedges have better dose coverage to the target volume than nonphysical wedges. This chapter aims to guide decision-making regarding the choice of wedge types in various clinical situations.

Keywords: physical wedge, nonphysical wedge, radiotherapy

1. Introduction

Wedged techniques are routinely used in external beam radiotherapy delivery to improve the dose distribution. In earlier years, physical wedges were typically constructed from high-density materials and fixed to certain wedge angles; they were standard accessories shipped with linear accelerators. Such wedges are usually mounted externally or internally in the gantry head of the linear accelerators. Nonphysical wedges, first proposed in the late 1970s by Kijewski et al., produce modulated dose distributions that were similar to those of physical wedges [1]. They rely on the dynamic movements of a pair of independent collimating jaws during treatment and have been widely implemented in modern radiotherapy machines. Both modalities possess unique advantages and limitations in terms of dosimetric characteristics, treatment accuracy, and efficiency.

In this chapter, we discuss and compare the clinical implementation and application of wedge techniques in radiation therapy.

2. Characteristics of physical or nonphysical wedges in clinical implementation

2.1. Fundamental properties of physical and nonphysical wedges

In radiation therapy, wedge filters are commonly used to improve dose uniformity toward the target volume [2]. A physical wedge is usually constructed from a high-density material, such as lead or steel, which attenuates the beam progressively across the entire field. A nonphysical wedge generates a sloping dose distribution by moving one of the jaws with variable speed, while the opposite jaw remains steady. Nonphysical wedges inherently have no beam attenuation or beam hardening effect and thus offer more flexibility than physical wedges [3, 4]. According to the International Commission on Radiation Units and Measurements, the wedge angle is defined as the angle at which an isodose curve is tilted at the central axis of the beam at a specified depth (usually 10 cm) [5].

Before deciding on physical or nonphysical wedges during clinical treatment planning, the treatment planning system (TPS) requires obtaining a number of measurements from each wedge system. In general, the TPS requires data on the percentage depth-dose (PDD), beam profiles, and wedge factors of the X-ray beams [6]. As an example, **Figure 1** shows the profile curve measurements when physical or nonphysical wedges at 30° and 60° were used (field size 10 × 10 cm^2).

The results show that nonphysical wedges have straighter profile curve lines than physical wedges, which are desirable in clinical practice. These results are consistent with those previously described [7, 8]. Ahmad et al. reported that differences in profiles between physical and nonphysical wedges were most evident in larger fields, shallow depths, thicker wedges, and when using a low-energy beam [8].

On the other hand, the presence of a wedge filter in the path of a radiation beam decreases its intensity; this must be taken into account when calculating treatment doses. When physical wedges were used, photon energy fluence is reduced in the wedged beam compared to the open beam; this effect is more pronounced when increasing the wedge angle [9]. It has also been shown that a physical wedge factor has a stronger depth dependence than a nonphysical wedge factor owing to beam hardening [2].

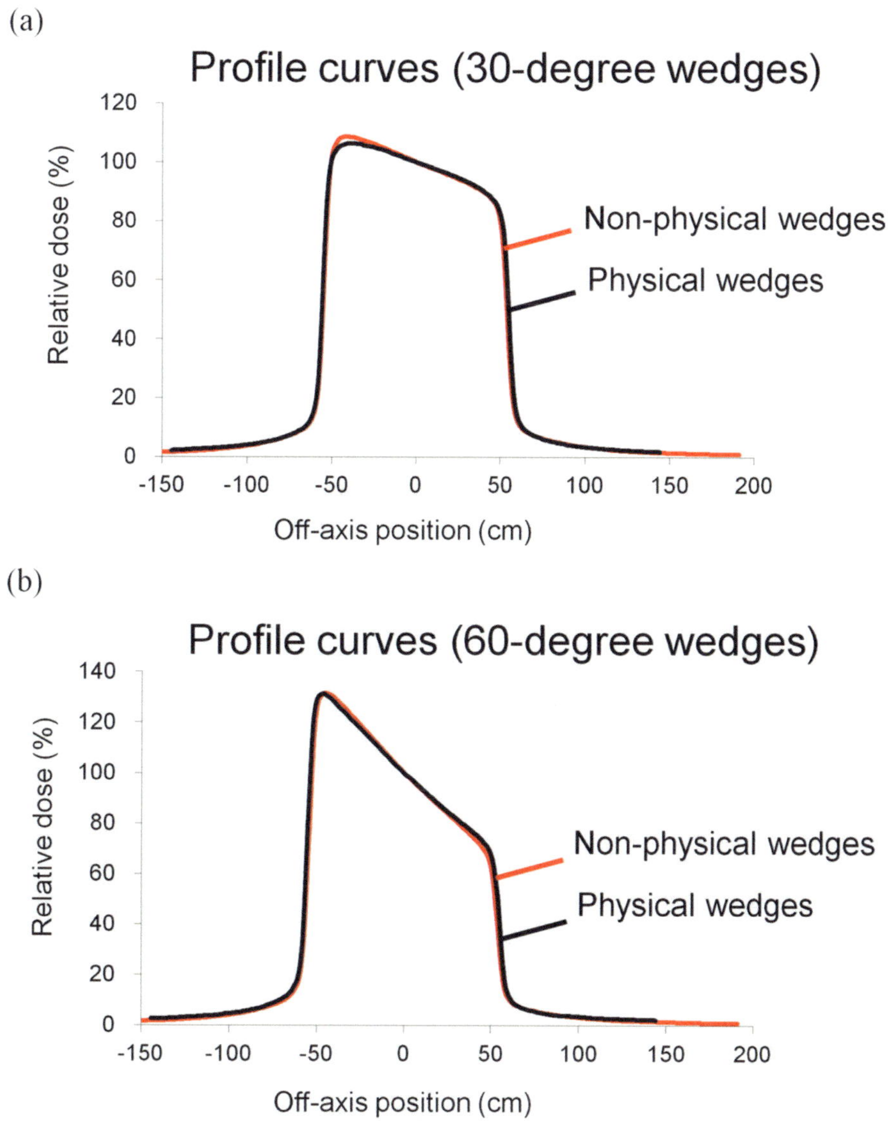

Figure 1. The profile curves of 10 MV X-ray beams using (a) 30° or (b) 60° of physical or nonphysical wedges under a source-surface distance of 100 cm and depth of 10 cm in water. The red line indicates profile curves of nonphysical wedges; the black line indicates that of physical wedges.

2.2. Comparison between calculation data and measurement data

Before wedge filters are installed in clinical practice, several measurements must be incorporated into the TPS for beam modeling. The modeling method for the TPS varies between manufacturers and also between calculation algorithms, as the mechanism of motion of the nonphysical wedges is different for every manufacturer. In this section, the Eclipse planning system (Varian Medical Systems, Palo Alto, CA, USA) and the Enhanced Dynamic Wedge (EDW, Varian Medical Systems, Palo Alto, CA, USA) are mainly described.

A physical wedge changes the beam energy fluence of the primary X-ray beam through the insertion of a metallic filter at the gantry head. This effect is modeled via a wedge transmission curve; specifically, depth doses, wedge profiles, and longitudinal profiles are used for such modeling. In the Eclipse system, the energy fluence of the primary X-ray beam is modeled as a two-dimensional spectrum that considers the mass-energy attenuation coefficient, which is calculated based on the wedge filter material and thickness. Furthermore, the physical wedge produces secondary radiation when interacting with the primary X-ray beam. Eclipse hence considers the wedge a source of scatter, and modeling is performed using a dual Gaussian plane. Moreover, when physical wedges are used in the Eclipse system, a separate electron contamination source model is applied to the calculation; it is necessary to verify the precision of the final model by comparing it to the acquired data before the wedge filters are installed in clinical practice.

Fogliata et al. compared the calculation models and measurement data using the analytical anisotropic algorithm (AAA) [10–13] and the Acuros XB (AXB) [14–16], which is built into Eclipse (version 10.0) [17]. Six and 15 MV X-rays were validated in their study; measurements were performed in water using the PTW-MP3 phantom with a 0.125 cm^2 cylindrical ionization chamber (Semiflex, PTW). Next, depth-dose curves were investigated for several field sizes. In the wedged field along the central axis, the difference in absolute dose between calculated vs. measured values revealed deviations (including standard deviations) smaller than 1%. Moreover, the profile curves were investigated in some field sizes at depths of d_{max}, 5, 10, 20, and 30 cm. In the central beam region, the average difference in profile curves between calculations and measurements was smaller than 1%, with a standard deviation lower than 1%. Output factor and monitor unit (MU) calculations were also investigated in some field sizes at a source-surface distance (SSD) of 90 cm and a depth of 5 cm in water. The difference between the calculated and measured MUs to deliver a fixed dose to the isocenter exhibited a maximum deviation of 0.2%. Therefore, when using AAA or AXB under reference conditions, it is possible to model correctly. However, when considering clinical use, validation in non-reference conditions is also necessary. Van Esch et al. validated depth-dose curves at SSDs of 80, 90, and 100 cm to verify the accuracy of modeling of the electron contamination as a function of source-to-skin distance [18]. For depth-dose curves involving different SSDs, they reported that the disagreement between calculated and measured data in the buildup region was high under conditions of higher energy and small SSD. In wedge profiles for 60° physical wedges using 18 MV for the selection of asymmetric fields (X = 15 cm, Y1 = 7.5 cm, Y2 = −5 cm), deviations up to 4% in the absolute dose at the center of the field were observed. Hence, accurate modeling using this method is difficult because the wedge produces numerous scattered photons and electrons. For tolerance settings at the time of modeling, please refer to Refs. [19, 20].

The nonphysical wedge produces a distribution similar to that of a physical wedge by moving the collimator jaw and/or modifying the dose rate. In the Varian EDW, only a single jaw is moved; moreover, the dose rate for the Siemens virtual wedge is varied. The EDW uses the segmented treatment table (STT) when planning the position of the moving jaw and corresponding doses. The golden STT (GSTT) is used for a wedge angle of 60°, which controls all other wedge fields (i.e., all the field sizes and the wedge angles) as well as the center axis dose of the open field [21]. In other words, EDW settings do not require any input data for beam configuration other than the open beam data. The movement of the collimator in the EDW affects the primary radiation and scatter components, as well as the backscatter of the collimator. Therefore, it is necessary to verify the accuracy of the modeling by comparing calculated estimates to the measured data.

For the EDW, Fogliata et al. also compared the calculations to the measurements using the AAA and AXB [17]. Moreover, depth-dose curves were investigated in field sizes of 20 × 20 cm^2. In wedge fields along the central axis, the difference in absolute dose between the calculations and measurements presented deviations (including standard deviations) smaller than 1%. Furthermore, profile curves were investigated in a field size of 20 × 20 cm^2 at depths of d_{max}, 5, 10, 20, and 30 cm. In the central beam region, the average differences of profile curves between calculations and measurements were smaller than 1%; standard deviations were lower than 1%. Furthermore, output factors and MU calculations were investigated in some field sizes at SSDs of 90 cm and a depth of 5 cm in water. The difference between the calculated and measured MUs when delivering a fixed dose to the isocenter presented a maximum deviation of 0.2%. Validation in a selection of asymmetric fields (X = 15 cm, Y1 = 7.5 cm, Y2 = −5 cm) indicated deviations up to 1.5% in the absolute dose at the center of the field [18]. Furthermore, in a Monte Carlo simulation study, the surface dose of TPS produced large errors of up to 40% compared to Monte Carlo simulation in depth-dose curves [22]. This was attributed to two reasons: First, the calculation of PDDs with TPS is based on ionization chamber measurement data; the measurements of this chamber could be affected by contaminated electrons produced by the moving collimators. Second, the measured surface dose may be averaged incorrectly owing to the erroneous calculation of the ion chamber volume because of the partial volume effect. Monte Carlo simulation indicated that there are significant TPS errors at the outer regions of the field; the maximum relative error of the position difference between TPS and the actual measurements is 20%. Lateral electronic disequilibrium exists in the penumbra regions of the dose profile, especially for smaller field sizes. As mentioned in the American Association of Physicists in Medicine report, TPS cannot accurately calculate backscatter, multiple scattering, or electron disequilibrium in AAA [23]. It is necessary to take into account the calculation precision in the region indicated by the black arrows in **Figure 2**.

3. Advantages and limitations of the wedge technique in clinical applications

3.1. Wedge property uncertainty during treatment

Tumor motion (i.e., intrafractional organ motion) is an important consideration during radiotherapy [24]. Intrafractional motion can be caused by the respiratory, skeletal muscular, cardiac, and gastrointestinal systems. Respiratory motion in particular affects all tumor sites in the thorax and abdomen; the disease of most relevance in this case is lung cancer, as shown in **Figure 3**. Of note, respiratory motion is just one potential source of error in radiotherapy [25]. Chen et al. reported that lung tumor motion varies from 0 to 5 cm [26]; Shirato et al. reported

(a)

(b)

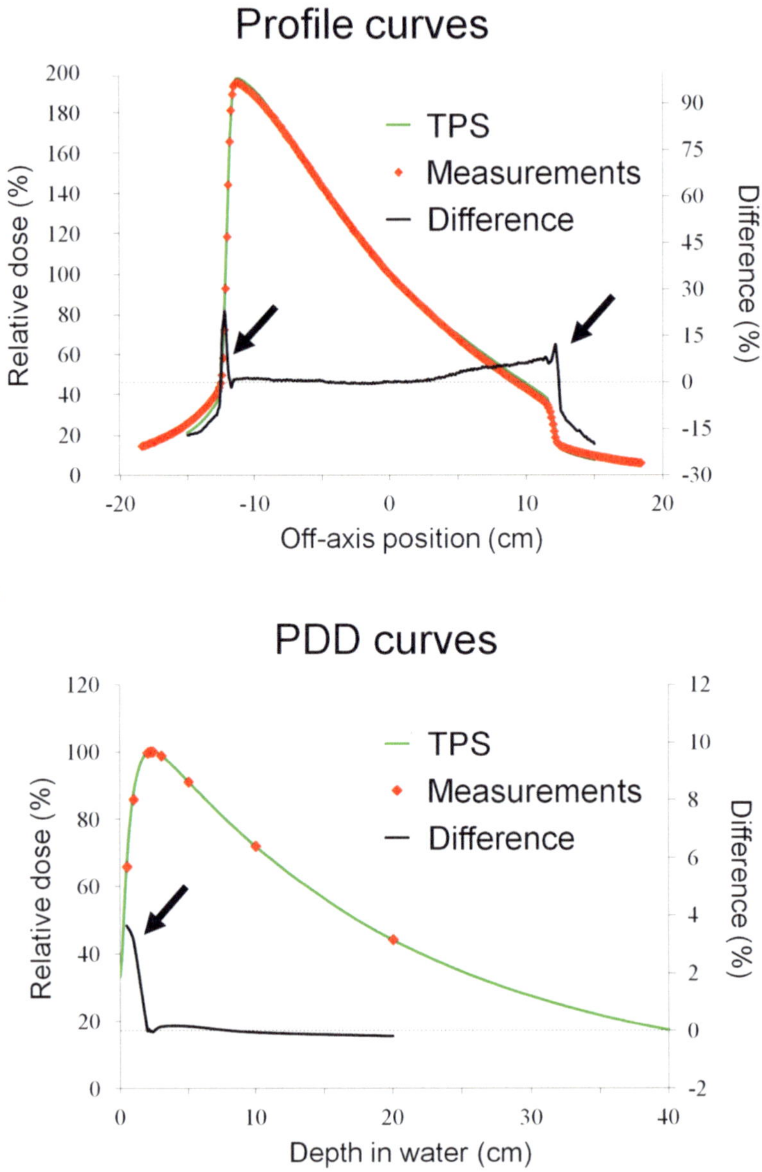

Figure 2. (a) Profile curves and (b) percentage depth-dose (PDD) curves of 10 MV X-ray beams in the treatment planning system (TPS) and measurements. The green line indicates TPS data, the red dots indicate measurement data, and the black line indicates the percentage of error between the TPS and actual measurements.

that the average amplitude of liver tumor motion was up to 1.9 cm [27], while Hamlet et al. reported that the larynx elevates approximately 2 cm while swallowing [28].

Intrafractional organ motion can result in two types of effect. The first is the "dose-blurring effect," which results in the over/under dosage of the tumor with radiation. The second is

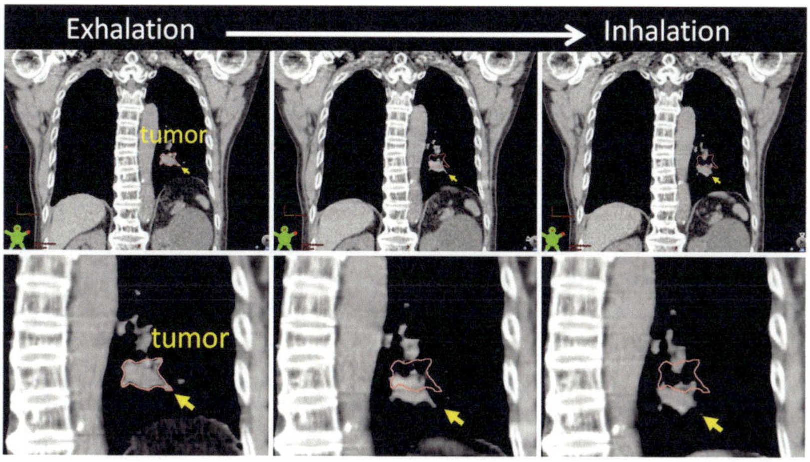

Figure 3. The change over time of tumor motion in the lung between exhalation and inhalation. The red line indicates the contour of the tumor during exhalation; the tumor moves up and down markedly during breathing.

termed the "interplay effect," which is only a problem in the case of dynamic delivery of intensity-modulated radiation therapy or dynamic treatments with nonphysical wedges. This effect is the result of interplay between the moving tumor and the motion of the radiation beam as defined by the nonphysical wedges [29, 30] and can result in dose discrepancy.

The respiratory-based interplay effects for nonphysical wedges have previously been studied; it was reported that approximately 50% of the organ receives a dose 5–15% higher than that prescribed when the collimator is moved from the caudal to the cranial direction. Conversely, collimator movement in the opposite direction results in under-dosing [29]. Moreover, Kakakhel et al. estimated the interplay effects for nonphysical wedges in a phantom study and reported that more than 90% of the area of the target region was covered by the prescribed dose when the phantom was rested. However, for a moving phantom, less than 70% of the target region was covered by the prescribed dose [24].

For the reasons stated above, nonphysical wedges should be considered with caution before utilization for treatment in cases of respiratory organ motion. On the other hand, physical wedges have limited field sizes, densities, and composition materials; hence, they create more low-energy electrons and photon-scattering radiation than nonphysical wedges [31]. Furthermore, the dose outside the field using nonphysical wedges is half that of physical wedges [32].

3.2. Appropriate choice whether physical or nonphysical wedge at several irradiation situations

The choice of physical vs. nonphysical wedges is critical in several clinical situations. As mentioned above, nonphysical wedges have more liabilities than physical wedges for the treatment of moving tumors. In contrast, physical wedges create more secondary radiation than nonphysical wedges. Petrovic et al. reported that the peripheral dose of the nonphysical wedge field is half that of the physical wedge field; this is owing to scatter outside the physical wedge field that arises from the interaction of the beam with the material of the physical wedge (such interactions include Compton scattering).

Clinically, this provides an advantage to the nonphysical wedge field [32]. The effect of secondary radiation outside the field is an important consideration for breast cancer treatment. For example, **Figure 4** shows how the low-dose area was expanded to the opposite breast when using physical wedges; such secondary radiation exposure may precipitate the development of another tumor. Warlic et al. reported that the average dose outside of the field with a nonphysical wedge was 2.7–2.8%, whereas the dose was 4.0–4.7% with a physical wedge. The nonphysical wedge is hence a practical advance that improves the dose distribution in patients undergoing breast conservation while simultaneously minimizing the dose to the contralateral breast, thereby reducing potential carcinogenic effects [33].

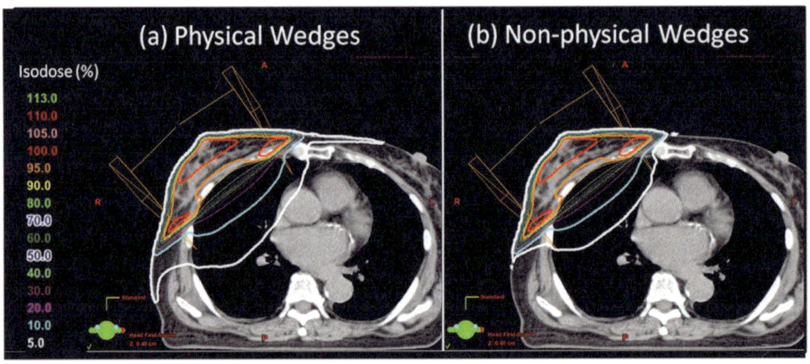

Figure 4. The dose distributions of radiotherapy in a breast cancer patient using (a) physical wedges or (b) nonphysical wedges. Each line indicates the dose corresponding to each treatment intensity planning.

Nonphysical wedges have significant benefits for both the therapists and patients. Saminathan et al. reported that the number of MUs used to deliver a particular dose using a nonphysical wedge field is less than that used for a physical wedge field [2]. Moreover, Njeh reported that using nonphysical wedges results in significant dose reductions to areas outside of the treatment field [34]. The reduction of MUs can also result in minimizing treatment times; this benefits patients who have worse performance statuses.

4. Conclusions

Each of the two wedge types, physical and nonphysical, has several characteristics that produce both advantages and disadvantages under specific conditions. Clinicians should choose between physical and nonphysical wedges with careful consideration to tumor motion, the effect of secondary radiation, and the performance status of the patient.

Author details

Hiroaki Akasaka*, Naritoshi Mukumoto, Masao Nakayama, Tianyuan Wang, Ryuichi Yada, Yasuyuki Shimizu, Saki Osuga, Yuki Wakahara and Ryohei Sasaki

*Address all correspondence to: akasaka@harbor.kobe-u.ac.jp

Division of Radiation Oncology, Kobe University Graduate School of Medicine, Kobe City, Hyogo, Japan

References

[1] Kijewski PK, Chin LM, Bjärngard BE. Wedge-shaped dose distributions by computer-controlled collimator motion. Med Phys. 1978;**5**:426–429.

[2] Saminathan S, Manickam R, Supe SS. Comparison of dosimetric characteristics of physical and enhanced dynamic wedges. Rep Pract Oncol Radiother. 2001;**17**:4–12. DOI: 10.1016/j.rpor.2011.06.007.

[3] Klein EE, Low DA, Meigooni AS, Purdy JA. Dosimetry and clinical implementation of dynamic wedge. Int J Radiat Oncol Biol Phys. 1995;**31**:583–592.

[4] Shih R, Lj XA, Hsu WL. Dosimetric characteristics of dynamic wedged fields: a Monte Carlo study. Phys Med Biol. 2001;**46**:N281–N292.

[5] Cherry P, Duxbury A, editors. Practical radiotherapy physics and equipment. New York, NY: Oxford University Press; 1998. 252 p.

[6] Caprile PF, Venencia CD, Besa P. Comparison between measured and calculated dynamic wedge dose distributions using the anisotropic analytic algorithm and pencil-beam convolution. J Appl Clin Med Phys. 2006;**8**;47–54.

[7] Avadhani JS, Pradhan AS, Sankar A, Viswanathan PS. Dosimetric aspects of physical and of Clinac 2100c linear accelerator. Strahlenther Onkol. 1997;**173**:524–528.

[8] Ahmad M, Hussain A, Muhammad W, Rizvi SQ, Matiullah. Studying wedge factors and beam profiles for physical and enhanced dynamic wedges. J Med Phys. 2010;**35**:33–41. DOI: 10.4103/0971-6203.57116.

[9] Geraily G, Mirzapour M, Mahdavi SR, Allahverdi M, Mostaar A, Masoudifar M. Monte Carlo study on beam hardening effect of physical wedges. Int J Radial Res. 2014;**12**:249–256. DOI: 10.1016/S0939-3889(15)70758-0.

[10] Ulmer W, Harder D. A triple Gaussian pencil beam model for photon beam treatment planning. Z Med Phys. 1995;**5**:25–30. DOI: 10.1016/S0939-3889(15)70758-0.

[11] Ulmer W, Harder D. Applications of a triple Gaussian pencil beam model for photon beam treatment planning. Z Med Phys. 1996;**6**:68–74. DOI: 10.1016/S0939-3889(15)70784-1.

[12] Ulmer W, Pyyry J, Waissl W. A 3D photon superposition/convolution algorithm and its foundation on results of Monte Carlo calculations. Phys Med Biol. 2005;**50**:1767–1790. DOI: 10.1088/0031-9155/50/8/010.

[13] Sievinen J, Ulmer W, Kaissl W. AAA photon dose calculation model in Eclipse™. Palo Alto (CA): Varian Medical Systems. 2005;**118**:2894.

[14] Vassiliev ON, Wareing TA, McGhee J, Failla G, Salehpour MR, Mourtada F. Validation of a new grid-based Boltzmann equation solver for dose calculation in radiotherapy with photon beams. Phys Med Biol. 2010;**55**:581–598. DOI: 10.1088/0031-9155/55/3/002.

[15] Fogliata A, Nicolini G, Clivio A, Vanetti E, Cozzi L. Dosimetric evaluation of Acuros XB advanced dose calculation algorithm in heterogeneous media. Radiat Oncol. 2011;**6**:82. DOI: 10.1186/1748-717X-6-82.

[16] Bush K, Gagne IM, Zavgorodni S, Ansbacher W, Beckham W. Dosimetric validation of Acuros XB with Monte Carlo methods for photon dose calculations. Med Phys. 2011;**38**:2208–2221. DOI: 10.1118/1.3567146

[17] Fogliata A, Nicolini G, Clivio A, Vanetti E, Mancosu P, Cozzi L. Dosimetric validation of the Acuros XB Advanced Dose Calculation algorithm: fundamental characterization in water. Phys Med Biol. 2011;**56**:1879–1904. DOI: 10.1088/0031-9155/56/6/022.

[18] Van Esch A, Tillikainen L, Pyykkonen J, Tenhunen M, Helminen H, Siljamäki S, Alakuijala J, Paiusco M, Lori M, Huyskens DP. Testing of the analytical anisotropic algorithm for photon dose calculation. Med Phys. 2006;**33**:4130–4148. DOI: 10.1118/1.2358333

[19] Fraass B, Doppke K, Hunt M, Kutcher G, Starkschall G, Stern R, Van Dyke J. American Association of Physicists in Medicine Radiation Therapy Committee Task Group 53: quality assurance of clinical radiotherapy treatment planning. Med Phys. 1998;**25**:1773–1829. DOI: 10.1118/1.598373.

[20] Mijnheer B, Olszewska A, Fiorino C, Hartmann G, Knöös T, Rosenwald JC, Welleweerd H. Quality assurance of treatment planning systems practical examples for non-IMRT photon beams (Vol. 1). Brussels: ESTRO; 2004. 96 p.

[21] Rodrigues C, Batel V, Germano S, Grillo IM, Pinto JL. Dosimetric study of enhanced dynamic wedges to clinical implementation into XiO treatment planning system. Electrónica e Telecomunicações. 2007;**4**:838–841.

[22] Chang KP, Chen LY, Chien YH. Monte Carlo simulation of linac irradiation with dynamic wedges. Radiat Prot Dosimetry. 2014;**162**:24–28. DOI: 10.1093/rpd/ncu211.

[23] American Association of Physicists in Medicine. Tissue inhomogeneity corrections for megavoltage photon beams: Report of Task Group No. 65. Madison, WI: Medical Physics Publishing; 2004. 135 p.

[24] Kakakhel MB, Kairn T, Kenny J, Seet K, Fielding AL, Trapp JV. Interplay effects during enhanced dynamic wedge deliveries. Phys Med. 2013;**29**:323–332. DOI: 10.1016/j.ejmp.2012.04.007.

[25] Keall PJ, Mageras GS, Balter JM, Emery RS, Forster KM, Jiang SB, Kapatoes JM, Low DA, Murphy MJ, Murray BR, Ramsey CR, Van Herk MB, Vedam SS, Wong JW, Yorke E. The management of respiratory motion in radiation oncology report of AAPM Task Group 76. Med Phys. 2006;**33**:3874–3900. DOI: 10.1118/1.2349696.

[26] Chen QS, Weinhous MS, Deibel FC, Ciezki JP, Macklis RM. Fluoroscopic study of tumor motion due to breathing: facilitating precise radiation therapy for lung cancer patients. Med Phys. 2001;**28**:1850–1856. DOI: 10.1118/1.1398037.

[27] Shirato H, Seppenwoolde Y, Kitamura K, Onimura R, Shimizu S. Intrafractional tumor motion: lung and liver. Semin Radiat Oncol. 2004;**14**:10–18. DOI: 10.1053/j.semradonc.2003.10.008

[28] Hamlet S, Ezzell G, Aref A. Larynx motion associated with swallowing during radiation therapy. Int J Radiat Oncol Biol Phys. 1994;**28**:467–470. DOI: 10.1016/0360-3016(94)90073-6.

[29] Pemler P, Besserer J, Lombriser N, Pescia R, Schneider U. Influence of respiration-induced organ motion on dose distributions in treatments using enhanced dynamic wedges. Med Phys. 2001;**28**:2234–2240. DOI: 10.1118/1.1410121.

[30] Isa M, Iqbal K, Afzal M, Buzdar S, Chow J. Physical and dynamic wedges in radiotherapy for rectal cancer: a dosimetric comparison. Med Phys. 2012;**39**:4636.

[31] Klein EE, Esthappan J, Li Z. Surface and buildup dose characteristics for 6, 10, and 18 MV photons from an Elekta Precise linear accelerator. J Appl Clin Med Phys. 2003;**4**:1–7. DOI: 10.1120/1.1520113.

[32] Petrovic B, Grzadziel A, Rutonjski L, Slosarek K. Linear array measurements of enhanced dynamic wedge and treatment planning system (TPS) calculation for 15 MV photon beam and comparison with electronic portal imaging device (EPID) measurements. Radiol Oncol. 2010;**44**:199–206. DOI: 10.2478/v10019-010-0037-5.

[33] Warlick WB, O'Rear JH, Earley L, Moeller JH, Gaffney DK, Leavitt DD. Dose to the contralateral breast: a comparison of two techniques using the enhanced dynamic wedge versus a standard wedge. Med Dosim. 1997;**22**:185–191.

[34] Njeh CF. Enhanced dynamic wedge output factors for Varian 2300CD and the case for a reference database. J Appl Clin Med Phys. 2015;**16**:5498.

Chapter 14

Motion Challenge of Thoracic Tumors at Radiotherapy by Introducing an Available Compensation Strategy

Ahmad Esmaili Torshabi and
Seyed Amir Reza Dastyar

Additional information is available at the end of the chapter

http://dx.doi.org/10.5772/67444

Abstract

In this chapter a description is explained about radiotherapy as common available method in treatment of thoracic tumors located at thorax region of patient body and move mainly due to respiration. In radiotherapy of dynamic tumors, the correct and accurate information of tumor position during the therapeutic irradiation determine the degree of treatment success. In this chapter we investigate quantitatively the effect of tumor motion on treatment quality by considering to possible drawbacks and errors at external surrogate's radiotherapy as clinical treatment modality. For this aim, tumor motion information of a group of real patients treated with Cybeknife Synchrony system (from Georgetown University Hospital) was taken into account. A fuzzy logic based correlation model was employed for tumor motion tracking. Final results represent graphically the amount of tumor motion estimated by our utilized correlation model on three dimensions with targeting error calculation. It's worth mentioning that each strategy that can improve targeting accuracy of dynamic tumors may strongly enhance treatment quality by saving healthy tissues against additional high dose. In this chapter we just tried to introduce readers with thoracic tumor motion error as challenging issue in radiotherapy and motion compensation solutions, implemented clinically up to now.

Keywords: radiotherapy, moving thoracic tumors, external surrogate's radiotherapy, correlation model, motion compensation

1. Introduction

Cancer is a range of diseases including abnormal cells that grow out of control. Cancerous cells can be formed in the tissues or organs of patient body, and the damaged cells can invade surrounding tissues. Among different types of cancers, some of them that are known as most common cancers such as lung, breast, and prostate cancers cause many deaths independent of human race or ethnicity. It should be noted that with early detection and treatment, most people continue a normal life [1, 2] .

There are three common available methods for treatment of different cancers known as surgery, chemotherapy, and radiotherapy alone or in combination mode as surgery-chemotherapy, surgery-radiotherapy, chemotherapy-radiotherapy, or surgery-chemotherapy-radiotherapy as the best treatment modality. Each treatment strategy depends on how the cancer is diagnosed and its stage. In clinical treatment, doctor will discuss with patients about which treatments are most suitable for them [1–7]. In the following, a description is explained about common treatment methods ranging from surgery to radiotherapy.

The first and oldest option of treatment modality for a variety range of cancers is surgery or operation that means to perform surgery. The type of surgery will depend on the type of each cancer. Surgery is usually followed by chemotherapy or radiotherapy in modern methods in order to enhance treatment quality. In this method, whole cancerous cells or lesion must be cut and removed. Moreover, surrounding cells around tumors that may potentially be cancerous cells are removed to avoid growing secondary tumors after operation. The tissue surrounding the tumor volume is called the margin. Removing this nearby margin depends directly on the medical doctor decision during surgery. All forms of surgery are considered as invasive procedures. With conventional surgery, the surgeon makes large incisions through skin, muscle, and sometimes bone. In some situations, surgeons can use surgical techniques that are less invasive. These less-invasive techniques may speed recovery and reduce pain afterward. At surgery strategy, in order to avoid growing secondary cancer, whole organ that include tumor cells are removed. For example, there are two main types of breast cancer surgery as: First mode, surgery to remove the cancerous cells, entitled as breast-conserving surgery, where just the tumor and a little surrounding breast tissue are removed. Second mode, surgery to remove the whole breast, is called a mastectomy. However, in some cases, a mastectomy can be implemented by reconstructive surgery to recreate a bulge replacing the removed breast.

Chemotherapy involves using anti-cancer or cytotoxic medication to kill the cancer cells. Chemotherapy is usually given as an outpatient treatment, which means patients will not have to stay in hospital overnight. The medications are usually given through a drip straight into the blood through a vein. Chemotherapy is also usually used after surgery to destroy any cancer cells that have not been removed. This strategy is called as adjuvant chemotherapy. In some cases, chemotherapy is done before surgery, which is often used to shrink big tumors as much as possible. Several different medications are used for chemotherapy depending on tumor type and its site. For example, the choice of medication and the combination will depend on the type of breast cancer and how much it is spread [3, 6, 7]. Some patients may have chemotherapy sessions once every 2–3 weeks, over a period of 4–8 months, to give the body a rest in between treatments time. The main side effects of chemotherapy are caused by their influence on normal, healthy cells, such as immune cells.

Radiotherapy is the use of ionizing radiation beams such as high-energy X-rays or charge particles for cancer treatment. The therapeutic ionizing beam is generated by means of machines called linear accelerator or cyclotron or synchrotron and can damage and destroy cancer cells within the area being irradiated. Radiotherapy is a very specialist treatment and is a common treatment for various ranges of cancer such as head and neck or thoracic tumors. In most cases, radiotherapy is given after surgery. This reduces the risk of cancer coming back by getting rid of any possible cancer cells that are still in the area. **Figure 1** shows schematically the performance of linear machine as particle accelerator for therapeutic beam generation and irradiation to the patient [4, 5, 8].

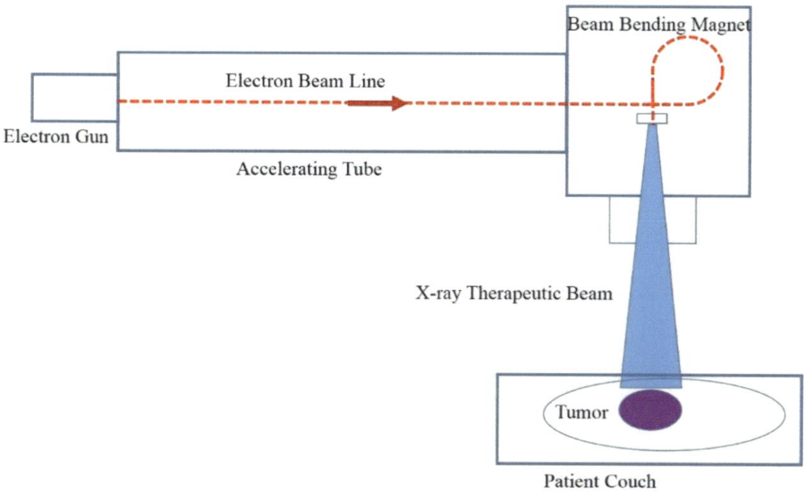

Figure 1. A schematic layout of linear accelerator and the process of therapeutic beam generation.

Ionizing rays are able to produce biological damages physically and chemically. They release their energy by colliding with cells. This can produce fast-moving electrons, which ultimately produce the biological damage to tissues. As seen in **Figure 2**, the therapeutic beam can directly break the DNA known as physical effect or prepare a toxic environment around the cancerous cell for killing them known as chemical effect.

It should be noted that healthy tissues surrounding the tumor volume are affected by ionizing radiation, but their cells can usually recover themselves better than cancer cells implementing proper treatment planning strategies.

In radiotherapy, the main principle is delivering the maximum dose onto tumor volume while keeping the normal nearby tissues save against the high dose at the same time. Treatments are usually given regularly over a period of time so that they have the greatest effect on the cancer cells [5]. Radiotherapy can also be given implanting radioactive seeds into tumor volume. This is called internal radiotherapy or brachytherapy. By this strategy, the normal cells will be saved against additional dose that may have side effects. In this technique, tumor accessibility is very important to implant radioactive seeds. Therefore, intra-cavity tumors are subjects for brachytherapy.

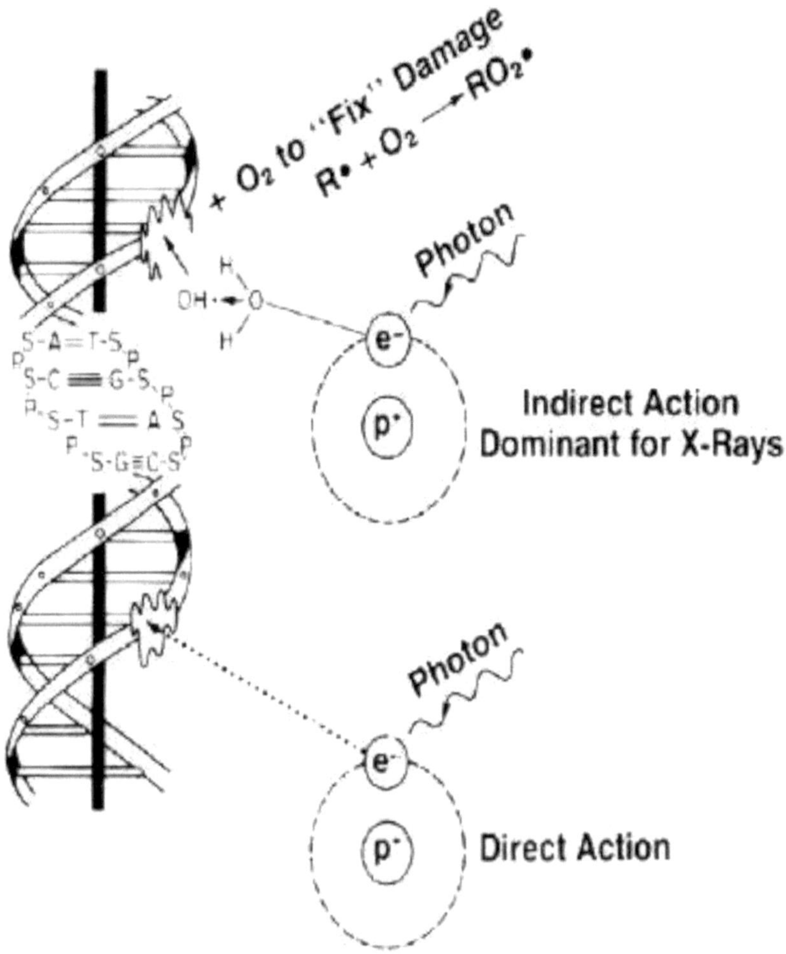

Figure 2. DNA damage of tumor cells by means of ionizing radiations.

Figure 3 represents various steps of a successful radiotherapy based on 2D or 3D treatment planning system for tumor definition and localization. For this aim, tomography images are utilized as first step of treatment process. Simulation step realizes the best area to be irradiated as target using high dose of irradiation while causing the fewest possible side effects considering critical organs or organs at risk (OAR). Moreover, patient positioning and verification is another important issue of radiotherapy that must be carefully considered [4].

In general, total tumors can be categorized into two groups as static and dynamic tumors. This dividing comes from physical motion properties of tumors that is highly important during patient positioning and verification. In modern radiotherapy, tumor motion property is highly effective on treatment quality and must be taken into account during treatment planning process. In radiotherapy of dynamic tumors, the correct and accurate information of tumor position during the therapeutic irradiation determine the degree of treatment success. Among total tumors, dynamic tumors have been located in thorax and abdomen regions of patient body

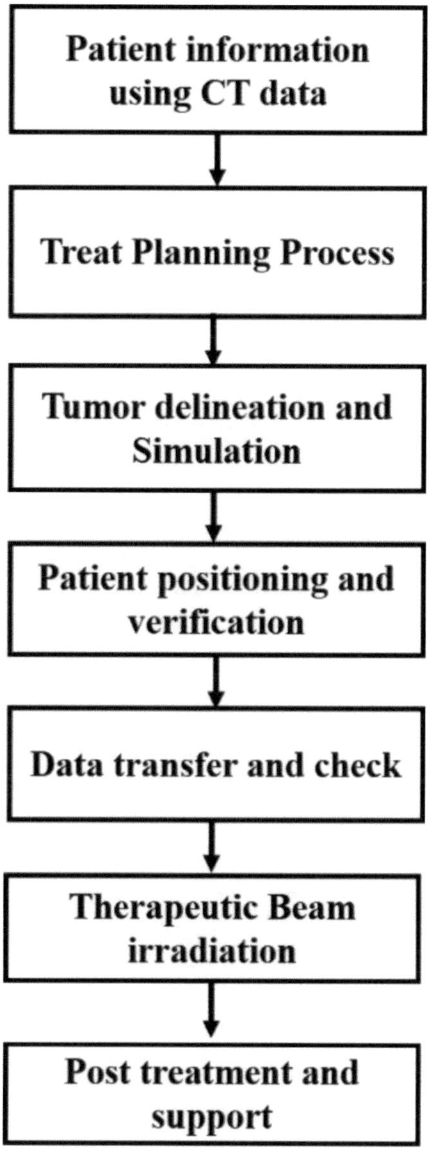

Figure 3. Block diagram of treatment process during radiotherapy.

move due to breathing cycle phenomena, heart beat, and gastrointestinal system motions. The first case has the most important effect on targeting accuracy in radiation treatment. This motions and/or possible deformation that are usually nonregular cause a constraint to achieve the accurate knowledge of tumor location during the treatment process. This nonregularity issue refers to variations on breathing motion amplitude and frequency, while these two parameters are highly variable at each time for each patient and therefore require caution at clinical settings. It is obvious that the parameters of breathing motion phenomena are different at each patient, and a sort of adaptive treatment planning must be depicted for each patient on a case by case basis, and this issue is problematic for operators and needs more accuracy at treatment planning process. This motion error that is known as intra-fractional organs motion error may lead to a significant uncertainty of tumor localization. Therefore, a great amount of over or under dosage is happened onto tumor, and healthy surrounding tissues may receive high dose that is far away from prescribed dose that has been determined before irradiation [8–14]. Apart from intra-fraction motion error, we face with another motion error known as inter-fraction motion that refers to patient body displacement on treatment couch. This motion error must be considered at patient positioning stage during patient setup in pretreatment time few minutes before irradiation starting. Our focus in this chapter is on intra-fraction motion error.

At radiotherapy of dynamic tumors using old strategy, considerable margins were added around the planning target volume as treatment site to cover whole tumor displacement and possible deformation (known as internal target volume), and therefore, normal tissues surrounding the target may irradiate unnecessarily. During the past decade, radiation treatment of moving tumors has been undergone major technological and methodological strategies. Such this development has been obtained by investments in research programs, computer development, and technology transfer from research to medicine, and generating of new generation therapy units dedicated on tumor motion tracking in real time. These assessments were motivated by the requirements to enhance radiotherapy quality in patients with dynamic thoracic tumors such as those with lung, liver, or pancreas cancers. Several strategies have been proposed to compensate the effect of motion error on planned dose such as breath-holding, respiratory motion-gating, and real-time tumor-tracking techniques [15–20].

In breath-holding technique, the goal is to immobilize the breast tumor by asking the patient to keep breathing in a specific level. Breath-holding technique requires cooperating patients that are problematic for patients with noncontrolled breathing [15, 17]. Respiratory-gated radiotherapy was proposed as another method to save normal surrounding tissue of dynamic region against additional high dose by irradiating the therapeutic beam only in a predefined phase of the breathing cycle [18, 19]. In real-time tumor-tracking technique, the irradiation beam is continuously repositioned dynamically to trace breast tumor motion in real time. In this method that is still under developing, the beam is always ON during a treatment fraction.

The developed technologies and methods for tumor tracking in X-ray radiotherapy can also be implemented for applications in hadron therapy using protons or heavier ions as therapeutic beams. Recent assessments show the using of particle therapy at worldwide in recent years, while 39 facilities were operational at the end of 2011, 33 with protons and six with carbon ions. Moreover, 20 new facilities are currently in the planning stage or under construction. As an example, hypo-fractionated particle therapy shows promising results in local control and overall survival in stage one of non–small lung cancer cells. Due to physical properties of charged particles, therapeutic beams can be steered by fast magnets to follow dynamic targets in real-time mode. Therefore, for treatment of moving tumors, charged particles such as protons and carbon ions have better geometrical and biological selectivity in regard with photon beam, and this useful property can improve tumor tracking and localization at clinical applications. At particle therapy, conventional dose delivery system is based on passive range modulation of the beam. Some scattering strategies are implemented to provide lateral beam flattering according to transverse size of tumor volume. Moreover, some passive devices such as ridge filters are used to make spread out Bragg peak (SOBP) as responsible to flat the beam longitudinally in direction of beam propagation inside tumor volume. Thus, 3D uniform dose can be generated onto tumor volume simultaneously. In particle therapy, the treatment of dynamic tumors can be taken into account on the basis of passive modulation technique or wobbling magnets performance.

In order to implement respiratory gated and real-time tumor-tracking radiotherapy techniques that mentioned above, tumor position information must be extracted as function of time during treatment. These strategies make use of time-resolved 4D imaging systems during treatment planning process in combination with technologies of image guiding. This solution enhances targeting accuracy during irradiation. Moreover, in treatment planning by using 4D computed tomography, images can highly improve target and sensitive organs around the tumors can be saved against additional doses accordingly in comparison with conventional radiotherapy. In other word, enlargement of margins around the dynamic tumors is significantly reduced using new technology considering tumor motion tracking.

Based on above descriptions, tumor motion monitoring requires additional imaging hard wares at treatment room to represent inter and intra fraction motions for patient geometrical setup in pre-treatment and real-time tumor tracking during treatment, respectively. Among several monitoring methods, some of clinically available techniques range from continuous X-ray imaging (i.e., fluoroscopy) to the use of external surrogates radiotherapy [20–33]. In an ideal form, the tumor motion would be observed continuously using fluoroscopic imaging system at external beam radiotherapy. This aim can also be achieved using cone beam computed tomography (CBCT) installed at radiotherapy treatment room. It is worth mentioning that with conventional megavoltage X-ray radiotherapy, inter-fraction daily variations can be obtained by time-resolved on-board images taken by CBCT that show respiratory-correlated tumor motion before treatment.

While tumor contrast is not proper during imaging of some organs by fluoroscopy or CBCT, a fiducial marker is implanted near or inside tumor volume representing a given point of that nonvisible tumor [8]. Therefore, internal clips represent tumor position with a 3D spatial point shown by x(t), y(t), and z(t) over treatment time.

During each irradiation fraction, implanted fiducial is traced by means of fluoroscopy imaging system, providing 3-dimensional (3D) coordinates at usually 30 frames per second. The tumor motion information is then utilized to turn the beam ON, while the tumor is in the desired place at radiotherapy based on respiratory motion-gated strategy. Apart from some advantageous points of using fluoroscopy imaging, this method would deliver significant imaging dose mainly at hypo-fractionated radiotherapy and radiosurgery [8, 9]. Therefore, a trade off must be taken into account between additional imaging dose and motion monitoring accuracy. As solution, using external surrogate's technique, the patient is kept away additional imaging dose versus fluoroscopy-based tumor motion monitoring.

At external surrogate's radiotherapy, the external rib cage and abdomen skin motion is synchronized and correlated with internal tumor motion by developing a proper correlation model in training step before the treatment. It should be mentioned that the external motion is traced by means of specific external markers placed on thorax region (rib cage and abdomen) of patient body and recorded by some monitoring systems such as infrared optical tracking (OTS) or laser-based systems. In contrast, the internal tumor motion is tracked using implanted internal clips inside or near the tumor volume and is visualized using orthogonal X-ray imaging system in snapshot mode. The generated correlation model can estimate the tumor motion from external markers data as input when internal marker data are out of access. The end result is a nonlinear mapping from the motion data of external markers as input to an output, which is the estimate of tumor position versus time. Recently, several respiratory motion prediction models have been developed in different mathematical approaches [34–37]. Since the breathing phenomena have inherently high uncertainty and therefore cause a significant variability in input/output data set, a mathematical model with highest accuracy may correlate input data with tumor motion estimation with less uncertainty error [8].

Since explaining all proposed strategies concerning tumor motion management is very extensive, we concentrated on external surrogate's radiotherapy in this chapter as clinical available strategy. Therefore, in this chapter, we quantitatively investigate the effect of motion error of thoracic tumors on treatment process at external surrogate's radiotherapy. To do this, the motion information of a group of real patients treated with Cyberknife Synchrony system (from Georgetown University Hospital) was taken into account, and the amount of possible errors of target localization was calculated using available statistical metrics [15].

2. Material and methods

The database utilized in this chapter consists of 10 patients treated with real-time compensation of tumor motion by means of the Synchrony® respiratory tracking module, as available in the Cyberknife® system. This system provides tumor tracking relying on external/internal correlation model between the motion of external infrared markers and of clips implanted near thoracic tumors. In this system, the correlation model will be constructed at the beginning of each treatment session and will be updated over the course of treatment. **Figure 4** depicts three-mentioned steps as model configuration, model performance, and model update during treatment. The model is built by means of training data set before starting the treatment. Training data include 3D external markers motion as model input and internal implanted clip as model output. When the model is made, it can be applied to estimate tumor motion as a function of time during the treatment. The model can also be updated and re-built as needed during the treatment with X-ray imaging representing the internal marker location. For model performance, the only input data including external markers motion are given, and the output is tumor motion estimation. The utilized model in this flowchart is based on fuzzy logic inference system that is robust enough for tumor motion prediction based on our previous studies [34–38].

Markers motion data set represents the position information of each marker as function of time. This data set is saved in matrix form for model construction and performance. **Figure 5** shows a matrix with n rows and nine columns including x, y, and z of three utilized external markers located on rib cage and abdomen regions. For model construction and performance, the motion data set should be firstly clustered. Motion data set is firstly arranged at two input and output matrices.

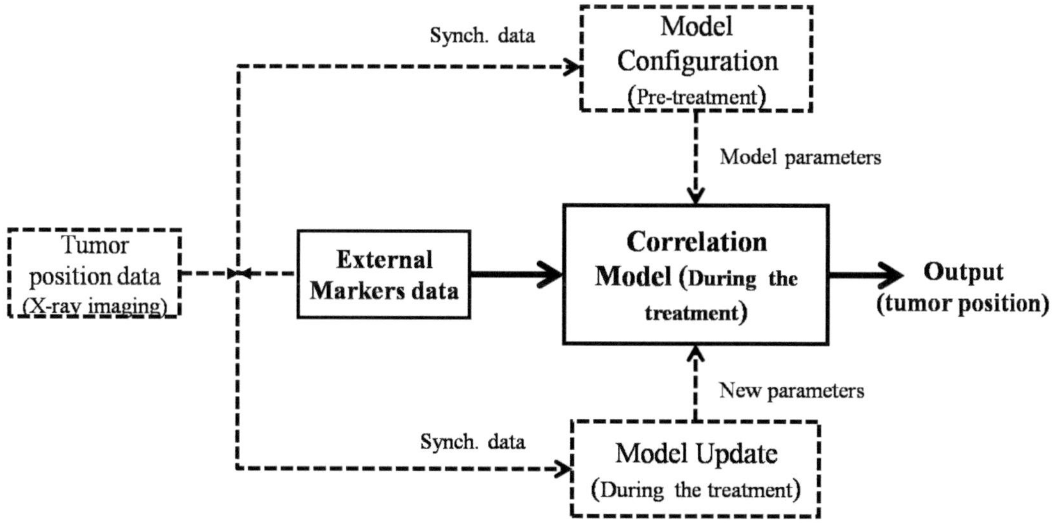

Figure 4. A block diagram of a correlation model including its construction, performance and update.

As mentioned before, the utilized correlation model is on the basis of fuzzy logic concept. In fuzzy logic, linguistic variables represent operating parameters to apply a more human-like way of thinking. Fuzzy logic works by means of if-then rule-based approach to solve a problem rather than attempting to model a system mathematically. Recently, the main features of fuzzy logic theory make it highly applicable in many systematic designs in order to obtain a better performance when data analysis is too complex or impractical for conventional mathematical models. Since breathing motion variability is remarkable, fuzzy logic-based correlation model may robust and can practically be applied on a real patient data set. In fuzzy logic-based systems, membership functions represent the magnitude of participation of each input, graphically. The proposed fuzzy correlation model involves data clustering for membership function generation, as inputs for fuzzy inference system section. Data clustering analysis is the organization of a collection of data set into clusters based on similarity. In the implemented fuzzy logic algorithm, data from all three external markers arranged in an input matrix with nine columns, and data

$$\text{External database} = \begin{pmatrix} X(t_1)_{M1} & Y(t_1)_{M1} & Z(t_1)_{M1} & X(t_1)_{M2} & Y(t_1)_{M2} & Z(t_1)_{M2} & X(t_1)_{M3} & Y(t_1)_{M3} & Z(t_1)_{M3} \\ X(t_2)_{M1} & Y(t_2)_{M1} & Z(t_2)_{M1} & X(t_2)_{M2} & Y(t_2)_{M2} & Z(t_2)_{M2} & X(t_2)_{M3} & Y(t_2)_{M3} & Z(t_2)_{M3} \\ X(t_3)_{M1} & Y(t_3)_{M1} & Z(t_3)_{M1} & X(t_3)_{M2} & Y(t_3)_{M2} & Z(t_3)_{M2} & X(t_3)_{M3} & Y(t_3)_{M3} & Z(t_3)_{M3} \\ \cdot & \cdot & \cdot & \cdot & \cdot & \cdot & \cdot & \cdot & \cdot \\ \cdot & \cdot & \cdot & \cdot & \cdot & \cdot & \cdot & \cdot & \cdot \\ \cdot & \cdot & \cdot & \cdot & \cdot & \cdot & \cdot & \cdot & \cdot \\ X(t_n)_{M1} & Y(t_n)_{M1} & Z(t_n)_{M1} & X(t_n)_{M2} & Y(t_n)_{M2} & Z(t_n)_{M2} & X(t_n)_{M3} & Y(t_n)_{M3} & Z(t_n)_{M3} \end{pmatrix}_{n\times 9}$$

Figure 5. X, Y and Z motion direction of three external markers inside matrix with n rows and nine columns.

from internal marker set in an output matrix with 1 column are clustered initially. Sugeno and Mamdani types of fuzzy inference systems configured by (1) data fuzzification, (2) *if-then* rules induction, (3) application of implication method, (4) output aggregation, and (5) defuzzification steps, utilized due to its specific effects on model performance. The proposed correlation model was developed in MatLab (The MathWorks Inc., Natick, MA) using the embedded toolboxes of fuzzy logic. **Figure 6** shows nine data points (small spots) of motion data set of one external marker clustered at three groups (large spots). The cluster centers (large spots) were distributed as an available mathematical method that works on the basis of data points' spatial distribution density. After data clustering, membership functions will be obtained using the information of clusters center. The mathematical information of these functions is used for defining the parameters of learning based inference system as correlation model.

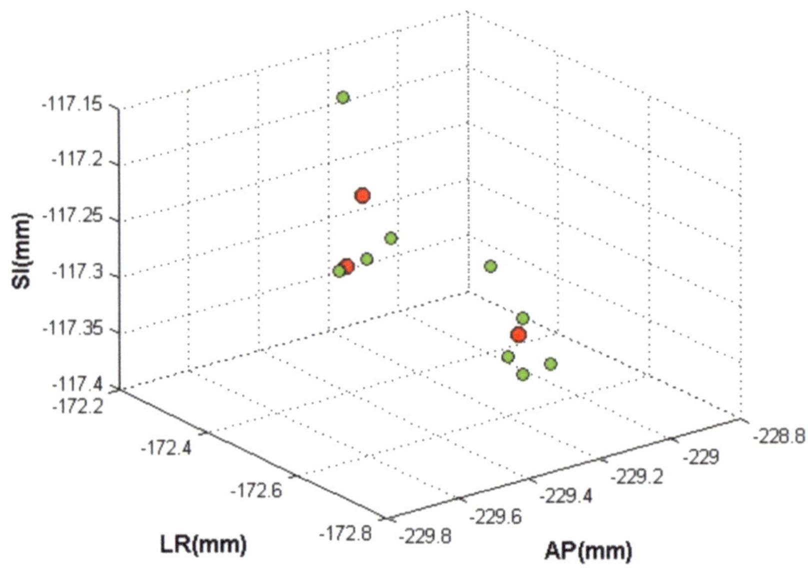

Figure 6. Nine data points (small spots) of motion data set of an external marker with three clusters (large spots).

For real-time tumor tracking, the correlation models should be executed without a significant delay such that on-time compensation strategy should be applied against tumor motion. Therefore, the execute time of each correlation model that strongly depends on the utilized mathematical procedures should be taken into account for clinical application.

3. Results

In order to show quantitatively the challenging issues of targeting accuracy concerning thoracic tumor, its motion and correlation model output of one lung patient were shown graphically. Moreover, root means square error (RMSE) was utilized as mathematic tool, and the average of RMSE over total patients used in this work was reported. **Table 1** illustrates the

Tumor location	P1	P2	P3	P4	P5	P6	P7	P8	P9	P10
	RLL	LLL	Pancreas	Right hilum	LLL	Chest wall	Liver	RUL	Left splenic bed	Left flank
Tumor motion on SI (mm)	31.1	11.6	15.8	18.2	23.8	2.6	18.7	4.0	2.0	3.0
Tumor motion on LR (mm)	5.0	6.1	15.9	12.4	3.1	3.2	3.3	1.8	3.5	2.2
Tumor motion on AP (mm)	3.8	10.2	12.0	7.7	1.8	7.7	7.8	6.4	4.3	2.4
External motion (mm)	3.4	4.4	3.3	1.4	2.7	1.9	5.5	5.8	6.0	1.6
Imaging points intervals (s), mean	66.9	81.7	55.8	73.7	65.1	63.6	64.5	97.6	81.7	58.1
Imaging points intervals (s), STD	33.1	32.1	33.0	38.2	32.0	31.7	29.1	44.1	32.8	26.0
Total treatment time (min)	78.0	68.1	90.1	61.4	68.3	59.4	41.9	70.0	61.3	69.7

Table 1. Motion features of tumors and external markers of selected patients with their treatment time.

motion information of 3D external markers and implanted clip inside tumor volume for 10 patients plus treatment time for each patient.

As seen in **Table 1**, tumors type include lung liver, pancreas, and chest wall. In this table, LLL, RLL, and RUL indicate left lower lung, right lower lung, and right upper lung, correspondingly. The average 3D RMSE over this patient group is 0.99 mm.

Figure 7 shows tumor motion in anterior posterior (AP), superior inferior (SI), and left right (LR) directions obtained from stereoscopic X-ray imaging regarding with correlation model output for a lung cancer patient. As seen in this figure, remarkable error belongs to tumor motion tracking at SI direction versus two other directions while the minimum similarity was happened in this direction. At both SI and LR directions, minimum targeting error is happening at middle part of total treatment time.

Figure 8 shows the tumor motion tracking of one patient with liver cancer over few minutes of treatment time on anterior posterior (AP) directions. The stereoscopic X-ray imaging points indicated by dark spots in these figures represent the exact position of tumor location at that time.

As seen in this figure, breathing condition is almost normal and tumor tracking is going well with least uncertainty error, and there is a close correlation among model output and real

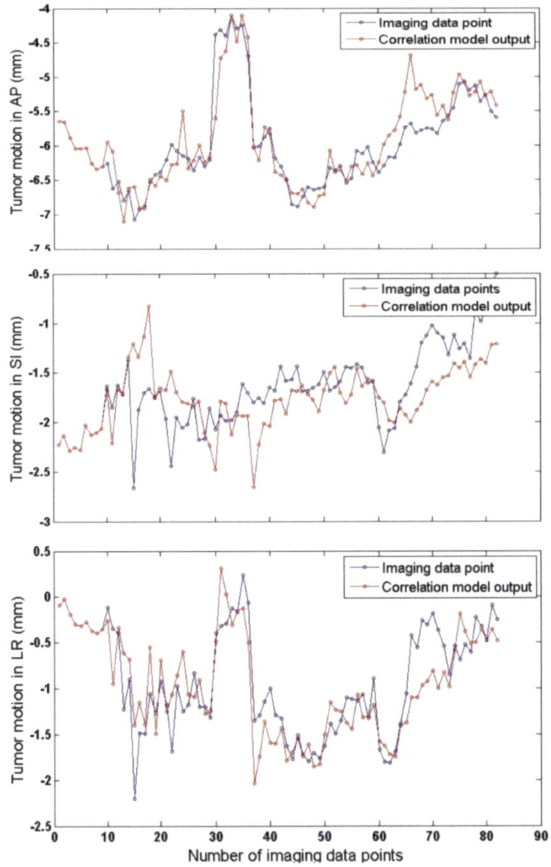

Figure 7. Lung tumor motion in anterior posterior (AP), superior inferior (SI) and left right (LR) directions obtained from stereoscopic X-ray Imaging in comparison with correlation model output.

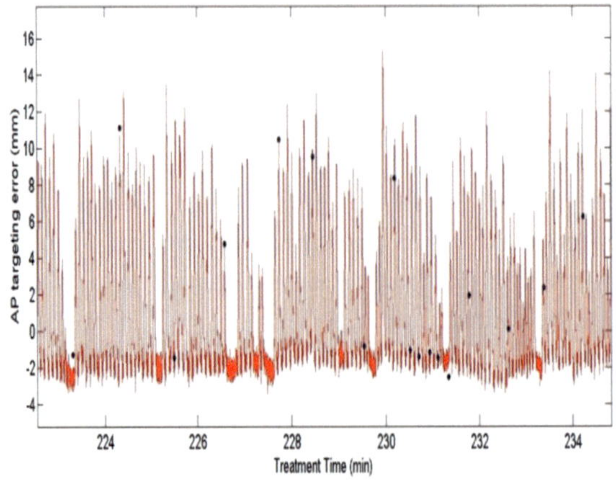

Figure 8. Motion prediction of a liver tumor by means of fuzzy-based correlation model over treatment time. Dark spots taken by stereoscopic system represent the exact position of the tumor.

position of tumor. For this patient, the calculated root mean square error (RMSE) is 1.7-mm 3D that represents tumor motion tracking is performing as well by means of utilized fuzzy-based prediction model. As noncontrol patient with large error, **Figure 9** represents targeting error of one worse patient with pancreas cancer with abnormal breathing motion variation at LR direction. As seen in this figure, tumor motion tracking is with large error; while at some times, the distance between imaging data point and the output of correlation model is significant. For example, third imaging point is far away from model output that represents motion tracking is not going well. This is nonnegligible targeting error that should be considered to be minimized.

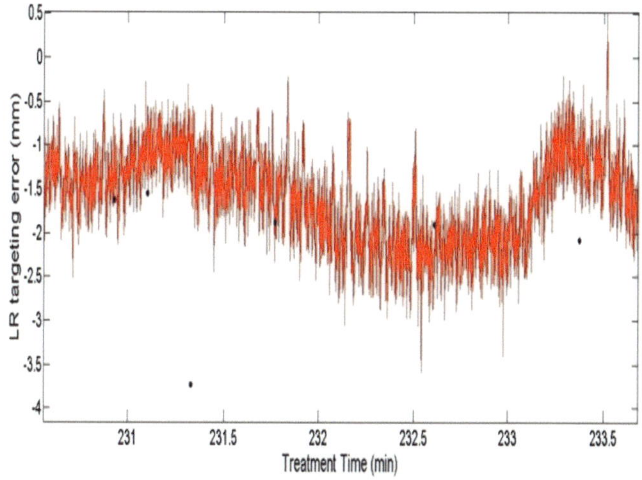

Figure 9. Motion prediction of a pancreas tumor by means of fuzzy-based correlation model over treatment time. Dark spots taken by stereoscopic system represent the exact position of tumor.

4. Discussion

Cancer disease is one of the most common reasons of death at worldwide. A number of treatments for cancer include surgery, chemotherapy, and radiotherapy. Radiation therapy is one of the most common treatments for some cancer cells. It uses X-rays, gamma rays, electron beams, or protons and heavy ions to physically and chemically damage DNA of cancer cells. Radiation can be given alone or used with other treatment modalities, such as surgery or chemotherapy. In principal, at radiation therapy, several strategies can be utilized to deliver high doses of radiation to the cancer cells as target while delivering minimum dose to the surrounding healthy tissues at the same time. The goal of radiation treatment is to damage cancer cells, with as little harm as possible to nearby healthy cells. By the way, nearby normal cells may also be affected by radiation, but they will recover and go back to work normal. Unlike chemotherapy, which exposes the whole body to cancer-fighting drugs, in most cases, radiation therapy is a local treatment.

In this chapter, we focused on radiation treatment of moving thoracic tumors located in thorax region of patient body and move mainly due to respiration. This motion will be problematic for tumor localization and its aligning against therapeutic beam. In old strategies, tumor volume at its total moving space entitled internal tumor volume was considered as target for irradiation. In this strategy, a remarkable dose is received by nearby normal tissues that may cause serious side effects. Then, several efforts were done for tumor motion error compensation as motion-gated radiotherapy or real-time tumor-tracking radiotherapy. At both latter strategies, tumor motion information should be extracted as a function of time during irradiation. In this chapter, we quantitatively assess the effect of tumor motion and possible drawbacks and errors at external surrogate's radiotherapy. For this aim, tumor motion information of a real patient treated with Cyberknife Synchrony system was taken into account. A fuzzy logic-based correlation model was developed to track tumor motion using motion data set of rib cage and abdomen region of patient. Final results represent graphically the amount of tumor motion estimated by utilized model on 3D with a calculated targeting error. In order to reduce such errors, more robust prediction models should be implemented. Moreover, the accuracy of model learning and its configuration at pretreatment step before therapeutic irradiation may reduce estimation error. At external beam radiotherapy of dynamic tumors, another issue that must be considered is due to patient displacement or inter-fractional motion error between each fractions of treatment process. In the modern radiotherapy, the success degree of a treatment strongly depends on the compensation of both inter- and intra-fraction motion errors.

5. Conclusion

At modern radiotherapy, the main aim is enhancing treatment quality by maximizing target localization and dose delivery accuracy onto tumor volume while minimizing the dose received by normal nearby tissues. Reaching to this aim can be problematic and difficult for thoracic tumors where these tumors move mainly due to respiration. Therefore, while tumor motion is an issue, target localization cannot be done carefully and an over-under dose my deliver onto tumor volume that will not be the prescribed dose simulated at treatment planning process. In order to compensate the effect of tumor motion error during therapeutic beam irradiation, several strategies have been implemented or under developing. Three major strategies are as follow: breath-holding technique as old method, respiratory-gated radiotherapy as current clinical available method, and real-time tumor tracking radiotherapy as under developing technique. In the latter case, the irradiation beam is continuously repositioned dynamically to trace breast tumor motion in real time. For both latter cases, the key component for reaching to our aim is to discover the information of tumor position versus time. To do this, some additional monitoring systems are required to track tumor motion as real time ranging from continuous X-ray imagers to the use of external markers or surrogates radiotherapy. In this chapter, we introduced readers with tumor motion as a challenging issue during radiotherapy and presenting external surrogates based radiotherapy as clinical implemented method at several radiotherapy centers or hospitals in the worldwide. In this work, we utilized a typical fuzzy logic-based correlation model to predict tumor motion due to the robustness and simplicity of this model that has been proved at our recent works. This method is still under assessment to minimize available uncertainty errors or to remove possible drawbacks. We had several comprehensive studies on different aspect of this strategy by introducing different prediction models for real-time tumor tracking, their mathematical structures, and the properties of motion data set as inputs of the prediction models [34–38].

Acknowledgements

The authors acknowledge Sonja Dieterich for providing access to the clinical database.

Author details

Ahmad Esmaili Torshabi* and Seyed Amir Reza Dastyar

*Address all correspondence to: ahmad4958@gmail.com

Medical Radiation Division, Department of Electrical & Computer Engineering, Graduate University of Advanced Technology, Kerman, Iran

References

[1] Hayden, EC. (2009). Cutting off cancer's supply lines. Nature. 458(7239):686–687.

[2] Maverakis E, Cornelius LA, Bowen GM, Phan T, Patel FB, Fitzmaurice S, He Y, Burrall B, Duong C, Kloxin AM, Sultani H, Wilken R, Martinez SR, Patel F. (2015). Metastatic melanoma—a review of current and future treatment options. Acta Derm Venereol. 95(5):516–524

[3] Mieog JSD, van der Hage JA, van de Velde CJH. (2007). Neoadjuvant chemotherapy for operable breast cancer. Br J Surg. 94(10):1189–1200.

[4] Wickberg A, Holmberg L, Adami H-O, Magnuson A, Villman K, Liljegren G. (2014). Sector resection with or without postoperative radiotherapy for stage I breast cancer: 20-year results of a randomized trial. J Clin Oncol. 32(8):791–797.

[5] Taylor CW, Nisbet A, McGale P, Darby SC. (2007). Cardiac exposures in breast cancer radiation therapy: 1950s–1990s. Int J Radiat Oncol Biol Phys. 69(5):1484–1495.

[6] Romond EH, Perez EA, Bryant J, Suman VJ, Geyer CE, Davidson NE, Tan-Chiu E, Martino S, Paik S, Kaufman PA, Swain SM, Pisansky TM, Fehrenbacher L, Kutteh LA, Vogel VG, Visscher DW, Yothers G, Jenkins RB, Brown AM, Dakhil SR, Mamounas EP, Lingle WL, Klein PM, Ingle JN, Wolmark N. (2005). Trastuzumab plus adjuvant chemotherapy for operable HER2-positive breast cancer. N Engl J Med. 353(16):1673–1684.

[7] Wagstaff AJ, Ibbotson T, Goa KL. (2003). Capecitabine: a review of its pharmacology and therapeutic efficacy in the management of advanced breast cancer. Drugs. 63(2):217–236.

[8] Riboldi M, Orecchia R, Baroni G. (2012). Real-time tumour tracking in particle therapy: technological developments and future perspectives. Lancet Oncol. 13(9):e383–e391.

[9] Riboldi M, Sharp G, Baroni G, Chen G. (2009). Four-dimensional targeting error analysis in image-guided radiotherapy. Phys Med Biol. 54(19):5995–6008.

[10] Cedric XY, Jaffray DA, Wong JW. (1998). The effects of intra-fraction organ motion on the delivery of dynamic intensity modulation. Phys Med Biol. 43(1):91–104.

[11] Seppenwoolde Y, Shirato H, Kitamura K, et al. (2002). Precise and real time measurement of 3D tumor motion in lung due to breathing and heartbeat, measured during radiotherapy. Int J Radiat Oncol Biol Phys. 53(4):822–834.

[12] Shirato H, Seppenwoolde Y, Kitamura K, Onimura R, Shimizu S. (2004). Intra-fractional tumor motion: lung and liver. Semin Radiat Oncol. 14(1):10–18.

[13] Stevens CW, Munden RF, Forster KM, et al. (2001). Respiratory-driven lung tumor motion is independent of tumor size, tumor location, and pulmonary function. Int J Radiat Oncol Biol Phys. 51(1):62–68.

[14] Wu J, Lei P, Shekhar R, Li H, Suntharalingam M, D'Souza WD. (2009). Do tumors in the lung deform during normal respiration? An image registration investigation. Int J Radiat Oncol Biol Phys. 75(1):268–275.

[15] Liu HH, Balter P, Tutt T, et al. (2007). Assessing respiration-induced tumor motion and internal target volume using four-dimensional computed tomography for radiotherapy of lung cancer. Int J Radiat Oncol Biol Phys. 68(2):531–540.

[16] Zhao JD, Xu ZY, Zhu J, et al. (2008). Application of active breathing control in 3-dimensional conformal radiation therapy for hepatocellular carcinoma: the feasibility and benefit. Radiother Oncol. 87(3):439–444.

[17] Cervino LI, Gupta S, Rose MA, Yashar C, Jiang SB. (2009). Using surface imaging and visual coaching to improve the reproducibility and stability of deep-inspiration breath hold for left-breast-cancer radiotherapy. Phys Med Biol. 54(22):6853–6865.

[18] McNair HA, Brock J, Symonds-Tayler JRN, et al. (2009). Feasibility of the use of the active breathing co ordinator™ (ABC) in patients receiving radical radiotherapy for non-small cell lung cancer (NSCLC). Radiother Oncol. 93(3):424–429.

[19] Kubo HD, Hill BC. (1996). Respiration gated radiotherapy treatment: a technical study. Phys Med Biol. 41(1):83–91.

[20] Vedam S, Keall P, Kini V, Mohan R. (2001). Determining parameters for respiration-gated radiotherapy. Med Phys. 28(10):2139–2146.

[21] Shirato H, Shimizu S, Kunieda T, et al. (2000). Physical aspects of a realtime tumor-tracking system for gated radiotherapy. Int J Radiat Oncol Biol Phys. 48(4):1187–1195.

[22] Murphy MJ. (2004). Tracking moving organs in real time. Semin Radiat Oncol. 14(1): 91–100.

[23] Shirato H, Shimizu S, Shimizu T, Nishioka T, Miyasaka K. (1999). Real time tumour-tracking radiotherapy. Lancet. 353(9161):1331–1332.

[24] Shimizu S, Shirato H, Kitamura K, et al. (2000). Fluoroscopic real-time tumor-tracking radiation treatment (RTRT) can reduce internal margin (IM) and set-up margin (SM) of planning target volume (PTV) for lung tumors. Int J Radiat Oncol Biol Phys. 48:166–167.

[25] Zhang T, Keller H, O'Brien MJ, Mackie TR, Paliwal B. (2003). Application of the spirometer in respiratory gated radiotherapy. Med Phys. 30(12):3165–3171.

[26] Balter JM, Wright JN, Newell LJ, et al. (2005). Accuracy of a wireless localization system for radiotherapy. Int J Radiat Oncol Biol Phys. 61(3):933–937.

[27] Hsu A, Miller N, Evans P, Bamber J, Webb S. (2005). Feasibility of using ultrasound for real-time tracking during radiotherapy. Med Phys. 32(6):1500–1512.

[28] Wu J, Dandekar O, Nazareth D, Lei P, D'Souza W, Shekhar R. (2006). Effect of ultrasound probe on dose delivery during real-time ultrasound-guided tumor tracking. Conf Proc IEEE Eng Med Biol Soc. 1:3799–3802.

[29] Yan H, Yin FF, Zhu GP, Ajlouni M, Kim JH. (2006). The correlation evaluation of a tumor tracking system using multiple external markers. Med Phys. 33(11):4073–4084.

[30] Nakamura K, Shioyama Y, Nomoto S, et al. (2007). Reproducibility of the abdominal and chest wall position by voluntary breathhold technique using a laser-based monitoring and visual feedback system. Int J Radiat Oncol Biol Phys. 68(1):267–272.

[31] Hughes S, McClelland J, Tarte S, et al. (2009). Assessment of two novel ventilatory surrogates for use in the delivery of gated/tracked radiotherapy for non-small cell lung cancer. Radiother Oncol. 91(3):336–341.

[32] Kirkby C, Murray B, Rathee S, Fallone B. (2010). Lung dosimetry in a linac-MRI radiotherapy unit with a longitudinal magnetic field. Med Phys. 37(9):4722–4732.

[33] Cervino LI, Du J, Jiang SB. (2011). MRI-guided tumor tracking in lung cancer radiotherapy. Phys Med Biol. 56(13):3773–3785.

[34] Torshabi AE, Pella A, Riboldi M, Baroni G. (2010). Targeting accuracy in real-time tumor tracking via external surrogates: a comparative study. Technol Cancer Res Treat. 9:551–562.

[35] Torshabi AE, Riboldi M, Imani Fooladi AA, Modarres Mosalla SM, Baroni G. (2013). An adaptive fuzzy prediction model for real time tumor tracking in radiotherapy via external surrogates. J Appl Clin Med Phys. 14:102–114.

[36] Torshabi AE. (2014). Investigation the robustness of adaptive neuro-fuzzy inference system for tracking of moving tumors in external radiotherapy. Australas Phys Eng Sci Med. 37:771–778.

[37] Ghorbanzadeh L, Torshabi AE, Soltani Nabipour J, Ahmadi Arbatan M. (2016). Development of a synthetic adaptive neuro-fuzzy prediction model for tumor motion tracking in external radiotherapy by evaluating various data clustering algorithms. Technol Cancer Res Treat. 15(2):334–347.

[38] Torshabi AE, Riboldi M, Pella A, Negarestani A, Rahnema M, Baroni G. (May 2011). A clinical application of fuzzy logic. Fuzzy Logic, INTECH open access publisher, ISBN 979-953-307-578-4, Slavka Krautzeka, Rijeka, Croatia, 2011.